Fetal

Pharmacology

Symposium on Fetal Pharmacology, Stockholm, 1971.

Fetal
Pharmacology

Edited by

Lars O. Boréus, M.D.
Karolinska Hospital
Stockholm, Sweden

Raven Press, Publishers ■ New York

International Standard Book Number 0-911216-32-4
Library of Congress Catalog Card Number 77-181301

Foreword

On behalf of the Board of Directors of the Foundation for Child Development (formerly the Association for the Aid of Crippled Children), I express gratitude to Dr. Lars Boréus, who so effectively organized the Symposium on Fetal Pharmacology in Stockholm in December 1971 and who subsequently edited this volume. Similarly, the Foundation is appreciative of the efforts of the members of the Symposium's Advisory Committee who delineated the main areas of interest for the program and identified the scientists best able to lead discussions in these areas.

It is our hope that this volume will provide an overview of present knowledge and an indication of the principal future needs of research and training in the important field of fetal pharmacology.

Robert J. Slater, M.D.
President,
Foundation for Child Development
New York City
August, 1972

Preface

Life does not begin at birth. Prenatally, we are exposed to a variety of chemicals and drugs inadvertently or deliberately administered to the pregnant woman. In rare instances the exposure results in a malformed child. These cases naturally attract wide attention, generate compassion, and stimulate further research. They also, unfortunately, lead many people to look on drug therapy during pregnancy with fear and suspicion. Indeed, it sometimes is forgotten that many fetuses and newborn infants owe their survival to the maternity care of which drug therapy frequently is an essential part.

Progress in prenatal drug therapy has been slow. New compounds often are furnished with warnings against their use by women of fertile age, and these compounds are therefore shunned by physicians. Widely publicized lawsuits have added to the sense of apprehension with which many view prenatal drug therapy. In recent years, a massive research program in teratology has not been able to dispel this pessimistic atmosphere. Instead, the complexity of conditions obtaining during embryonic-fetal life has become increasingly apparent to investigators, and a reliable animal test system for teratogenicity in man still seems out of reach.

This volume represents an attempt to reverse the tendency toward overemphasis of the negative aspects of drug therapy in pregnancy. Here the fetus is looked upon as a potential patient. Basic pharmacological principles have been applied, and opportunities as well as risks considered. The approach has been stimulated by recent advances in clinical pharmacology in general, and in the technology of fetal monitoring, chemical microanalyses of drugs, and improved prenatal diagnostic methods in particular.

The sponsors of this volume, the Foundation for Child Development (formerly the Association for the Aid of Crippled Children) in New York and the Karolinska Institutet in Stockholm have perceived the importance of fetal pharmacology in future medical research. They made it possible to bring together, in December 1971 in Stockholm, many outstanding scientists for the conference on which this volume is based. It is the hope of all those involved in the volume that it will help to focus attention on the necessity for an intense, multidisciplinary attack on the problem of the safe use of drugs in the pregnant woman and on the problems of the pharmacology of the fetus itself.

Lars O. Boréus, M.D.
Karolinska Institutet
Stockholm
August, 1972

CONTENTS

SESSION II: DRUGS AND AUTONOMIC FUNCTION

Contents

SESSION III: DRUG METABOLISM

SESSION IV: DEVELOPMENT OF DEVELOPMENTAL PHARMACOLOGY

Contents

SESSION V: DRUGS AND THE BLASTOCYST

CLOSING SESSION

Contributors and Participants

H. Andersen
Children's Hospital
Fuglebakken
Copenhagen, Denmark

S. Aronsson
Department of Pediatrics
Lund Hospital
S221 85
Lund, Sweden

C. Beling
The New York Hospital-Cornell Medi-
cal Center
525 East 68th Street
New York, New York 10021

U. Borell
Department of Obstetrics
Karolinska Hospital
S-104 01 Stockholm 60, Sweden

L. O. Boréus
Department of Clinical Pharmacology
Karolinska Hospital
S-104 01 Stockholm 60, Sweden

M. Bradbury
Department of Physiology
St. Thomas's Hospital
London SE1, England

H. E. Brøndsted
Institute of Physiology
University of Aarhus
Aarhus, Denmark

R. Caldeyro-Barcia
Centro Latinoamericano de Perinato-
logia y Desarrollo Humano
Hospital de Clinicas
Piso 16
Montevideo, Uruguay

H. Davson
University College of London
Gower Street
London WC1E 6BT, England

G. S. Dawes
University of Oxford
Nuffield Institute of Medical Research
Osler Road
Headington, Oxford OX3 9DS, Eng-
land

E. W. Dempsey
Department of Anatomy
Columbia University
630 West 168th Street
New York, New York 10032

J. Drabkova
Department of Anesthesiology
Charles University
U nemocnice 2
Prague 2, Czechoslovakia

J. Elis
Czechoslovak Academy of Sciences
Institute of Pharmacology
Albertov 4
Prague 2, Czechoslovakia

xiii

Contributors

S. Fabro
Department of Pharmacology
George Washington University
    School of Medicine
1331 H Street N. W.
Washington, D.C. 20005

B. Falck
Department of Anatomy and Histology
University of Lund
Biskopsg 5
S-223 62 Lund, Sweden

J. R. Fouts
Pharmacology and Toxicology Branch
National Institute of Environmental
    Health Sciences
National Institutes of Health
Research Triangle Park, North Car-
    olina 27709

F. Fuchs
The New York Hospital-Cornell Medi-
    cal Center
525 East 68th Street
New York, New York 10021

G. Gennser
Department of Obstetrics
Malmö General Hospital
S-214 01 Malmö, Sweden

W. L. Hayton
School of Pharmacy
State University of New York at Buffalo
Buffalo, New York 14222

A. Hervonen
Department of Anatomy
University of Helsinki
Siltavuorenpenger, Helsinki, Finland

R. M. Hill
Department of Pediatrics
St. Luke's Episcopal Hospital
Houston, Texas 77025

B. Holmstedt
Department of Toxicology
Karolinska Institute
S-104 01 Stockholm 50, Sweden

E. C. Horning
Institute for Lipid Research
Baylor College of Medicine
Texas Medical Center
Houston, Texas 77025

M. G. Horning
Institute for Lipid Research
Baylor College of Medicine
Texas Medical Center
Houston, Texas 77025

A. Ingelman-Sundberg
Department of Obstetrics
Sabbatsbergs Hospital
S-113 82 Stockholm, Sweden

A. Jost
Laboratory of Comparative Physiology
Faculty of Sciences
University of Paris VI
9 Quai St. Bernard
Paris Ve, France

M. R. Juchau
Department of Pharmacology, SH-20
University of Washington
Seattle, Washington 98105

L. Kanerva
Department of Anatomy
University of Helsinki
Siltavuorenpenger, Helsinki, Finland

Contributors

A. G. Karczmar
Department of Pharmacology and Experimental Therapeutics
Loyola University Medical Center
2160 South First Avenue
Maywood, Illinois 60153

C. Kellogg
Department of Pharmacology
University of Gothenburg
S-400 33 Gothenburg 33, Sweden

S. Kety
Psychiatric Research Laboratory
Massachusetts General Hospital
Boston, Massachusetts 02114

K. S. Larsson
Teratology Laboratory
Karolinska Institute
S-104 01 Stockholm 60, Sweden

H. Lemtis
Abt. für experimentelle Gynäkologie
Frauenklinik
Klinikum Steglitz
Hindenburgdamm 30,
D-1 Berlin 45, Germany

G. Levy
Department of Biopharmaceutics
School of Pharmacy
State University of New York at Buffalo
Buffalo, New York 14222

J. Lind
Department of Pediatrics
Karolinska Hospital
S-104 01 Stockholm 60, Sweden

P. Lundborg
Department of Pharmacology
University of Gothenburg
S-400 33 Gothenburg 33, Sweden

C. Lutwak-Mann
Unit of Reproductive Physiology and Biochemistry
University of Cambridge
Downing Street
Cambridge, England

J.-P. Maltier
Laboratory of Comparative Physiology
University of Paris VI
9 Quai Saint-Bernard
Paris Ve, France

T. Mann
Unit of Reproductive Physiology & Biochemistry
University of Cambridge
Downing Street
Cambridge, England

W. G. McBride
Women's Hospital
Crown Street
Surry Hills, Sidney, N.S.W. Australia

B. L. Mirkin
Division of Clinical Pharmacology
Departments of Pharmacology and Pediatrics
University of Minnesota
Minneapolis, Minnesota 55455

D. Neubert
Pharmakologisches Institut der Freien Universität
Thielallee 69/73
D-1 Berlin 33, Germany

O. Nilsson
Department of Anatomy
University of Uppsala
Uppsala, Sweden

Contributors

H. Nishimura
Department of Anatomy
Faculty of Medicine
University of Kyoto
Sakyo-ku
Kyoto, Japan

J. Nowlin
Institute for Lipid Research and De-
partment of Pediatrics
Baylor College of Medicine
Houston, Texas 77025

S. Orrenius
Department of Forensic Medicine
Karolinska Institute
S-104 01 Stockholm 60, Sweden

C. Owman
Department of Anatomy and Histology
Division of Histology
Biskopsg 5
S-223 62 Lund, Sweden

R. Paoletti
Universita di Milano
Istituto di Farmacologia e di Farma-
cognosia
Via A Del Sarto 21
I-20129 Milan, Italy

C. Petter
Laboratory of Comparative Physiology
University of Paris VI
9 Quai Saint-Bernard
Paris Ve, France

A. Rane
Department of Pharmacology
Karolinska Institute
S-104 01 Stockholm 60, Sweden

N. Räihä
Children's Hospital
Stenbäcksgaten 11
Helsinki 29, Finland

N. R. Saunders
Department of Physiology
University College London
London WC1, England

P.-Y. Schifferli
Centro Latinoamericano de Perinato
logia y Desarrollo Humano
Hospital de Clinicas
Montevideo, Uruguay

F. Sjöqvist
Division of Clinical Pharmacology
Department of Pharmacology
Medical School
S-581 85 Linköping, Sweden

R. J. Slater
Foundation for Child Development
345 East 46th Street
New York, New York 10017

S. J. Strada
Laboratory of Preclinical Pharmacol-
ogy
National Institute of Mental Health
Saint Elizabeths Hospital
Washington, D.C. 20032

C. Stratton
Institute for Lipid Research and De-
partment of Pediatrics
Baylor College of Medicine
Houston, Texas 77025

C. A. Swinyard
New York University Medical Center
400 East 34th Street
New York, New York 10016

G. Telegdy
Department of Physiology
University Medical School
Pecs, Hungary

Contributors

K. Teramo
Department of Obstetrics
University of Helsinki
Helsinki 29, Finland

A. Tissari
Department of Pharmacology
University of Helsinki
Siltavuorenpenger 10
Helsinki 17, Finland

S. Ullberg
Department of Toxicology
University of Uppsala
S-751 23 Uppsala 1, Sweden

B. Uvnäs
Department of Pharmacology
Karolinska Institute
S-104 01 Stockholm 60, Sweden

A. Wilson
Institute for Lipid Research and De-
partment of Pediatrics
Baylor College of Medicine
Houston, Texas 77025

B. Weiss
National Institute of Mental Health
Division of Special Mental Health Re-
search, I.R.
Saint Elizabeths Hospital
Washington, D.C. 20032

D. M. Woodbury
Department of Pharmacology
University of Utah College of Medicine
Salt Lake City, Utah 84112

Fetal Pharmacology, edited by L. Boréus
Raven Press, New York © 1973

Drug Distribution in Pregnancy

Bernard L. Mirkin

*Division of Clinical Pharmacology, Departments of Pharmacology & Pediatrics,
University of Minnesota, Health Sciences Center, Minneapolis, Minnesota 55455*

GENERAL CONSIDERATIONS

Pharmacologic contamination of fetal and neonatal environments by maternally administered drugs has been a source of increasing concern during the past decade. The frequency with which therapeutic agents (prescribed and nonprescribed) are administered during pregnancy appears to be quite high; a recent study has shown that 92% of the subjects in a control population of pregnant females received at least one drug during gestation, whereas 4% received 10 or more (Peckham and King, 1963). In a majority of the cases cited, the therapeutic agents were used to treat maternal illnesses or symptoms which were generally unrelated to maintenance of the pregnancy. Since the therapeutic criteria governing the use of drugs in these situations are oriented essentially to maternal needs, they do not necessarily take cognizance of the fact that nearly all of the drugs thus administered can cross the placenta and ultimately enter the fetal milieu.

The effect of a given drug on fetal development or reactivity is determined to a large extent by whether the agent is utilized chronically throughout gestation or only acutely at parturition. Administration of a pharmacologic agent during the initial trimester of gestation can lead to diverse teratologic effects which may be classified as either morphologic (e.g., genital masculinization induced by progestational steroids; abnormal

1

dentition by tetracyclines) or nonmorphologic (e.g., high incidence of behavioral and neurological abnormalities in the offspring of epileptic mothers receiving diphenylhydantoin; enhancement of fetal enzyme activity secondary to induction by maternally administered drugs). In contrast, drugs given to the mother at parturition tend to produce more immediate and generally transient effects in the fetus which may under some circumstances persist into neonatal life. The drugs most commonly used at this stage of gestation are central nervous system depressants (barbiturates, local anesthetics, analgesics), neuromuscular blocking agents (succinylcholine, curare), and autonomic agents (atropine, scopolamine).

A comprehensive list of drugs commonly used in human obstetrics and the adverse effects apparently associated with their administration is presented in Table 1. The magnitude of this compilation underscores the necessity of informing those practitioners who must prescribe drugs for pregnant women about the potential hazards which may accrue from such utilization.

TRANSPLACENTAL PASSAGE AND FETAL LOCALIZATION OF DRUGS

Transplacental passage

Many factors appear to influence the placental transfer of pharmacologically active molecules. Characteristics of the placenta and drugs traversing it which seem to be significant in modulating transplacental passage are listed below:

Lipid solubility. The permeability of the placenta appears greatest for compounds possessing a high degree of lipid solubility or a large partition coefficient (organic solvent-water). It is commonly assumed that the placental membranes are lipoprotein in nature and therefore resemble other biological membranes delimiting body compartments. Although some generalizations referable to placental transfer can be derived from systematic analyses performed in other biological model systems (e.g., gastrointestinal tract, renal tubule, central nervous system), it is apparent that the placenta constitutes a biological membrane possessing unique characteristics of its own.

Degree of ionization. Drug molecules tend to penetrate biological membranes more rapidly in their unionized state (Mayer, Maickel, and Brodie, 1959). It should be noted that drugs such as the salicylates which are 100% ionized at pH 7.4 cross the placental membranes quite rapidly where-

TABLE 1. *Adverse effects in the human fetus and neonate attributed to maternally administered drugs.*

Agent	Fetal or Neonatal Effect
Antihypertensives	
thiazides	electrolyte imbalance
	thrombocytopenia (?)
reserpine	nasal stuffiness, hypothermia
nitrites	methemoglobinemia
ganglionic blockers	paralytic ileus
Central nervous system depressants	
chlorpromazine	sedation, retinopathy
chlordiazepoxide	neonatal depression
narcotic analgesics	neonatal depression
	"withdrawal symptoms"
local anesthetics	fetal bradycardia and acidosis,
	neonatal depression
thalidomide	skeletal anomalies
barbiturate sedatives	neonatal bleeding dyscrasia, increased
	rate of neonatal drug metabolism
Anti-bacterials	
tetracycline	abnormal dentition
streptomycin, gentamycin	deafness (8th nerve toxicity)
nitrofurantoin	hemolysis
chloramphenicol	cardiovascular collapse,
	"gray syndrome"
penicillin (high conc.)	convulsions
sulfonamides	hyperbilirubinemia
Hormones	
androgens	virilization of female
oral progestins	
estrogens	feminization of male
Miscellaneous	
thiouracil	goiter
salicylates	neonatal hemorrhage
quinine	thrombocytopenia, deafness
coumadin anticoagulants	hemorrhage
chloroquine	retinopathy

as their rate of penetration into the central nervous system is significantly retarded (Oh and Mirkin, 1971).

Molecular weight. Compounds with a molecular weight of less than 600 readily traverse the placenta, whereas those exceeding 1,000 are relatively impermeable.

Placental blood flow. The transfer of highly lipid-soluble drugs across the placenta appears to be proportional to placental flow. This is analagous to the relationship observed between the uptake of volatile anesthetic agents, pulmonary blood flow, and alveolar ventilation; in that transfer, an increase in alveolar ventilation is associated with a greater uptake of highly lipid-soluble volatile anesthetics.

Placental metabolism of drugs. Numerous aromatic oxidase reactions (hydroxylation, demethylation, N-dealkylation) can be carried out under *in vitro* conditions by placental homogenates. The significance of these reactions under *in vivo* conditions is not yet clearly defined (Juchau, 1972).

Aging of placenta. The permeability and rate of diffusion of molecules is altered as the placenta matures due to a decrease in thickness of the trophoblastic epithelium (Strauss, Goldenberg, Hirata, and Okudaira, 1965). Despite this observation, several studies suggest that drugs cross the rodent placenta more rapidly in the first trimester than in the last (see section III).

Upon traversing the placenta, pharmacologically active molecules may be localized in specific fetal tissues or body compartments, excreted into the amniotic fluid and uterine lumen of rodents, metabolized to some extent by fetal liver, or returned to the maternal circulation via retrograde feto-placental transfer. Some of the basic biochemical and physiologic characteristics of the fetus which appear to determine ultimately the disposition of drugs transferred across the placenta are discussed below.

The permeability of specialized membranes such as those present in the hemato-encephalic barrier, renal tubule, and yolk sac markedly influences drug distribution in the fetus. The blood-brain barrier is highly permeable in the early development of many mammalian species so that the fetal brain may be exposed to extremely high concentrations of a given drug during intrauterine existence. Since the fetal brain contains a high percentage of water and has a low myelin content, its affinity for lipophillic drugs is decreased, a factor which may serve to offset the high permeability observed during ontogenesis.

Selective uptake of drugs by fetal tissues may be attributable to one of several processes such as nonspecific lipid solubility. This would explain why certain organs with a relatively high lipid content (e.g., adrenal gland, ovary, and liver) are able to concentrate a wide variety of pharmacologic agents. Specific cellular constituents also play an important role in the tissue sequestration of drugs by providing discrete binding sites for particular exogenously administered molecules or endogenously occurring substrates. A catecholamine-binding protein has been identified within the adrenergic neuron which appears at a specific time in ontogenesis prior to which no catecholamines are bound (Mirkin, 1972); similarly, the uptake and binding of organic anions (bilirubin) by hepatic parenchymal cells seems to require a special transfer protein (Levi, Gatmatain, and Arias, 1970). In this category may also be included those enzyme-substrate interactions involving drugs and drug-metabolizing enzymes which are present in the liver, placenta, and adrenal gland. It should be noted that the binding capacity and/or affinity of fetal plasma proteins for certain drugs appears to be significantly less than that of maternal plasma, and this may markedly alter the quantity of free drug available for tissue distribution (Shoeman, Kauffman, Azarnoff, and Boulos, 1972). Another factor which may influence selective tissue uptake is the capacity of the yolk sac, with its endodermal lining resembling the microvilli and endoplasmic reticulum of the liver, to metabolize and secrete drugs into the uterine lumen of the rat. It is still unresolved if the yolk sac exerts an important role in eliminating drugs from the developing human fetus, but any compromise of its apparent function would appear to have a potentially deleterious effect on fetal drug disposition (Waddell, 1972).

The distribution of fetal circulation is probably of great importance in determining the relative concentrations of drug presented to a given anatomical region in the fetus. After a drug crosses the placenta to enter the umbilical vein, 60 to 85% of the flow in the umbilical vein enters the liver via the portal vein, and about 15 to 40% passes directly through the liver via the ductus venosus into the inferior vena cava. Consequently, a very large proportion of the drug initially present in the umbilical vein may be selectively taken up by the liver and achieve concentrations exceeding those obtained in any of the other fetal organs. In addition, the concentration of drug in the inferior vena cava is also decreased by venous drainage from the lower limbs and abdominal viscera. Upon the drug's reaching the left atrium, further dilution occurs via the superior vena cava which drains the cephalic regions of the fetus and enters the left atrium through the foramen ovale. These dilutional tendencies diminish the blood levels of drug reaching the left ventricle, lungs, and central nervous system so that they are similar to those of the ascending aorta, whereas the liver, adrenal gland, and kidney are perfused by blood containing concentrations equivalent to that in the descending aorta (Dawes, 1968). A summary of the factors which appear to influence the transplacental passage and fetal distribution of drugs is presented in Table 2.

Unfortunately, there exists very little information with which to evaluate critically the influence of the aforementioned factors on drug distribution in the feto-placental unit. A review of the many investigations pertaining to

TABLE 2. *Determinants of drug disposition in the feto-placental unit.*

A. *Factors Which May Influence the Transplacental Passage of Drugs*
   1. lipid solubility
   2. degree of ionization
   3. molecular weight
   4. placental blood flow
   5. placental metabolism of drugs
   6. aging of placenta

B. *Factors Which May Influence the Distribution of Drugs in the Fetus*
   1. permeability of specialized membranes
   2. selective tissue uptake of drug
        nonspecific lipid solubility
        specific binding to cellular constituents
            binding protein
            enzyme-substrate interaction
        active secretion by yolk sac [rodents; human (?)]
   3. distribution of fetal circulation

the placental transmission of drugs (more than 650 articles in the period 1969–1971) quickly reveals that most studies merely contain data describing maternal and fetal drug levels in blood samples obtained under poorly controlled experimental conditions. Relatively few pharmacokinetic studies have been published describing the distribution of a drug in specific maternal and fetal tissues at systematically selected time periods. The acquisition of data relating to drug distribution in the fetus has necessitated the development of rather unique and innovative investigative approaches. Several types of *in vivo* pharmacokinetic models have been devised in which the distribution of a maternally administered agent can be quantitatively or qualitatively determined at a fixed time period. Some of these procedures are applicable only to subhuman species whereas others may also be utilized in the human. In the former category are total body radioautography (Ullberg, 1959) and chronic indwelling catheterization of the fetal and maternal circulations. The total body radioautographic technique, which has been used primarily with small rodents, permits a comparative evaluation of drug distribution throughout the entire body mass of both mother and fetus. It is qualitative or at best semi-quantitative in nature unless each tissue section is assayed specifically for unmetabolized and metabolized drug. Information suitable for pharmacokinetic analyses has been obtained with chronic indwelling catheters which allow acquisition of maternal and fetal blood specimens at specific time intervals after maternal drug administration. These data have been used to determine the rates and extent of biotransformation of drugs entering the fetal circulation, and the penetration rate constants of drugs into different tissues or body compartments (particularly where a comparison of transfer across the blood-brain barrier and the placenta are desired), as well as to analyze the regional distribution of fetal circulation.

Most human investigations of placental drug transfer have been carried out under conditions where the agent(s) to be investigated have been utilized for maternal therapy or where therapeutic abortion is planned and an experimental drug may be administered (under certain circumstances) to the mother prior to or during the procedure. In the light of these restrictions, therefore, it is not difficult to understand why pharmacokinetic data in the human have been limited primarily to arterio-venous umbilical vessel gradients with relatively meager information regarding fetal tissue levels. Within the past few years, however, human abortus specimens have become more readily available, and, consequently, the opportunities for obtaining kinetic data on the distribution and concentration of drugs in fetal tissues appear to be significantly enhanced.

An excellent model demonstrating the systematic application of several investigative techniques to a problem in clinical pharmacology is provided by the following studies on diphenylhydantoin (DPH).

1. Total body radioautography was utilized to determine the distribution of ^{14}C-DPH in maternal and fetal tissues of the mouse over a 24-hr time period (Waddell and Mirkin, 1972). These studies were combined with thin-layer radiochromatography so that the relative concentration of ^{14}C-DPH and its metabolites in each tissue section were assayed. The highest concentrations of ^{14}C-DPH were found in the liver, heart, adrenal cortex, ovary (corpora lutea), and kidneys. ^{14}C-DPH constituted 95 to 99% of the isotope present in these tissues with minor quantities (1 to 5%) of ^{14}C-parahydroxydiphenylhydantoin also detected.

2. The pharmacokinetics of DPH has been investigated in larger rodent species so that actual tissue concentrations of drug can be determined as well as rates of elimination and transfer from one tissue compartment to another. The maternal and fetal tissue distribution of DPH following its administration (25 mg/kg i.v.) to pregnant rats is shown in Fig. 1. Each tissue was ranked according to its drug concentration 1 hr after injection, and the following pattern was observed (highest to lowest concentration): maternal liver, maternal and fetal heart, placenta, fetal liver, maternal and fetal brain, plasma. The ratio of fetal brain to fetal liver (FB/FL) concentration

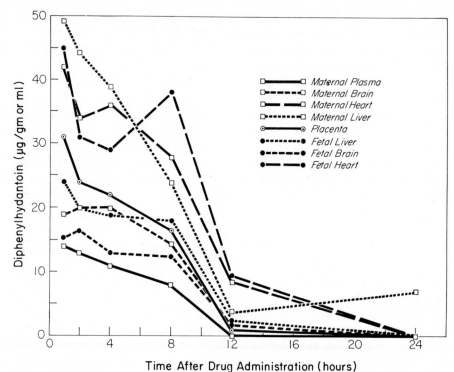

FIG. 1. Pharmacokinetic analysis of diphenylhydantoin in tissues of the maternal and fetal rat. Diphenylhydantoin (25 mg/kg i.v.) administered on the 20th gestational day. Ordinate: DPH (μg/g or ml). Abscissa: hours after drug administration.

of DPH was compared to that of maternal brain to maternal liver (MB/ML); the fetal ratio of 0.6 at 1 hr was closer to unity than was the maternal ratio of 0.4. These data suggest that DPH may preferentially distribute into fetal brain despite the apparent similarity in DPH concentrations of both fetal and maternal brain when expressed on a milligram/gram basis. The fetal clearance of DPH after a single maternal i.v. dose parellels that of the mother with no evidence of any fetal accumulation or lag phase.

3. A recent study utilizing in-dwelling catheterization techniques has confirmed the transplacental passage of DPH in goats and has demonstrated that the binding of DPH to maternal plasma proteins is greater than to fetal plasma proteins. This may significantly influence the quantity of free drug available for transplacental passage

and fetal distribution (Shoeman et al., 1972).

4. The placental transfer of DPH in the human has been investigated in subjects receiving the drug chronically for seizure disorders and in those receiving it acutely, prior to therapeutic intervention. The distribution pattern of DPH in human fetal specimens obtained after a single maternal i.v. dose is similar to that found in the mouse and rat in that the highest concentrations of DPH are present in liver, heart, and adrenal gland (Mirkin, 1971). Subjects receiving DPH throughout gestation had umbilical artery and vein concentrations of DPH which were virtually identical to those of maternal plasma. DPH was identified in the plasma of these neonates up to the 5th postpartum day with an estimated mean plasma half-life of 60 to 70 hr. Relatively large concentrations of *para*-hydroxy-DPH-glucuronide but virtually no DPH or *para*-hydroxy-DPH was present in the urine of neonates whose mothers had received DPH therapy during gestation (Mirkin and Reynolds, *in preparation*).

Although this series of investigations does provide a reasonable model for demonstrating the predictive value of data obtained in subhuman species, it should be emphasized that such extrapolations are hazardous and ultimately require experimental confirmation in the human.

DISTRIBUTION OF SPECIFIC DRUGS IN MATERNAL AND FETAL TISSUE

The information relevant to drug disposition in the maternal-placento-fetal unit can generally be considered as either qualitative or quantitative in nature. Although the amounts of substantive data in this area are not voluminous, several of the more pertinent and recent contributions have been selected for discussion.

Qualitative data

Numerous pharmacologic investigations utilizing total body radioautographic techniques have been published, and a massive quantity of qualitative information relative to drug disposition in the maternal-feto-placental unit has accumulated (Table 3). These data indicate that the fetal distribution of most drugs tends to parallel that of the mother, although in nearly all instances the maternal liver concentration greatly exceeded the fetal liver. Some drugs such as meprobamate, sulfapyridine, and urea appear to dis-

TABLE 3. *Radioautographic analysis of drug distribution in maternal and fetal tissues.*

Drug	Liver	Bile	Lung	Intestine	Adrenal	Urine	Fat	Reference
14C-Amitriptyline	+[a]		+	++		+		Cassano (1968)
14C-Chlordiazepoxide	+			++				Placidi et al. (1968)
35S-Chlorpromazine	+		+	++		+		Sjöstrand et al. (1965)
14C-Cortisone					+			Hanngren et al. (1964)
14C-DDT	+++			+++			++	Bäckström et al. (1965)
14C-Dieldren	+++		++	+++			++	Bäckström et al. (1965)
14C-Diethylstilbestrol	+		++	+				Bengtsson et al. (1963)
14C-Imipramine			+			+		Cassano et al. (1966)
3H-Meprobamate								Ewaldsson (1963)
14C-Phenobarbital	+	+		+				Waddell (1971)
35S-Thiopental							+	Cassano et al. (1967)

[a] Represents tissue with highest concentrations of radioactivity following maternal administration of isotope.

tribute in a fairly uniform manner with no apparent predilection for a specific maternal or fetal tissue. In contrast, agents such as amitriptyline, chlordiazepoxide, chlorpromazine, cortisone, DDT, dieldrin, diethylstilbestrol, imipramine, phenobarbital, DPH, and numerous other agents appear to distribute more selectively in both maternal and fetal tissues.

Quantitative data

Drugs acting on the autonomic nervous system

(1) *Atropine*. Fetal plasma levels of ^{3}H-atropine 20 min after an intravenous injection to pregnant women (gestational ages ranging from 10 to 17 weeks) were one-half those of maternal plasma (Kivalo and Saarikoski, 1970). The largest total concentration of ^{3}H-atropine was found in the placenta and liver; the distribution of ^{3}H-atropine in fetal tissues, expressed in terms of concentration per gram tissue (nC/g), was as follows: liver 2.52; placenta 1.68; heart 1.23; kidney 1.0; brainstem 0.32; and cerebrum 0.27. Thus, the ^{3}H-atropine concentration of central nervous system tissue was about 25% that of myocardial tissue at this time. Based on the assumption that both fetal effectors (CNS and heart) possess similar thresholds to the anticholinergic actions of atropine, these data suggest that the fetal tachycardia commonly observed after maternal administration of atropine reflects a greater influence on peripheral rather than central vagal activity.

The distribution and excretion of ^{14}C-atropine has been described in mice and the following tissue distribution noted (highest to lowest concentration): gallbladder, urinary bladder, kidneys, liver, adrenal gland, and central nervous system (Gosselin, Gabourel, Kalser, and Wills, 1955). Other studies have indicated that the greatest concentrations of ^{14}C-atropine have been found in the liver with virtually no activity detectable in the brain 2 hr after administering the drug (Evertbusch and Geiling, 1956).

(2) *Pyridostigmine*. Maternal blood, placental, and fetal concentrations of ^{14}C-pyridostigmine peaked 15 min after an intramuscular injection to the mother (Roberts, Thomas, and Wilson, 1970). The concentration of drug in the placenta was equivalent to that of maternal blood, whereas the fetal concentration was markedly lower than either of these tissues. Relative tissue concentrations at this time interval were as follows: maternal blood, 28.9 μg/100 ml; placenta, 18.2 μg/100 g; and fetus, 0.86 μg/100 g. The fetal distribution of 3-hydroxy-N-methyl-pyridinium, a metabolite of pyridostigmine, differed from the parent compound in that the fetus had concentrations

of the metabolite which were three to four times greater than maternal blood or placental tissue. This distinction in the tissue distribution of metabolite indicates that either the metabolite is transferred across the placenta to a greater extent than the parent compound or that pyridostigmine is rapidly and extensively metabolized by fetal tissues.

The clinical significance of the above observations is such that it may explain the onset of neonatal myasthenia (about 40 cases in the past 25 years) which has been reported after administration of anticholinesterase agents to pregnant women afflicted with myasthenia gravis. A recent, excellently documented case clearly demonstrates that a woman receiving pyridostigmine did transfer the drug to the fetus, thereby producing a significant decrease in fetal plasma cholinesterase activity (Blackhall, Buckley, Roberts, Roberts, Thomas, and Wilson, 1969). The placental transfer of pyridostigmine and its main metabolite in the pregnant rat reinforces the view that neonatal myasthenia in the human may be iatrogenically induced in females given anticholinesterase agents during gestation.

(3) *Nicotine.* The passage of ^{14}C-nicotine, its metabolites cotinine, γ-(3-pyridyl)-γ-oxo-N-methylbutyramide, and hydroxycotinine, and two unknown metabolites across the placenta and their localization in mice has been documented (Tjälve, Hanson, and Schmiterlöw, 1968). The placenta retained nicotine and impeded its transfer into the fetal circulation, so that fetal concentrations were rather low. The nicotine which entered the fetal circulation was concentrated in the lungs, trachea, adrenals, kidney, and intestine. Significantly, very little nicotine was present in the fetal liver, an observation which parallels that in the maternal liver which also appears to accumulate minimal quantities of nicotine. In contrast, cotinine, the main metabolite of nicotine, does traverse the placenta readily and is distributed rather ubiquitously. These data clearly reveal major differences in the transfer rates of nicotine across the blood-brain barrier and the placental membranes.

(4) *Catecholamines; angiotensin II.* The transfer of catecholamines from the maternal circulation to the fetus has been investigated in pregnant rats administered ^{3}H-norepinephrine intravenously. Assay of the adrenal, heart, and spleen 5, 30, and 60 min thereafter revealed no ^{3}H-norepinephrine in these tissues, whereas relatively large concentrations were present in the placenta. Recent studies carried out in pregnant dogs have also failed to detect any significant transplacental passage or fetal uptake of maternally administered ^{3}H-norepinephrine (Mirkin, 1971, *unpublished data*). A comparable investigation with ^{14}C-DL-norepinephrine has been performed in the

human (Sandler, Ruthven, Contractor, Wood, Booth, and Pinkerton, 1963). Quantities ranging from 2 to 18% (n = 3) of a maternally administered isotopic dose were detected in cord sera, whereas fetal heart sera contained 0.6 to 2.2%. The procedure used to assay for norepinephrine did not exclude contamination with some catechol acids; consequently, the proportion of transferred isotope which actually constituted ^{14}C-DL-norepinephrine remains uncertain. Since the placenta possesses considerable monoamine oxidase activity, it is quite probable that catecholamines undergo extensive oxidative deamination at this site.

Similar observations have been made with respect to angiotensin II in that placental transfer was not discernible when angiotensin II was given (i.v.) to pregnant monkeys. However, administration directly into the fetal circulation produced a marked vasopressor response in the fetus (Behrman and Kittinger, 1968). It would appear, therefore, that catecholamines and other vasopressor substances influence fetal homeostasis not by penetration into the fetal circulation but rather by a direct influence on the uterine circulation leading to a reduction in uterine blood flow and fetal asphyxia (Adamsons, Mueller-Heubach, and Meyers, 1971).

Drugs acting on the central nervous system

(1) *Anticonvulsant agents (diazepam, diphenylhydantoin).* Investigations utilizing ^{14}C-diazepam in the pregnant monkey have demonstrated a rapid transfer across the placenta with significant uptake and prolonged retention of this compound (and metabolites) in fetal cerebellum, spinal cord, and peripheral nerves (Idänpään-Heikkilä, Taska, Allen, and Schoolar, 1971*b*). Recent studies in man have shown that ^{14}C-diazepam and its metabolites are rapidly transferred across the human placenta with much greater concentrations present in cord blood (47.5 ng/ml) than maternal blood (25.6 ng/ml) one hour after administration. Fetal tissue concentrations of diazepam and metabolites also peaked at this time. The highest levels were observed in the fetal liver, brain and gastrointestinal tract. The metabolism of diazepam by fetal liver microsomes was minimal, constituting about 3% of the added substrate; no metabolism was noted in homogenates prepared from human placenta, fetal brain or fetal small intestine (Idänpään-Heikkilä, Jouppila, Puolakka, and Vorne, 1971*a*).

The distribution of DPH in human and subhuman fetal tissues has been described in section II (Mirkin, 1971; Waddell and Mirkin, 1972).

(2) *Morphine.* Generalized depression of the central nervous system

has been frequently observed in neonates following delivery from mothers who have received analgesics prior to parturition. Data describing the fetal tissue distribution of morphine are scanty and have been restricted primarily to animal studies with ^{3}H-dihydromorphine (Sanner and Woods, 1965). These studies demonstrated that maternal plasma levels of ^{3}H-dihydromorphine were two-and-one-half times greater than fetal levels 30 min, 1, and 2 hr after a subcutaneous dose; fetal brain concentrations were three times greater then maternal at each of the time intervals indicated. Conjugated ^{3}H-dihydromorphine was not detectable in maternal brain until 16 hr after administration, whereas small quantities were recovered from fetal brain within 2 hr. It is apparent, therefore, that the fetal distribution of ^{3}H-dihydromorphine and its metabolites differs significantly from that of the adult.

Similar studies have been carried out in which the maternal and fetal distribution of ^{3}H-dihydromorphine in tolerant and nontolerant pregnant rats was compared (Yeh and Woods, 1970). The maternal plasma concentrations of ^{3}H-dihydromorphine in tolerant rats were lower and the fetal plasma levels higher than in nontolerant maternal and fetal controls. The rate of removal of ^{3}H-dihydromorphine from its site of injection was more rapid in tolerant animals, as were the apparent transfer rates of ^{3}H-dihydromorphine into maternal brain, fetal plasma, and fetal brain. These data are consistent with the concept that tolerance increases the rate of transfer of ^{3}H-dihydromorphine across the placenta and perhaps other biological membranes.

(3) *Non-volatile anesthetic agents (thiopental, ketamine).* Numerous publications have shown that thiopental readily crosses the placenta to achieve significant concentrations in umbilical venous blood (Crawford, 1956; Flowers, 1963; Finster, Mark, and Morishima, 1966). The relative distribution of thiopental in fetal tissues of the pregnant guinea pig 2 min after a maternal dose (35 mg/kg i.v.) is as follows (μg/g tissue): liver 66; skeletal muscle 32; heart 28; spinal cord 28; kidney 19; spleen 19; brain 17; and lung 17. The fetal liver concentration was approximately two to four times greater than that found in other fetal organs (Finster, Morishima, Mark, Perel, Dayton, and James, 1967).

Human subjects presenting with a diagnosis of fetal anencephaly have been given thiopental and their fetal tissues analyzed for this compound. The fetal distribution of thiopental (μg/g tissue) in two cases is presented below (Case I, 1½ hr after thiopental; Case II, 2½ hr after thiopental): subcutaneous fat (88, 43); liver, left lobe (65, 43); lung (25, 14); kidney (16, 11); pancreas (15, 14); spleen (15, 11); spinal cord (11), heart (10,

10) and skeletal muscle (9). The blood levels (μg/ml) for these respective cases were: maternal vein (19, 19), umbilical vein (11, 14), and umbilical artery (10, 12). An interesting aspect of this study was the segmental sequestration of thiopental in the middle lobe of the fetal liver when injected via the umbilical vein which primarily perfuses this portion of the liver. The quantity of thiopental in the middle lobe was nearly one-half of the injected dose and approximately four times greater than the left lobe. These observations suggest that the fetal liver initially takes up large quantities of transplacentally passed drugs, thereby shielding the remaining fetal tissues (particularly the central nervous system) from overwhelming gradients and perhaps toxic influences of these agents (Finster et al., 1967).

The dissociative anesthetic ketamine, a phencyclidine derivative, has been utilized in obstetrical anesthesia and its fetal distribution characterized in four abortus specimens (see Table 4). The data available from preliminary studies demonstrate an accumulation of ketamine in the placenta with concentrations in fetal plasma and brain tending to approximate those of maternal plasma (Cumming, 1971, *unpublished data*).

(4) *Local anesthetics (mepivacaine, lidocaine, prilocaine).* The administration of local anesthetics during obstetrical procedures has been associated with adverse effects such as fetal depression (Shnider and Way, 1968), fetal bradycardia (Sjövall, Trolle, Boe, and Vara, 1967; Gordon, 1968) and stimulation (Finster, Poppers, Sinclair, Morishima, and Daniel, 1965). Although the absorption and placental transfer of local anesthetic agents from a variety of maternal sites of administration (caudal, epidural, paracervical) has been demonstrated in the human, virtually no information exists about the distribution of such agents in fetal tissues. In one study, the maternal venous plasma level of mepivacaine 30 min after administration was 2.9 μg/ml with concentrations of 1.9 and 1.4 μg/ml noted in the umbilical vein and artery, respectively (Morishima, Daniel, Finster, Poppers, and James, 1966). The only quantitative data relative to the distribution of local anesthetic agents in fetal tissues are from studies carried out in pregnant rats administered ^{14}C-lidocaine (Katz, 1968; Katz, Gershwin, and Hood, 1968) and ^{14}C-prilocaine (Katz, 1969). The relative distribution pattern of these agents in maternal tissues 1 min after an intravenous dose was as follows (in descending order of magnitude): kidney, liver, brain, blood, muscle. The tissue concentration ratios of blood to placenta and blood to fetus were 0.26 and 0.31, respectively, 1 min after drug administration. These values were significantly higher than observations made 5, 15, and 60 min thereafter. In contrast, the placenta to fetus ratio of 1.2 remained

TABLE 4. *Distribution of ketamine in human fetal[a] and maternal tissues.*

Case No.	Total Ketamine[b] Dose (mg/kg)	Time After Last Dose (min)	Maternal Plasma (μg/ml)	Placenta (μg/g)	Fetal Plasma (μg/ml)	Fetal Liver (μg/g)	Fetal Brain (μg/g)
1	1.5	4	no sample	3.8	no sample	no sample	1.8
2	3.0	30	0.32	no sample	0.36	no sample	0.55
3	3.8 (2 doses) (1st—2.3 mg/kg) (2nd—1.5 mg/kg)	24	0.6	6.5	0.46	2.2	1.45
4	4.0 (2 doses) (1st—3.0 mg/kg) (2nd—1.0 mg/kg)	6	1.85	1.2	no sample	0.15	0.5

[a] All specimens were obtained from gestations of 10 to 14 weeks duration.
[b] Ketamine administered parenterally into maternal circulation at time of therapeutic abortion.

constant over the entire period, suggesting that the fetus and placenta achieve an early equilibrium state which is not markedly influenced by variations in maternal blood concentration.

Psychopharmacologic agents

(1) Δ^9-*tetrahydrocannabinol* (Δ^9-*THC;* Δ^9-*THC-*^{3}*H*). The major psychoactive component of Cannabis, Δ^9-THC, has been shown to exert teratogenic effects in the pregnant hamster (Geber and Schramm, 1969a), rabbit (Geber and Schramm, 1969b), and rat (Persaud and Ellington, 1968). The placental transfer of Δ^9-THC-^{3}H has been studied in the pregnant hamster. Its presence in the fetus was detected 15 min after an intraperitoneal injection, and peak fetal concentrations were noted 30 min thereafter. A marked placental uptake of Δ^9-THC-^{3}H was observed so that placental concentrations were two to three times greater than fetal at comparable time periods (Idänpään-Heikkilä, Fritchie, Englert, Ho, and McIsaac, 1969). The fetal concentrations of Δ^9-THC-^{3}H were substantially greater than those of maternal plasma and brain at 15, 30, and 120 min. Maternal administration of Δ^9-THC-^{3}H during the first trimester (6th day of gestation) produced fetal concentrations of Δ^9-THC-^{3}H which were about three times greater than those obtained after administration in the last trimester (15th day of gestation), suggesting a greater permeability to this compound early in gestation. The radioactive material assayed in the placenta and fetus contained 55 and 25% of its activity, respectively, in the form of nonmetabolized Δ^9-THC-^{3}H, with the remainder consisting of various metabolites.

(2) *Lysergic acid diethylamide* (LSD; ^{14}C-LSD). The distribution of ^{14}C-LSD has been studied in the pregnant mouse; this compound was found to be present in fetal tissues 5 min after a maternal injection (Idänpään-Heikkilä and Schoolar, 1969). Greater than 70% of the radioactive material in the placenta and fetal tissues consisted of ^{14}C-LSD. The distribution pattern in the fetus was similar to that of the mother with the following tissue concentration gradient (descending order): lungs, liver, intestine, brain, heart. Since maternal and fetal blood contained extremely low concentrations of ^{14}C-LSD, the very rapid transport of this compound from vascular compartments to an extravascular site has been proposed. The placental transfer of ^{14}C-LSD appeared to be more rapid with a higher percentage of the administered dose present in the fetus (2.4%) when the drug was administered early rather than late in gestation. These data are similar to the observations noted previously with Δ^9-THC-^{3}H (see above).

(3) *Chlorpromazine and metabolites.* Analyses performed on fetal and maternal plasma have demonstrated the presence of chlorpromazine and 7-hydroxychlorpromazine following the intramuscular injection (50 to 100 mg) of chlorpromazine to mothers at parturition. Maternal urine contained chlorpromazine and 25 metabolites, whereas chlorpromazine and 21 metabolites were isolated from neonatal urine. Dihydroxy metabolites and non-metabolized chlorpromazine were found in amniotic fluid as well as maternal and neonatal urine (O'Donoghue, 1971). The origin of the metabolites in the urine of the neonate has been investigated by comparing the urine of untreated neonates delivered from treated mothers (those receiving chlorpromazine) with the urine of neonates administered chlorpromazine but delivered from untreated mothers (not receiving chlorpromazine). The urine from the former (untreated) group contained a number of conjugated metabolites which did not appear in urine of the latter (treated) group of neonates. These data suggest that the five conjugated metabolites of chlorpromazine found in the urine of untreated neonates delivered from treated mothers are probably formed in the maternal system and that the placenta is permeable not only to the parent compound chlorpromazine, but apparently to many of its metabolites.

Phenothiazine compounds have been shown to be capable of inducing severe retinopathy in the human. This is morphologically characterized by a migration of pigment granules from degenerated retinal pigment epithelium into the receptor layer of the retina (Bernstein and Ginsberg, 1964). Autoradiographic studies in pregnant mice receiving ^{35}S-chlorpromazine have demonstrated that significant amounts of radioactivity attributable to chlorpromazine persist in ocular tissue for periods up to 5 months after the drug had disappeared from other fetal tissues (Ullberg et al., 1970).

Drugs acting on the myocardium

(1) *Digitoxin.* The placental transfer of ^{14}C-digitoxin has been studied in pregnant rats and guinea pigs (Okita, Gordon, and Geiling, 1952). This compound and its metabolic products cross the placenta of both species with a much greater percentage of a maternally administered dose appearing in the fetuses of the guinea pigs ($22 \pm 2\%$) than in the rat ($0.65 \pm 0.03\%$). The metabolite-to-digitoxin ratio in the fetal guinea pig was about 47, whereas that of the fetal rat was approximately 15, implying that digitoxin metabolites found in the maternal system readily cross the placenta or that fetal tissues are able to metabolize digitoxin actively. The concentration of

digitoxin and its metabolites in the fetal heart exceeded that of the maternal heart by twofold.

In the human, less than 1% of a maternally injected dose of ^{14}C-digitoxin was detected in the fetus as unchanged digitoxin and less than 3.5% as its metabolite (Okita, Plotz, and Davis, 1956). The concentration of ^{14}C-digitoxin and metabolites in human fetal tissues obtained 3 to 5 hr after maternal administration of this drug was as follows (in descending order): kidney, heart, liver, lung, intestine, brain. The tissues from first-trimester fetuses contained higher concentrations of cardiac glycoside than corresponding tissues taken from older fetuses.

(2) *Digoxin.* The transplacental passage of digoxin has been studied with immunoassay techniques, and the rapid movement of this glycoside across the placenta has been demonstrated in rats and humans. Pharmacokinetic investigations in the rat were designed to allow a comparison of maternal and fetal serum digoxin levels at specific time periods after a maternal injection (0.1 mg/kg i.v.) The maternal and fetal serum digoxin concentrations obtained in this study are presented below [time after injection of digoxin to mother in minutes (min); serum digoxin concentration expressed as ng/ml; each value represents mean of two individual experiments]:

2 min (Mat. 251, Fetal 42); 5 min (Mat. 262, Fetal 52); 10 min (Mat. 134, Fetal 49); 20 min (Mat. 120, Fetal 18); 40 min (Mat. 69, Fetal 12); 80 min (Mat. 60, Fetal 8); 160 min (Mat. 34, Fetal 17); and 320 min (Mat. 19, Fetal 5) (Mirkin and Singh, 1972).

The serum digoxin concentrations of maternal and umbilical cord sera have been determined in two women receiving digoxin therapy during their gestations. In Case 1, the maternal digoxin concentration at parturition was 0.7 ng/ml, the cord sera level 1.4 ng/ml, and the neonatal sera (2 hr post-delivery) 0.54 ng/ml. The maternal sera of Case 2 contained 1.6 ng/ml of digoxin at parturition and 1.4 ng/ml on the third post-partum day. Cord sera had a concentration of 1.0 ng/ml whereas the neonatal digoxin level at 24 hr was 1.2 ng/ml, at 48 hr 0.86 ng/ml, and at 72 hr 0.83 ng/ml (Singh and Mirkin, *in preparation,* and *unpublished*).

Drugs acting on the endocrine system

(1) *Corticosterone; cortisone.* The passage of adrenal cortical steroids across the placenta has been demonstrated in the mouse (Hanngren, Hans-

son, Sjoqvist, and Ullberg, 1964) and rat (Zarrow, Philpott, and Denenberg, 1970). ^{14}C-4-Corticosterone given intravenously was present in each maternal and fetal tissue analyzed (skeletal muscle, liver, central nervous system, and plasma), with the highest fetal concentrations contained in liver and skeletal muscle. The relative activity ratio of fetal plasma to muscle was approximately one, and, when compared with the maternal plasma to muscle ratio of five, suggested an impaired ability of fetal muscle to bind corticosterone. Comparable ratios for fetal liver and muscle were 1.5 in the fetus, 8.6 in the 2-day-old rat, and 51 in the adult female. These data demonstrate substantial differences in the hepatic binding capacity of fetal, neonatal, and adult liver.

(2). *3-beta-Hydroxysteroid dehydrogenase inhibitor (isoxazole; ^{14}C-isoxazole).* Administration of ^{14}C-isoxazole to pregnant rats was characterized by a significant inhibition of the adrenal dehydrogenase system and concentration of ^{14}C-isoxazole in the fetal adrenal gland, testes, intestine, and liver, in descending order of concentration. The persistent and selective retention of ^{14}C-isoxazole by enzyme-containing tissues of the fetal rat (Goldman and Kenneck, 1970) in conjunction with its lack of uptake by ovarian tissue supports the hypothesis that dehydrogenase activity is absent in the fetal rat ovary and does not appear until the 9th day of neonatal life (Goldman and Kohn, 1970). A marked increment in adrenal cortical tissue mass was noted in rats receiving the dehydrogenase inhibitor. This observation also correlates directly with studies demonstrating the discrete localization of isoxazole only in tissues possessing active dehydrogenase systems.

Environmental pollutants and food additives

(1) *Halogenated hydrocarbon insecticides (DDT, DDE, benzene hexachlorophene, dieldrin).* The concentrations of DDT and DDE in human maternal blood, umbilical cord blood, amniotic fluid, placental tissue, and vernix caseosa have been recently determined (O'Leary, Davies, Edmundson, and Reich, 1970). The presence of DDT in blood is generally associated with a recent exposure, whereas the detection of DDE reflects chronic, long-term exposure to DDT (Edmundson, Davies, Nachman, and Roeth, 1969). DDE was present in the tissues of all the pregnant women studied (n=152), and the levels in maternal blood were significantly greater than those of cord blood or amniotic fluid. In contrast, the DDE concentrations of vernix caseosa were significantly higher than placental concentrations and contained the highest concentrations detected in any of the tissues examined. The fetal dis-

tribution of DDT and DDE in the human was not investigated, and the possibility of achieving extremely high concentrations in fetal lipids with high turnover rates must be considered. The storage of halogenated insecticides in the lipids of pregnant and nonpregnant women has been investigated, and it is interesting to note that lower concentrations of DDT were present (1.6 ppm) in pregnant women than nonpregnant ones (3.4 ppm). A similar pattern was noted for other metabolites of DDT, benzene hexachlorophene (lindane), and dieldrin. This difference in tissue concentration suggests that pregnant women may metabolize these compounds more rapidly than nonpregnant females (Polishuk, Wassermann, Wassermann, Groner, and Lazarovici, 1970).

(2) *2,3,5-Triiodobenzoic acid.* The compound 2,3,5-triiodobenzoic acid may constitute a significant environmental pollutant capable of inducing teratologic malformations in mice and rats (Nelson, 1969). This compound and its metabolites 2,5-diiodobenzoic and 3,5-diiodobenzoic acid rapidly cross the placenta, achieving fetal to maternal blood plasma ratios of 0.85 to 0.98 within 2 hr. The distribution of these compounds in fetal tissue appears homogenous, although fetal liver concentrations are higher than most other fetal tissues (McDowell, Landolt, Kessler, and Shaw, 1971).

(3) *Cyclamates (cyclohexylamine sulfamic acid).* Maternal administration of ^{14}C-cyclohexylamine sulfamic acid (^{14}C-cyclamate) prior to therapeutic abortion produced fetal blood concentrations which were about 25% of maternal levels at each of the time periods investigated (Pitkin, Reynolds, and Filer, 1970). ^{14}C-Cyclamate concentrations in fetal spleen, pancreas, kidney, lung, and skin exceeded those of fetal blood but were appreciably lower than concentrations in fetal liver. These studies were carried out in first trimester gestations and clearly demonstrate the ease with which cyclamates may cross the placenta during this stage in development.

SUMMARY

I have attempted in this chapter to identify and analyze those factors which appear to exert a significant influence upon placental transfer and fetal drug localization. It is essential to note that each of these processes is operating concurrently so that multiple kinetic events are occurring in both maternal and fetal environments. An attempt to summarize and schematically depict current concepts of drug disposition in a model of the maternal-placento-fetal unit is presented in Fig. 2. It is apparent that the many gaps

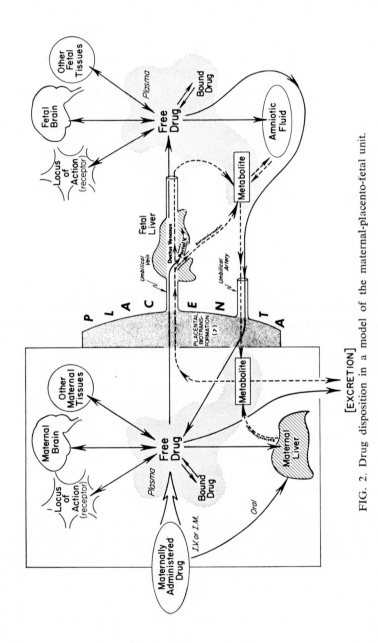

FIG. 2. Drug disposition in a model of the maternal-placento-fetal unit.

which exist in our knowledge must be filled before we can successfully design pharmacologically active molecules possessing maximal therapeutic efficacy and minimal toxicity for the fetus.

ACKNOWLEDGMENT

This work was partially supported by U.S. Public Health Service Grants from the Pharmacology-Toxicology Program (GM 15477) and from the Clinical Pharmacology Program (GM 01998), of the National Institute of General Medical Sciences.

REFERENCES

Adamsons, K., Mueller-Heubach, E., and Meyers, R. E. (1971): Production of fetal asphyxia in the rhesus monkey by administration of catecholamines to the mother. *American Journal of Obstetrics and Gynecology*, 109:248-262.

Bäckström, J., Hansson, E., and Ullberg, S. (1965): Distribution of C^{14}-DDT and C^{14}-dieldren in pregnant mice determined by whole-body radioautography. *Toxicology and Applied Pharmacology*, 7:90-96.

Behrman, R. E., and Kittinger, G. W. (1968): Fetal and maternal responses to *in utero* angiotensin infusions in *Macaca mulatta*. *Proceedings of the Society for Experimental Biology and Medicine*, 129:305-308.

Bengtsson, G., and Ullberg, S. (1963): The autoradiographic distribution pattern after administration of diethylstilbesterol compared with that of natural estrogens. *Acta Endocrinologica*, 43:561-570.

Bernstein, H. N., and Ginsberg, J. (1964): The pathology of chloroquine retinopathy. *Archives of Ophthalmology*, 71:238-245.

Blackhall, M. I., Buckley, G. A., Roberts, D. V., Roberts, J. B., Thomas, B. H., and Wilson, A. (1969): Drug-induced neonatal myasthenia. *Journal of Obstetrics and Gynaecology of the British Commonwealth*, 76:157-162.

Cassano, G. B. (1968): An autoradiographic study of the distribution of drugs acting on the central nervous system in the whole body and brain. *Journal of Nuclear Biology and Medicine*, 12:13-24.

Cassano, G. B., Ghetti, B., Gliozzi, E., and Hansson, E. (1967): Autoradiographic distribution study of "short acting" and "long acting" barbiturates: ^{35}S-thiopentone and ^{14}C-phenobarbitone. *British Journal of Anesthesiology*, 39:11-20.

Cassano, G., and Hansson, E. (1966): Autoradiographic distribution studies in mice with C^{14}-imipramine. *International Journal of Neuropsychiatry*, 2:269-278.

Crawford, J. S. (1956): Some aspects of obstetrical anesthesia. *British Journal of Anesthesia*, 28:146-154.

Dawes, G. S. (1968): *Foetal and Neonatal Physiology*. Year Book Medical Publishers, Chicago.

Edmundson, W. F., Davies, J. E., Nachman, G. A., and Roeth, R. L. (1969): *p, p'*-DDT and *p, p'*-DDE in blood samples of occupationally exposed workers. *Public Health Reports of the United States Public Health Service*, 84:53-58.

Evertbusch, V., and Geiling, E. M. K. (1956): Studies with radioactive atropine: Distribution and excretion patterns in the mouse. *Archives Internationales de Pharmacodynamie et de Thérapie*, 105:175-192.

Ewaldsson, B. (1963): Autoradiographic studies on the distribution of H^3-meprobamate in the body. *Archives Internationales de Pharmacodynamie et de Thérapie*, 142:163-169.

Finster, M., Mark, L. C., and Morishima, H. O. (1966): Plasma thiopental concentrations in the newborn following delivery under thiopental-nitrous oxide anesthesia. *American Journal of Obstetrics and Gynecology*, 95:621-629.

Finster, M., Morishima, H. O., Mark, L. C., Perel, J. M., Dayton, P. G., and James, L. S. (1967): Tissue thiopental concentrations in the fetus and newborn. *Anesthesiology*, 28:248-249.

Finster, M., Poppers, P. J., Sinclair, J. C., Morishima, H. O., and Daniel, S. S. (1965): Accidental intoxication of the fetus with local anesthetic drug during caudal anesthesia. *American Journal of Obstetrics and Gynecology*, 92:922-924.

Flowers, C. E. (1963): Factors related to the placental transfer of thiopental in the hemochorial placenta. *American Journal of Obstetrics and Gynecology*, 85:646-658.

Geber, W. F., and Schramm, L. C. (1969a): Teratogenicity of marihuana extract as influenced by plant origin and seasonal variation. *Archives Internationales de Pharmacodynamie et de Thérapie*, 177:224-230.

Geber, W. F., and Schramm, L. C. (1969b): Effect of marihuana extract on fetal hamsters and rabbits. *Toxicology and Applied Pharmacology*, 14:276-282.

Goldman, A. S., and Kenneck, C. Z. (1970): Persistence of label in rat offspring after maternal administration of a ^{14}C-labeled inhibitor of 3-beta-hydroxysteroid dehydrogenase. *Endocrinology*, 86:711-716.

Goldman, A. S., and Kohn, G. (1970): Rat ovarian 3-beta-hydroxysteroid dehydrogenase: normal developmental appearance in tissue culture. *Proceedings of the Society for Experimental Biology and Medicine*, 133:475-478.

Gordon, H. R. (1968): Fetal bradycardia after paracervical block. *New England Journal of Medicine*, 279:910-914.

Gosselin, R. E., Gabourel, J. D., Kalser, S. C., and Wills, J. H. (1955): The metabolism of C^{14}-labelled atropine and tropic acid in mice. *Journal of Pharmacology and Experimental Therapeutics*, 115:217-229.

Hanngren, A. E., Hansson, S., Sjöqvist, E., and Ullberg, S. (1964): Autoradiographic distribution studies with ^{14}C-cortisone and ^{14}C-cortisol. *Acta Endocrinologica*, 47:95-104.

Idänpään-Heikkilä, J., Fritchie, G. E., Englert, L. F., Ho, B. T., and McIsaac, W. M. (1969): Placental transfer of tritiated-1-$\triangle^9$-tetrahydrocannabinol. *New England Journal of Medicine*, 281:330.

Idänpään-Heikkilä, J. E., Jouppila, P. I., Puolakka, J. O., and Vorne, M. S., (1971a): Placental transfer and fetal metabolism of diazepam in early human pregnancy. *American Journal of Obstetrics and Gynecology*, 109:1011-1016.

Idänpään-Heikkilä, J., and Schoolar, J. (1969): LSD: Autoradiographic study on the placental transfer and tissue distribution in mice. *Science*, 164:1295-1297.

Idänpään-Heikkilä, J. E., Taska, R. J., Allen, H. A., and Schoolar, J. C. (1971b): Placental transfer of diazepam-C^{14} in mice, hamsters and monkeys. *Journal of Pharmacology and Experimental Therapeutics*, 176:752-757.

Juchau, M. R. (1972): Mechanisms of drug biotransformation reactions in the placenta. *Federation Proceedings*, 31:48-52.

Katz, J. (1968): The distribution of ^{14}C-labelled lidocaine injected intravenously into the rat. *Anesthesiology*, 29:249-253.

Katz, J., Gershwin, M. E., and Hood, W. L. (1968): The distribution of C^{14}-lidocaine in the rat using whole body autoradiography. *Archives Internationales de Pharmacodynamie et de Thérapie*, 175:339-346.

Katz, J. (1969): An autoradiographic study of placental transmission of labelled prilocaine in the rat. *British Journal of Anesthesiology,* 41:929-932.

Kivalo, I., and Saarikoski, S. (1970): Quantitative measurements of placental transfer and distribution of radioactive atropine in fetus. *Annales Chirurgiae et Gynaecologiae Fenniae,* 59:80-84.

Levi, A. J., Gatmatain, B. S., and Arias, I. M. (1970): Deficiency of hepatic organic anion-binding protein, impaired anion uptake and "physiologic" jaundice in newborn monkeys. *New England Journal of Medicine,* 283:1136-1139.

Mayer, S., Maickel, R., and Brodie, B. B. (1959): Kinetics of penetration of drugs and other foreign molecules into cerebrospinal fluid and brain. *Journal of Pharmacology and Experimental Therapeutics,* 127:205-211.

McDowell, R. W., Landolt, R. R., Kessler, W. V., and Shaw, S. M. (1971): Placental transfer of 2,3,5-triiodobenzoic acid in the rat. *Journal of Pharmaceutical Sciences,* 60:695-699.

Mirkin, B. L. (1971): Diphenylhydantoin: Placental transport, fetal localization, neonatal metabolism and possible teratogenic effects. *Journal of Pediatrics,* 78:329-337.

Mirkin, B. L. (1972): Ontogenesis of the adrenergic nervous system. *Federation Proceedings,* 31:65-74.

Mirkin, B. L., and Singh, S. (1972): Placental transfer and pharmacokinetics of digoxin in the pregnant rat. *Proc. 5th Int. Congress on Pharmacology.*

Morishima, H. O., Daniel, S. S., Finster, M., Poppers, P. J., and James, L. S. (1966): Transmission of mepivacaine hydrochloride across the human placenta. *Anesthesiology,* 27:147-154.

Nelson, B. (1969): Herbicides: Order on 2,4,5-T issued at unusually high level. *Science,* 166:977-979.

O'Donoghue, S. E. F. (1971): Distribution of pethidine and chlorpromazine in maternal fetal and neonatal biological fluids. *Nature,* 229:124-125.

Oh, Y., and Mirkin, B. L. (1971): Transfer of drugs into the central nervous system and across the placenta: A comparative study utilizing aminopyrine (A), diphenylhydantoin (D), sodium salicylate(s) and mecamylamine (M). *Federation Proceedings,* 30:2034.

Okita, G. T., Gordon, R. B., and Geiling, E. M. K. (1952): Placental transfer of radioactive digitoxin in rats and guinea pigs. *Proceedings of the Society for Experimental Biology and Medicine,* 80:536-538.

Okita, G. T., Plotz, E. J., and Davis, M. E. (1956): Placental transfer of radioactive digitoxin in pregnant women and its fetal distribution. *Circulation Research,* 4:376-380.

O'Leary, J. A., Davies, J. E., Edmundson, W. F., and Reich, G. A. (1970): Transplacental passage of pesticides. *American Journal of Obstetrics and Gynecology,* 107:65-68.

Peckham, C. H., and King, R. W. (1963): A study of intercurrent conditions observed during pregnancy. *American Journal of Obstetrics and Gynecology,* 87:609-624.

Persaud, T. V. N., and Ellington, A. C. (1968): Teratogenic activity of cannabis resin. *Lancet,* II:406-407.

Pitkin, R. M., Reynolds, W. A., and Filer, L. J. (1970): Placental transmission and fetal distribution of cyclamate in early human pregnancy. *American Journal of Obstetrics and Gynecology,* 108:1043-1050.

Placidi, G. F., and Cassano, G. B. (1968): Distribution and metabolism of ^{14}C-labelled chlordiazepoxide in mice. *International Journal of Neuropharmacology,* 7:383-389.

Polishuk, Z. W., Wassermann, M., Wassermann, D., Groner, Y., and Lazarovici, S. (1970): Effects of pregnancy on storage of organochlorine insecticides. *Archives of Environmental Health,* 20:215-217.

Roberts, J. B., Thomas, B. H., and Wilson, A. (1970): Placental transfer of pyridostigmine in the rat. *British Journal of Pharmacology and Chemotherapy,* 38:202-205.

Sandler, M., Ruthven, C. R. J., Contractor, S. F., Wood, C., Booth, R. T., and Pinkerton, J. H. M. (1963): Transmission of noradrenaline across the human placenta. *Nature*, 197:598.

Sanner, J. H., and Wood, L. A. (1965): Comparative distribution of tritium-labelled dihydromorphine between maternal and fetal rats. *Journal of Pharmacology and Experimental Therapeutics*, 148:176-184.

Shnider, S. M., and Way, E. L. (1968): Plasma levels of lidocaine in mother and newborn following obstetrical conduction anesthesia: Clinical applications. *Anesthesiology*, 29:951-958.

Shoeman, D. W., Kauffman, R. E., Azarnoff, D., and Boulos, B. M. (1972): Placental transfer of diphenylhydantoin in the goat. *Biochemical Pharmacology*, 21:1237-1243.

Sjöstrand, S. E., Cassano, G. B., and Hansson, E. (1965): The distribution of ^{35}S-chlorpromazine in mice studied by whole body radioautography. *Archives Internationale de Pharmacodynamie et de Thérapie*, 156:34-47.

Sjövall, A., Trolle, D., Boe, F., and Vara, P. (1967): Studies of the effect of anesthetics on foetus. Part I. The effect of paracervical block with mepivacaine upon foetal acid-base values. *Acta Obstetrica et Gynecologica Scandinavica*, 46:Suppl. 2.

Strauss, L., Goldenberg, N., Hirota, K., and Okudaira, Y. (1965): Structure of the human placenta. In: *Proceedings: Symposium on the Placenta, Its Form and Functions, Birth Defects Original Article Series*, Vol. 1, National Foundation-March of Dimes, Washington, D.C.

Tjälve, H., Hansson, E., and Schmiterlöw, C. G. (1968): Passage of C^{14}-nicotine and its metabolites into mice foetuses and placentae. *Acta Pharmacologica et Toxicologica*, 26:539-555.

Ullberg, S. (1959): Autoradiographic studies on the distribution of labelled drugs in the body. *Progress in Nuclear Energy*, 2:29-35.

Ullberg, S. Lindquist, N. G., and Sjostrand, S. E. (1970): Accumulation of chorioretinotoxic drugs in the fetal eye. *Nature*, 227:1257-1258.

Waddell, W. J. (1972): Localization and metabolism of drugs in the fetus. *Federation Proceedings*, 31:52-62.

Waddell, W. J., and Mirkin, B. L. (1971): Distribution and metabolism of diphenylhydantoin-C^{14} in fetal and maternal tissues of the pregnant mouse. *Biochemical Pharmacology*, 21:547-552.

Yeh, S. Y., and Woods, L. A. (1970): Maternal and fetal distribution of H^{3}-dihydromorphine in the non-tolerant rat. *Journal of Pharmacology and Experimental Therapeutics*, 174:9-13.

Zarrow, M. X., Philpott, J. E., and Denenberg, V. H. (1970): Passage of ^{14}C-corticosterone from the rat mother to the foetus and neonate. *Nature*, 226:1058-1059.

DISCUSSION

LIND: Are your observations valid for the whole pregnancy or for the term of pregnancy? What kind of interaction do we have in early pregnancy compared with late pregnancy?

MIRKIN: The rodent studies were performed on pregnant rats at the 20th day of gestation. It is not clear whether this reflects the situation as it exists early in gestation. Some very fragmentary data suggest a more rapid transfer in rats studied about the 15th day of gestation.

DAWES: Do you accept the assumption implicit in the last section of your paper that transfer of a drug into the placental tissue is equivalent to transplacental transfer?

MIRKIN: The placental rate constants for the transfer of drugs into the placenta do not categorically reflect placental transfer. This was apparent during the study of a homologous series of sulfa drugs in which some compounds with high penetration rate constants manifest a relatively low degree of placental transfer.

DAWES: Have you come across any drug that is actively transferred across the placenta, as are the amino acids?

MIRKIN: We have not studied any drugs which are actively transferred.

KARCZMAR: Did you study any quarternary compounds?

MIRKIN: No.

ELIS: I would like to make a remark to the question of drug distribution at different stages of pregnancy. We studied the sodium salicylate maternal/fetal ratio in rats and women. After the dose of 50 mg/kg of sodium salicylate administered orally on the 16th and 20th day of gestation to rats we found that the salicylic acid level 3 hours later in placenta was about 60% and the level in the fetus about 50% of the level found in maternal blood. The same results were observed in women in the 8th, 10th, and 40th weeks of pregnancy when 50 mg/kg of sodium salicylate was administered orally and the salicylic acid level was determined 3 hours later. Thus, the ratio for salicylic acid between maternal and fetal blood is practically the same in pregnant women and rats. This supports the old view of Rattner et al. (1928) that the penetration of drugs through the placenta may be the same in rodents and in man in spite of the difference in the structure of the placenta.

HOLMSTEDT: I think it is important already in the beginning of this symposium that we get the following facts straightened out. (1) Is the anatomy, physiology, and biochemistry of the placenta in various species similar to such a degree that results obtained in one species have relevance for another? (2) Can results obtained with drug administration in animals at all be extrapolated to humans?

MIRKIN: I don't believe that the kinetic constants will prove similar for man and animal, but perhaps meaningful predictive data can be developed which may prove applicable to the human.

SJÖQVIST: What is the lower sensitivity range of your assay method for diphenylhydantoin?

MIRKIN: The assay utilized was that of Dill et al. which can determine concentrations ranging as low as 0.5 to 1.0 μg/ml plasma.

Fetal Pharmacology, edited by L. Boréus
Raven Press, New York © 1973

Pharmacokinetic Aspects of Placental Drug Transfer

Gerhard Levy and William L. Hayton

School of Pharmacy, State University of New York at Buffalo, Buffalo, New York

INTRODUCTION

There are very few opportunities to study the kinetics of drug transfer across the placenta in humans during the early stages of pregnancy, i.e., in the most critical period for the production of fetal anomalies. It is particularly important, therefore, to maximize the information output of such studies. As has been pointed out, any substance given to the mother, if present in sufficient quantity in the maternal circulation, can and will reach the fetus (Ginsburg, 1968). This raises the questions of how much drug reaches the fetus, how rapidly it enters the fetal circulation, and how long it remains in the fetus. Depending on whether a drug acts by a reversible mechanism (such as central nervous system depression) or by producing an irreversible effect (such as teratogenicity), it may be important to focus either on the time course of drug concentrations in the fetus (Levy and Gibaldi, 1972) or on the total drug level-time integral (Jusko, 1972). The ratio of the total area under the drug concentration vs. time curve for the fetus to that of the mother may well serve as an index of relative exposure of the fetus to a drug taken by the mother. For example, the data reported by Depp, Kind, Kirby, and Johnson (1970) show an essentially identical time

29

course of methicillin concentrations in maternal and fetal serums following intravenous administration to the mother; this represents an index of relative exposure equal to unity. The same study showed that dicloxacillin concentrations in the fetal serum were much lower at all times than in the maternal serum. The index of relative exposure for dicloxacillin is less than 0.2 as calculated from the published data. Drugs which are intended to reach the fetal circulation should have a high index of relative exposure; drugs which could harm the fetus and are intended for the mother only should have a low index of relative exposure.

Studies of placental drug transfer in humans during the early stages of pregnancy are complicated not only by the limited availability of subjects and by legal and ethical restrictions. There is the additional complication from the pharmacokinetic point of view in that only a one-point determination of drug concentration in the fetus is ordinarily feasible in humans. The pharmacokinetic characterization of placental drug transfer is, therefore, based usually on a composite of data obtained from different subjects at different times. A meaningful pharmacokinetic analysis of such data is extremely difficult and cannot be very definitive. At this time, pharmacokinetics can serve most effectively as an aid in designing protocols so that the information to be obtained from placental transfer studies can be maximized. Computer simulations have, therefore, been carried out to determine the time course of drug concentrations in mother and fetus under various conditions.

MULTI–COMPARTMENT PHARMACOKINETIC MODELS

Some drugs are so rapidly distributed in the body upon reaching the bloodstream that the body acts like a single compartment with respect to these drugs and may be characterized as such for pharmacokinetic purposes. Other drugs, being less rapidly distributed, confer on the body the pharmacokinetic characteristics of a multi-compartment model (Gibaldi, Levy, and Weintraub, 1971). The mother and fetus can be viewed, in the most simple terms, as a two-compartment system. More complex pharmacokinetic models can represent the mother as a multi-compartment system; a compartment representing a drug-eliminating placenta may be added; the fetus as well as the mother may be assumed to excrete and/or metabolize a drug. These different pharmacokinetic models yield different types of drug concentration vs. time patterns in mother and fetus, as well as different fetal:maternal concentration ratio vs. time curves. Experimental protocols should be designed on the basis of these considerations.

SINGLE–COMPARTMENT MOTHER AND FETUS

In single-compartment simulations, the apparent volume of distribution of the maternal compartment is 20 volume units and that of the fetus is 0.002 volume units, a 10,000:1 ratio which is consistent with the relative body weights of mother and fetus after 2 to 3 months of gestation. In this and the following simulations, it will be assumed that all distribution, transfer, and elimination processes are apparent first-order, with rates (dA/dt) equal to the product of rate constant (k) and the amount of drug (A) in the originating compartment:

$$dA/dt = - kA$$

Clearances between mother and fetus are assumed to be equal in both directions:

$$k_{MF} \, V_M = k_{FM} \, V_F$$

where k_{MF} is the rate constant for drug transfer from mother to fetus, k_{FM} the rate constant for drug transfer from fetus to mother, and V_M and V_F the apparent volumes of distribution of the mother and fetus compartments, respectively. If plasma protein binding differs significantly between mother and fetus, the assumption of equal clearance in both directions is not valid and the model has to be modified accordingly unless all concentration terms are corrected for protein binding.

The upper left panel in Fig. 1 shows the time course of drug concentrations in mother and fetus following rapid intravenous injection of 1,000 dosage units of a drug, assuming the fetus to be rapidly accessible ("shallow"). The fetal:maternal drug concentration ratio rapidly reaches a constant value of near unity (upper right panel, Fig. 1). Constant-rate infusion of 2,000 dosage units over four time units yields the concentration and concentration ratio curves shown in the lower half of Fig. 1. This rapid equilibration to a fetal:maternal concentration ratio of about one has been found, for example, with thiopental (Moya and Thorndike, 1962).

Figure 2 is another simulation of a one-compartment mother and fetus, except that the fetus is much more slowly accessible ("deep"). The slow equilibration between the two compartments is not evident in the drug concentration curve for the mother because of the very small apparent volume

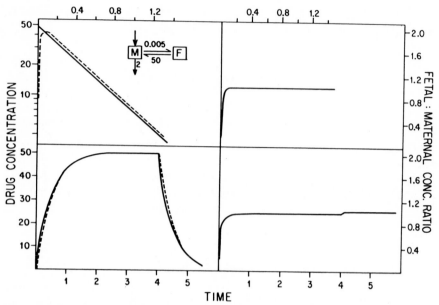

FIG. 1. Simulated time course of drug concentrations in mother (M) and fetus (F), each having the pharmacokinetic characteristics of a single compartment. The fetus compartment is "shallow." *Upper left:* Time course of drug concentrations in mother (——) and fetus (----) following rapid intravenous injection of the drug. *Upper right:* Fetal:maternal drug concentration ratio after rapid injection. *Lower left:* Time course of drug concentrations in mother and fetus following constant rate infusion for 4 time units. *Lower right:* Fetal:maternal drug concentration ratio during and after infusion. The parmacokinetic model is shown in the upper left panel; the numbers are apparent first-order rate constants in reciprocal time units.

of distribution of the fetus. The fetal:maternal drug concentration ratio after rapid injection approaches a value of two; it should be noted that this ratio is lower during infusion (when distribution is on-going continuously) than post-infusion. This is true generally; concentration ratios between compartments observed during constant rate drug infusion reflect an entirely different pharmacokinetic situation than the post-distributive concentration ratios attained some time after drug administration (Gibaldi, 1969). Examples of drugs showing fetal:maternal drug concentration ratios greater than unity are saccharin (Pitkin, Reynolds, Filer, and Kling, 1971), diazepam (Idänpään-Heikkilä, Jouppila, Poulakka, and Vorne, 1971), and cephalothin (MacAuley and Charles, 1968).

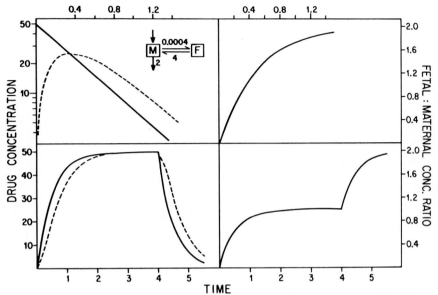

FIG. 2. As in Fig. 1, except that the fetus compartment is relatively "deep."

TWO–COMPARTMENT MOTHER AND FETUS

In two-compartment simulations, the mother is represented as a two-compartment system, consisting of a central compartment (M) which includes the blood plasma and the site of drug elimination, and a peripheral or "tissue" compartment (T). The two compartments are assumed to have the same apparent volume of distribution (10 volume units each), and the ratio between the sum of the apparent volumes of both maternal compartments (20 volume units) and that of the fetus (0.002 volume units) is 10,000:1. Drug is administered as 1,000 dose units by rapid intravenous injection or as a constant rate infusion of a total of 2,000 dose units into the central compartment of the mother.

Figure 3 represents a system in which the fetus is a "shallow" compartment while the maternal tissue compartment is "deep." A semilogarithmic plot of drug concentration in the central compartment of the mother and in the fetus vs. time is curved owing to slow distribution of drug into the tissue compartment. Tetracycline concentrations in maternal and fetal serum show such curvature (LeBlanc and Perry, 1967). Figure 4 depicts a similar

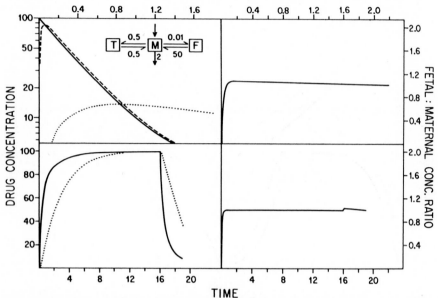

FIG. 3. Simulated time course of drug concentrations in the central (M) and "tissue" (T) compartments of the mother and in the fetus (F). M, ——; T, · · ·; F, - - - -. Rapid injection (*above*) and constant-rate infusion for 16 time units (*below*). Tissue is "deep"; fetus is "shallow." The concentration in F practically coincides with that in M during and after infusion.

system except that the fetus is "deep" and the maternal tissue compartment is more shallow than in the previous example. The fetal:central compartment concentration ratio is well above unity in the post-distributive phase. The post-distribution fetal:maternal central compartment drug concentration ratio eventually reaches a constant value of 1.265. This ratio is attained 2.9 time units after rapid injection and 2.4 time units after the end of infusion. More important, the drug concentration in the central compartment is 3.01 and 10.7 concentration units, respectively, at these times. This difference can be much more pronounced, depending on the apparent volume and "depth" of the compartments. Constant-rate infusion makes it possible to reach the steady state at higher drug concentrations than would be attained by rapid injection. The drug concentration in the central compartment of the mother may be so low at the steady state after rapid injection that precise assays are impossible. For example, an apparent steady state between maternal and fetal cephalothin concentrations in the blood is reached only when the maternal cephalothin concentration has decreased to about one-tenth of its initial level after intramuscular administration

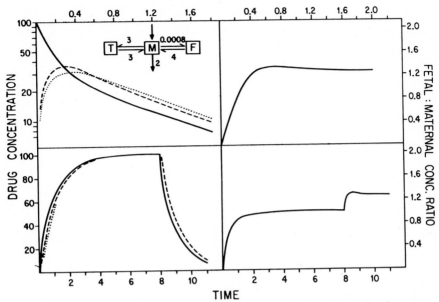

FIG. 4. As in Fig. 3, except that the fetus compartment is "deep" and the tissue compartment is more "shallow" than in Fig. 3. Constant rate infusion for 8 time units.

(Sheng, Huang, and Promadhattavedi, 1964). It may be useful to administer such a drug by constant-rate infusion so that the steady state is reached at drug concentrations which are well above assay limits.

Figure 5 represents a pharmacokinetic model consisting of a maternal central compartment, a relatively "deep" maternal tissue compartment, and a "deep" fetus compartment. Of particular interest is the pronounced maximum in the fetal:maternal central compartment drug concentration ratio some time after injection or infusion, and the fact that this ratio is well above unity. This pattern has been observed with ampicillin (Perry and LeBlanc, 1967) and gentamycin (von Kobyletzki, 1967). A comparison of Figs. 4 and 5 shows the pronounced effect of the rate constants for drug distribution between the maternal central and tissue compartments on the rate of attainment of the steady state.

DRUG ELIMINATION BY THE PLACENTA OR FETUS

There is considerable evidence that the human placenta and fetus are capable of metabolizing some drugs. The effects of these processes are

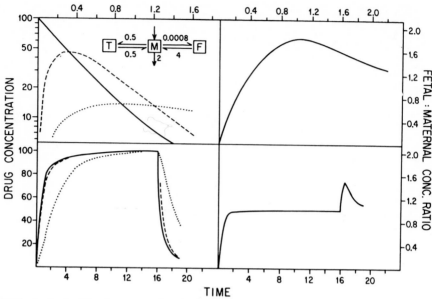

FIG. 5. As in Fig. 3, except that both tissue and fetus compartments are relatively "deep." Constant rate infusion for 16 time units.

simulated in Fig. 6, which shows in the upper panel the time course of drug concentrations in mother and fetus, and in the lower panel the fetal: maternal drug concentration ratio as a function of time after rapid intravenous injection of a drug. The pharmacokinetic model consists of a maternal compartment with an apparent volume of distribution (V_d) of 20 volume units, a placenta (P) compartment $(V_d = 0.008)$, and a fetus compartment $(V_d = 0.002)$. It is assumed that 1,000 dosage units of drug are injected rapidly into the maternal compartment. The following conditions were simulated.

Case	K_{el-F}	K_{el-P}	K_{el}	K_{PM}	K_{MP}	K_{PF}	K_{FM}
A	0	0	2	5,000	2	2.5	10
B	20	0	2	5,000	2	2.5	10
C	0	1,000	2	5,000	2	2.5	10

The rate constants were chosen rather arbitrarily in the absence of definitive information, with clearances between compartments being identical in both directions. Drug excretion and/or metabolism by the fetus has no discernible effect on drug concentrations in the mother because of the small apparent volume of the fetal compartment, but the fetal:maternal

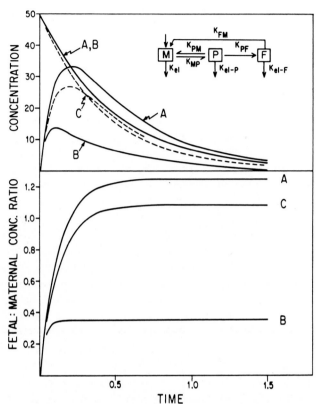

FIG. 6. Effect of drug elimination (metabolism and/or excretion) by the fetus (F) or placenta (P) on drug concentrations in the fetus and mother and on the fetal:maternal drug concentration ratio after a rapidly injected dose. *A:* no elimination by P or F; *B:* elimination by F but not by P; *C:* elimination by P but not by F. The continually descending curves in the upper panel represent the concentrations in M; the ascending and then descending curves represent drug concentrations in F.

drug concentration ratio is decreased appreciably. Drug metabolism by the placenta also decreases this ratio relative to the case where neither placenta nor fetus eliminates the drug.

There is evidence which suggests that the newborn infant (and therefore presumably the fetus at term) can metabolize lidocaine quite well. Consistent with this assumption and with the pharmacokinetic predictions is the fact that the fetal:maternal lidocaine plasma concentration ratio is well below unity following single and repeated injections (Shnider and Way, 1968; Fox, Houle, Desjardins, and Mercier, 1971) even though there appears to be no difference in the protein binding of the drug in maternal and fetal plasma.[1] Examples of such differences in plasma protein binding have been reported, and these can, of course, account for maternal:fetal drug concentration ratios other than unity.

CONCLUSIONS

The pharmacokinetic considerations presented here indicate the need to characterize fully the kinetics of drug distribution and elimination in the mother even if only a single-point determination can be made in the fetus. Fetal:maternal drug concentration ratios must be determined over a considerable period of time to attain a constant value if the maternal tissues and/or the fetus are "deep" compartments. Constant-rate infusions may cause this steady-state condition to be attained at higher concentrations than rapid injections, and this may permit more accurate determinations of these ratios. The ratio of fetal:maternal areas under the drug concentration curve from the time of drug administration to the time when all of the drug has been eliminated can serve as an index of relative exposure of the fetus to the drug. It would be best to determine this index on the basis of the concentrations of free (i.e., not plasma protein bound) rather than total drug. The significance of the index is affected, however, by the binding characteristics of the drug in the maternal and fetal tissues. The index is most representative of relative exposure to the drug if the apparent volume of distribution, in milliliters per kilogram of body weight, is essentially identical in mother and fetus. It is not sufficient and certainly not very informative to determine only if a drug is or is not transferred across the placenta or even to determine the rate of this process. Only a measure of relative exposure (which is a function of placental transfer in *both* directions, distribution of drug in the mother and the fetus, and placental and fetal drug elimination kinetics) will provide a meaningful basis for determining the potential effects on the fetus of drugs given to the mother during gestation.

ACKNOWLEDGMENT

This investigation was supported in part by U.S. Public Health Service research grant GM 19568.

---

[1] More recent studies indicate that, contrary to the findings of Shnider and Way (1968), lidocaine is bound much less extensively in umbilical than in maternal plasma and that the fetal:maternal concentration ratio can be rationalized on this basis (Tucker, Boyes, Bridenbaugh, and Moore 1970).

REFERENCES

Depp, R., Kind, A. C., Kirby, W. M., and Johnson, W. (1970): Transplacental passage of methicillin and diceoxacillin into the fetus and amniotic fluid. *American Journal of Obstetrics and Gynecology*, 107:1054-1057.

Fox, G. S., Houle, G. L., Desjardins, P. D., and Mercier, G. (1971): Intrauterine fetal lidocaine concentrations during continuous epidural anesthesia. *American Journal of Obstetrics and Gynecology*, 110:896-899.

Gibaldi, M. (1969): Effect of mode of administration on drug distribution in a two-compartment open system. *Journal of Pharmaceutical Sciences*, 58:327-331.

Gibaldi, M., Levy, G., and Weintraub, H. (1971): Drug distribution and pharmacologic effects. *Clinical Pharmacology and Therapeutics*, 12:734-742.

Ginsburg, J. (1968): Breakdown in maternal protection: drugs. *Proceedings of the Royal Society of Medicine*, 61:1244-1247.

Idänpään-Heikkilä, J. E., Jouppila, P. I., Poulakka, J. O., and Vorne, M. S. (1971): Placental transfer and fetal metabolism of diazepam in early human pregnancy. *American Journal of Obstetrics and Gynecology*, 109:1011-1016.

Jusko, W. J.: Pharmacodynamic principles in chemical teratology: Dose-effect relationships. *Journal of Pharmacology and Experimental Therapeutics* (*in press*).

LeBlanc, A. L., and Perry, J. E. (1967): Transfer of tetracycline across the human placenta. *Texas Reports on Biology and Medicine*, 25:541-545.

Levy, G., and Gibaldi, M. (1972): Pharmacokinetics of drug action. *Annual Review of Pharmacology*, 12:85–98.

MacAulay, M. A., and Charles, D. (1968): Placental transfer of cephalothin. *American Journal of Obstetrics and Gynecology*, 100:940-946.

Moya, F., and Thorndike, V. (1962): Passage of drugs across the placenta. *American Journal of Obstetrics and Gynecology*, 84:1778-1798.

Perry, J. E., and LeBlanc, A. L. (1967): Transfer of ampicillin across the human placenta. *Texas Reports on Biology and Medicine*, 25:547-551.

Pitkin, R. M., Reynolds, W. A., Filer, L. J, and Kling, T. G. (1971): Placental transmission and fetal distribution of saccharin. *American Journal of Obstetrics and Gynecology*, 111:280-286.

Sheng, K. T., Huang, N. N., and Promadhattavedi, V. (1964): Serum concentration of cephalothin in infants and children and placental transmission of the antibiotic. *Antimicrobial Agents and Chemotherapy*, 200-206.

Shnider, S. M., and Way, E. L. (1968): The kinetics of transfer of lidocaine (Xylocaine®) across the human placenta. *Anesthesiology*, 29:944-950.

Tucker, G. T., Boyes, R. N., Bridenbaugh, P. O., and Moore, D. C. (1970): Binding of anilide-type local anesthetics in human plasma: II. Implications in vivo, with special reference to transplacental distribution. *Anesthesiology*, 33:304-314.

von Kobyletzki, D. (1967): Experimentelle Untersuchungen zur Diaplazentaren Passage von Gentamycin. *International Journal of Clinical Pharmacology*, 2:116-119.

DISCUSSION

DAWES: What is the physiological counterpart or explanation of a "deep" fetus? Do you believe fetuses are normally "deep" or "shallow"?

LEVY: A "deep" compartment is relatively slowly penetrable. A compartment can be "deep" with respect to one drug and "shallow" with respect to another.

Fetal Pharmacology, edited by L. Boréus
Raven Press, New York © 1973

Ultrastructure of the Placenta: Consequences for Drug Distribution

Edward W. Dempsey

Department of Anatomy, Columbia University, College of Physicians and Surgeons, New York, New York 10032

Despite its obvious intervention between the circulatory systems of the mother and fetus, the placenta has received curiously little attention until recently. In a monograph published by the Association for the Aid of Crippled Children in 1959, the staff made a comprehensive study of the literature related to the placenta and fetal membranes and were able to find only about 2,700 references. It is interesting that so accurate an observer as Leonardo failed to depict the human placenta correctly (Boyd and Hamilton, 1970). There are remarkable differences in the disposition of the maternal and fetal elements of the placentas in various viviparous species. The confusion resulting from these differences greatly delayed proper recognition of the trophoblast's function in the transmission of metabolites to and from the fetus, and has probably been one factor in discouraging biological scientists from undertaking extensive studies of the organ. Even today, pathologists pay scant attention to the placenta in most births, dissuaded perhaps by the fact that viable babies, even though dysmature, may often be associated with frankly abnormal placentas.

In lower viviparous vertebrates, the yolk sac fuses with the chorion to form the primary placental connection. Such a placenta, when vascularized, becomes known as the *choriovitelline placenta,* and forms a transitional functional structure in many mammals. Indeed, in rabbits and other species it has important functions in transmitting antibodies from the mother to the fetus (Brambell, 1970). Although the yolk sac is often said to be a vestigial, rapidly disappearing structure in the human, Amoroso (*personal communication*) has shown that it frequently lies buried in the discoid mass of the placenta, persisting until at least the second trimester.

The definitive placenta in higher mammals, including man, is vascularized from the allantois, and is therefore described as the *chorioallantoic placenta*. A histological classification of such placentas in a variety of mammals was proposed by Grosser (1927). This system was based upon an assumed function of the placenta in impeding the transmission of substances in proportion to the number and kind of layers interposed between the mother and fetus. This classification is obviously deficient in many respects. It is more appropriate for mature than for young placentas. It refers only to the chorioallantoic and not to the choriovitelline placenta; yet the yolk-sac placenta has important functions and presence in many species including primates. It implies that transmission is passive, whereas it is now known that active transport processes exist. Perhaps its most damaging attribute has been the degree to which it has misled many uncritical investigators who, without personal and detailed knowledge of placental structure, have used the simplistic notions of Grosser as evidence to support their own theories of the fetal-maternal exchange process. I shall attempt to show that it is also incomplete and misleading in that it neglects two important aspects of placental ultrastructure, namely, erosion and pinocytosis by the trophoblast.

The importance of properly recognizing the morphological structure of placental barriers was heavily underscored in the aftermath of the thalidomide tragedy, when countless babies were born with congenital malformations now known to have been caused by a drug used by their mothers. Efforts to produce experimentally in pregnant animals the teratogenic results of thalidomide failed in the commonly used laboratory rodents; only in monkeys were the characteristic abnormalities produced. Indeed, even in the primate *Galago,* no abnormalities were seen (Wilson, 1969). This idiosyncrasy became less puzzling when it was shown that *Galago,* unlike other primates, has an epitheliochorial placenta, more similar to that of ungulates than to the hemochorial placenta of man (Dempsey, 1969). That the ultrastructure of other primate placentas should be investigated and correlated with their ability to transmit drugs and other metabolites is strongly suggested by this and by the recent finding of Jollie (*unpublished*) that in the marmoset, a platyrrhine monkey, the trophoblast is also different in ultrastructure from the situation in the Old World primates.

For many years, physiologists assumed that placental transfer was accomplished by the simple process of diffusion, in accordance with the Grosser scheme (Flexner, 1954). Indeed, this view is still held as the most probable means for transport of gases and electrolytes. However, an increasing amount of evidence now supports the view that phagocytosis and pinocytosis—histiotrophic nutrition—are much more prominent and sustained activities of trophoblast than was previously thought. In the first *Macy Conference on Gestation,* both Wislocki (1954) and Amoroso (1954) stated that phagocytosis had been observed only in the early stages of implantation in humans. However, a year later Boyd (1955) mentioned the frequent occurrence of phagocytosis in the basic trophoblast, and in 1957 Luse presented convincing phase-contrast and electron-microscopic evidence of phagocytosis in yolk-sac epithelium. Many such observations have been reported since then: in studying human placentas, Muir (1966) described the phagocytic uptake of iron-dextran particles by term placental trophoblast; transmission and scanning electron-microscopic observations indicative of phagocytic absorption have been reported by Dempsey, Lessey, and Luse (1970) and by Dempsey and Luse (1971). In considering the transport of passive immunity from mother to fetus, Brambell (1970) rejected the hypothesis of diffusion on the ground that only an active, cellular process could discriminate between related antibodies to the observed degree. He concluded that uptake by pinocytosis must be considered the most likely mechanism, and that selective destruction of the absorbed antibodies in the pinocytic vesicles (electron microscopists would refer to lysosomes) could account for the failure of some antibodies to reach the fetus although they had been absorbed by the placental cells. We may fairly conclude, therefore, that active, cellular processes are involved in the uptake of many biologically active molecules and that equally active processes determine their intracellular destruction, transformation, or transference across the placental barrier.

Notwithstanding the fact that the placenta is involved with active absorptive and selective transport mechanisms, recent observations have cast doubt on the completeness of the trophoblastic barrier. Light microscopists have long known that villi to which fibrin clots are adherent may lack a syncytial layer. However, little physiological significance has been attached to such villi; in general, they have been considered as degenerative structures not involved in transport. Electron micrographs of such regions are now available, demonstrating that maternal fibrin and leucocytes may completely displace the trophoblast and rest directly upon its basement membrane. Thus, in such areas, the only cellular element separating fetal and maternal blood is the fetal endothelium (Dempsey et al., 1970; Dempsey and Luse, 1971).

Such areas are not too uncommonly encountered in transmission electron micrographs of specimens obtained early in pregnancy (5th to 12th week of gestation). However, the sampling error is very great in electron microscopy since the large magnifications employed permit examination of only minute areas. The application of scanning electron microscopy to the placenta allowed observation of much larger areas and revealed that such fibrin clots commonly occur in young placentas (Dempsey and Luse, 1971). Recently, we have also found many areas in villi from full-term placentas which have been denuded of trophoblast. It would appear, therefore, that we must now consider it probable that diffusion into the fetal connective tissue spaces occurs throughout pregnancy. It remains, however, to determine quantitatively its significance.

REFERENCES

Amoroso, E. C. (1954): The functional role of the placenta. In: *Transactions of the First Conference on Gestation.* Josiah Macy, Jr. Foundation, New York.

Boyd, J. D. (1955): Morphology and physiology of the uteroplacental circulation. In: *Transactions of the Second Conference on Gestation.* Josiah Macy, Jr. Foundation, New York.

Boyd, J. D., and Hamilton, W. J. (1970): *The Human Placenta.* W. Heffer and Sons, Ltd., Cambridge.

Brambell, F. W. R. (1970): *The Transmission of Passive Immunity from Mother to Young.* American Elsevier, New York.

Dempsey, E. W. (1969): Comparative aspects of the placental barrier. In: *Proceedings of the Second International Workshop in Teratology.* Igaku Shoin Ltd., Tokyo.

Dempsey, E. W., Lessey, R. A., and Luse, S. A. (1970): Electron microscopic observations on fibrinoid and histiotroph in the junctional zone and villi of the human placenta. *American Journal of Anatomy,* 128:463-484.

Dempsey, E. W., and Luse, S. A. (1971): Regional specializations in the syncytial trophoblast of early human placentas. *Journal of Anatomy,* 108:545-561.

Flexner, L. B. (1954): The functional role of the placenta. In: *Transactions of the First Conference on Gestation.* Josiah Macy, Jr. Foundation, New York.

Grosser, O. (1927). *Fruhentwicklung, Eihautbildung und Placentation des Menschen und der Säugetiere.* Bergman, Munich.

Luse, S. A. (1957): The morphologic manifestations of uptake of materials by the yolk-sac of the pregnant rabbit. In: *Transactions of the Fourth Conference on Gestation.* Josiah Macy, Jr. Foundation, New York.

Muir, A. R. (1966): On the phagocytosis of iron-dextran by the human phasmoditrophoblast. *Journal of Obstetrics and Gynecology of the British Commonwealth,* 73:966-972.

Villee, C. A. (1960): *The Placenta and Fetal Membranes.* Williams and Wilkins, Co., New York.

Wilson, J. G. (1969): Teratological and reproductive studies in non-human primates. In: *Proceedings on the Second International Workshop in Teratology.* Igaku Shoin, Ltd., Tokyo.

Wislocki, G. B. (1954): The functional role of the placenta. In: *Transactions of the First Conference on Gestation.* Josiah Macy, Jr. Foundation, New York.

DISCUSSION

Uvnäs: Do you think that the reason why bushbabies do not show teratological damages is simply explained by differences between their placental structures?

Dempsey: It may be. The facts are that the two placentas are different and their responses are different. It is also true that other species, with different placental barriers, also do not exhibit teratological damage after administration of thalidomide.

Paoletti: What are the changes in phagocytic activity and fibrin clots observed in human placenta during the later stages of pregnancy?

Dempsey: We have not yet studied these changes in detail. My impression is that phagocytosis decreases and that clot formation, with attendant damage to the trophoblast, increases with advancing gestation age.

Räihä: It has been shown recently by de la Chapelle and co-workers that fetal leucocytes can be found in considerable amounts in the maternal circulation in human pregnancy. Could the mechanism of this transfer be explained on the basis of your morphological data on the placenta?

Dempsey: Yes, I think that villi are often broken off and carried in the maternal blood to form pulmonary emboli. The placental ends of such broken villi could easily bleed directly into the intervillous space, thus accounting for the presence of fetal leucocytes and erythrocytes in the maternal blood.

Mirkin: What characteristics distinguish the human placenta from a semipermeable membrane? Would you comment on these processes described and their potential influence on placental transfer?

Dempsey: The placenta exhibits phagocytosis and pinocytosis. Maternal plasma is sequestered into trophoblastic vacuoles and absorbed from them (or digested in them). Localized areas exist in which the trophoblast is lacking so that the only cellular barrier between the two circulations is the fetal endothelium. And lastly, a yolk sac exists for at least an important part of gestation. Because of its importance in lower mammals, its function in human gestation should at least be assessed.

Fetal Pharmacology, edited by L. Boréus
Raven Press, New York © 1973

Comparative Study on Maternal-Embryonic Transfer of Drugs in Man and Laboratory Animals

Hideo Nishimura

Department of Anatomy, Faculty of Medicine, Kyoto University, Kyoto, Japan

Conventional testing of new drugs in laboratory animals occasionally reveals its teratogenicity when a high dose is administered during early pregnancy. When the metabolism of that drug is similar in man and that animal species, a question may arise: Is the distribution pattern of the drug in human pregnancy comparable to that occurring in the teratological animal experiment? Because of ethical considerations, however, we are unable to use pregnant women for testing maternal-embryonic transfer of a new drug. Therefore, we have investigated a possibility of predicting the transfer of a new drug to human embryos on the basis of the animal and human data obtained with some drugs used clinically in pregnancy. That is, if the data show that the ratio of the drug level in maternal blood to that in embryos is similar in man and a given animal, we may be able to predict a level of a new drug in human embryos from the known drug level in the human blood by extrapolation of the animal data on maternal-embryonic transfer of the respective drug.

This chapter, which is a first step along this line, deals with the comparative studies on placental transfer of two drugs in early pregnancy of rodents and man. Although the results obtained so far could not be generalized to other drugs, the data may be useful in view of the vulnerability of early embryos. It should be noted that only a few investigations on transfer of drugs to early embryos have been reported (caffeine in man: Goldstein and Warren, 1961; ampicillin in man: Müller and Patsch, 1968; tetrahydrocannabinol in golden hamster: Idänpään-Heikkilä, Fritchie, Englert, Ho, and McIsaac, 1969; cyclamate in man: Pitkin, Reynolds, and Filer, 1970; sulfonamides in man: Kobyletzki, Morvay, and Gellen, 1971; diazepam in mouse: Idänpään-Heikkilä, Taska, Allen, and Schoolar, 1971).

PLACENTAL TRANSFER OF THIOPENTAL TO EARLY EMBRYOS

First, we studied the maternal-embryonic transfer of the anesthetic thiopental after a single injection to mice and women in early pregnancy. Maternal blood and whole embryos from 50 ICR-JCL mice at 14 days of gestation and from 120 women, whose pregnancy was interrupted for socioeco-

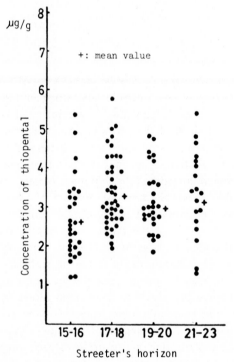

FIG. 1. Concentration of thiopental in human embryos at various developmental stages (5 to 10 min after injection of 300 mg).

nomic reasons at the second or third month, were used. All tissues were assayed after freezing at −20°C for a few weeks. It is known from thin-layer chromatography studies that the metabolic patterns of this drug in both species are about similar (Uno, 1969). We measured the amount of thiopental in the tissues of both species by Brodie's spectrophotometric method as modified by Uno.

The developmental stage of human embryos ranged from Streeter's horizon XV to XXIII (Streeter, 1948, 1951). However, as shown in Fig. 1, no noticeable stage difference was found in thiopental concentration measured several minutes after maternal injection. Therefore, we put together all the data obtained with such human embryos.

Figure 2 shows the concentration of thiopental in sequential maternal blood samples and embryos of mice following its maternal intravenous in-

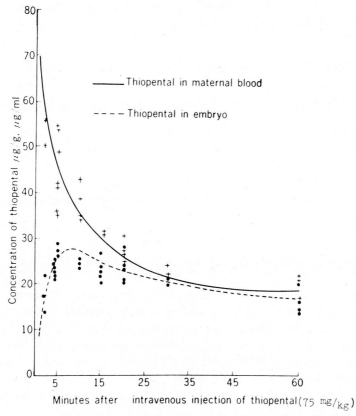

FIG. 2. Levels of thiopental in maternal blood and embryo (mouse).

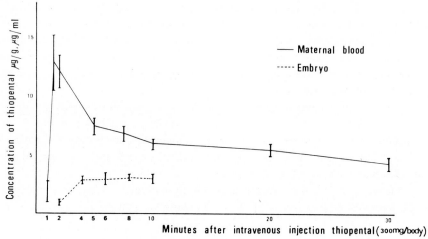

FIG. 3. Levels of thiopental in maternal blood and embryo (human).

jection at just sufficiently anesthetic dosage (75 mg/kg). This demonstrates that the drug level in embryos reaches a maximum after several minutes and that the concentration in the embryo is always lower than that in maternal blood.

Figure 3 shows the result of a similar study with the pregnant women injected intravenously with the anesthetic dosage (300 mg). The following similarities between data of the two species may be pointed out: (1) the highest drug level in embryos appears several minutes after the injection, and (2) the drug level in embryos is always lower than that in maternal blood.

PLACENTAL TRANSFER OF SULFAMETHOPYRAZINE TO EARLY EMBRYOS

Next, we made a similar comparative study with sulfamethopyrazine (SMP)[1], given orally to rats and women in early pregnancy. Maternal blood and whole embryos from 30 Sprague-Dawley rats at 12 days of gestation and from 15 women at second or third month of pregnancy were used. SMP was assayed by Bratton-Marshall's method on the tissues which had been frozen at $-20°C$ for a few weeks.

We measured the amounts of both free and total SMP in rat embryos

---

[1] Generously supplied by Eizai Co. Ltd. (Tokyo).

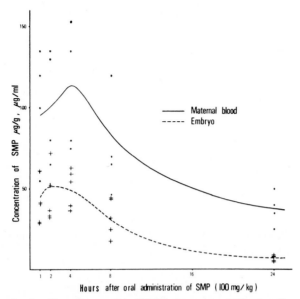

FIG. 4. Levels of sulfamethopyrazine (SMP) in maternal blood and embryo (rat).

from five mothers at 1 to 24 hr after the maternal drug intake, as well as in seven comparable human embryos. The results indicated that the amount of conjugated form of this drug is very small in embryos of both species. Therefore, the further assay was done for only free SMP.

Figure 4 shows the result in rats after a single maternal dose of SMP at 100 mg/kg which is about 10 times the dose in clinical use. It is seen that the drug level in embryos is always lower than that in maternal blood.

It should be added that another study with seven pregnant rats given 100 mg/kg SMP consecutively on gestational days 7 through 13 revealed no teratogenicity or lethality of the embryos.

Table 1 shows the preliminary result of the comparable study on placental transfer of SMP in pregnant women. It can be seen that in six out of eight cases the drug concentration in the embryo was far lower than that in the maternal blood. However, in two cases the reverse was found. Hence, a conclusive interpretation must await further investigation with more cases where the same and single dose is given at fixed intervals before the interruption of pregnancy. However, if we compare these human data with the values in rats shown in Fig. 4, it appears that the concentration of this drug in human embryos after its clinical use is far lower than the peak concentration in rat embryos after its maternal application at sub-teratogenic dose.

TABLE 1. *Placental transfer of sulfamethopyrazine (SMP) given orally to women in in 5 to 8 week pregnancy.*

Case	Dosage (mg) [interval after application (hr)]	Maternal blood (μg/ml)	Embryo (μg/g)
		Concentration of SMP	
A	200 [1]	15	0
B	200 [1]	19	0
C	200 [2]	15	2.4
D	200 [2]	10	18.8
E	200 [15] + 100 [4]	5	9.6
F	200 [24] + 200 [16]	20	4.9
G	200 [48] + 200 [24] + 100 [1]	33	8.6
H	200 [48] + 200 [24] + 100 [1]	36	2.1

This finding appears to be in accord with the clinical experience that the drug produces no adverse effects in human embryos.

ACKNOWLEDGMENT

This study was supported by a grant from the Association for the Aid of Crippled Children, New York. We are indebted to several obstetricians in Kinki, Chuba and Kanto areas for their help in supplying the human specimens.

The work was done in collaboration with Toyozo Uno, Shikibumi Kitazawa, and Yutaka Saito, in Faculty of Pharmaceutical Sciences, Kyoto University, and Takashi Tanimura, Yasuko Noguchi, and Junkichi Tomoyama, in Department of Anatomy, Faculty of Medicine, Kyoto University.

REFERENCES

Goldstein, A., and Warren, R. (1961): Passage of caffeine into human gonadal and fetal tissue. *Biochemical Pharmacology,* 11:166-168.

Idänpään-Heikkilä, J., Fritchie, G. E., Englert, L. F., Ho, B. T., and McIsaac, W. M. (1969): Placental transfer of tritiated-1-Δ^9-tetrahydrocannabinol. *New England Journal of Medicine,* 281:330.

Idänpään-Heikkilä, J., Taska, R. J., Allen, H. A., and Schoolar, J. C. (1971): Placental transfer of diazepam-^{14}C in mice, hamsters and monkeys. *Journal of Pharmacology and Experimental Therapeutics,* 176:752-757.

Kobyletzki, D. von, Morvay, J., and Gellen, J. (1971): Untersuchungen zur Pharmakokinetik von 7 Sulfonamiden in der Frühschwangerschaft beim Menschen. *Archiv für Gynäkologie,* 209:440-451.

Müller, R., and Patsch, R. (1968): Placentapassage von Ampizillin in die Frucht zur Behandlung von Listerioseinfektionen in der Schwangerschaft. *Archiv für Gynäkologie,* 206:98-106.
Pitkin, R. M., Reynolds, W. A., and Filer, L. J. (1970): Placental transmission and fetal distribution of cyclamate in early human pregnancy. *American Journal of Obstetrics and Gynecology,* 108:1043-1050.
Streeter, G. L. (1948): Developmental horizons in human embryos. Description of age groups XV, XVI, XVII and XVIII, being the third issue of a survey of the Carnegie collection. *Contributions to Embryology,* 32:133-203.
Streeter, G. L. (1951): Developmental horizons in human embryos. Description of age groups XIX, XX, XXI, XXII and XXIII, being the fifth issue of a survey of the Carnegie collection. *Contributions to Embryology,* 34:165-196.
Uno, T. (1969): Spectrophotometric assay of drugs in tissues. In: *Methods for Teratological Studies in Experimental Animals and Man,* edited by H. Nishimura and J. R. Miller. Igaku Shoin Ltd., Tokyo.

DISCUSSION

RÄIHÄ: Dr. Nishimura, do you have any information concerning the intactness of the placental circulation in your studies on drug transfer in the human embryo? We have shown recently (Rudolph et al., Pediat. Res. 5:452, 1971) that umbilical blood flow may be markedly decreased in the exteriorized human fetus although blood gases may appear to reflect good physiological function. This affects placental transfer studies.

NISHIMURA: We have no information on this point. Since the developmental stage of embryonic specimens in our study was from 5 to 8 weeks estimated fertilization age, it was technically difficult for the collaborating obstetricians to examine the placental circulation.

CALDEYRO-BARCIA: How do you explain the very marked individual differences in the concentration ratio embryo/maternal blood one hour after injection?

NISHIMURA: One of the reasons for such marked individual differences in our study with sulfamethopyrazine could be that the dose of the drug was not always the same in all cases. So, conclusive interpretation must await further studies where the same dose is given at various intervals before the interruption of pregnancy.

FABRO: How did you collect the human embryo? It is difficult at 8 to 12 weeks of pregnancy to obtain a specimen which is free of maternal blood and endometrium.

NISHIMURA: The method involves curettage and evacuation of the uterine contents. Several hundred obstetricians have been collaborating with us, and a number of them have the skill to obtain occasionally intact specimens. We asked these doctors to provide such specimens. In compliance with our request, they rinsed and blotted the embryos to remove maternal blood and other tissues. The specimens were then frozen and stored until the assay was initiated.

Fetal Pharmacology, edited by L. Boréus
Raven Press, New York © 1973

Autoradiography in Fetal Pharmacology

Sven Ullberg

Department of Toxicology, Uppsala University, Uppsala, Sweden

When problems which concern the uptake and distribution of drugs in the fetus are studied in experimental animals, the use of radioactively labeled substances offers many advantages compared with other methods. There is, for instance, no difficulty in distinguishing an injected substance from substances which are normally present in the body. Tracer techniques are also very generally applicable, since most compounds of pharmacological and toxicological interest can be labeled with ^{14}C or ^{3}H or some other suitable radioisotope. Radiometric analysis can be combined with microseparation of possible drug metabolites. In addition, very accurate quantitative data can be obtained by using pulse-counting equipment, such as a liquid scintillation spectrometer.

A disadvantage of being limited to determination of the concentration in biological samples is, however, that this does not permit a localization to defined structures. More detailed information can be obtained by using a method which involves a visual observation of the distribution pattern such as autoradiography. A limited number of substances can also be localized in tissue sections because they fluoresce in ultraviolet light (Fig. 3).

Sections from small tissue pieces can be used, but more comprehensive information can be obtained by using whole-body sections. Such sections can be prepared without the risk of redistributing soluble compounds in the tissues (Ullberg, 1954).

In our laboratory we seldom remove the fetuses before studying them by autoradiography. In experiments with mice, we generally section the whole pregnant animal. The concentration in the fetal and maternal tissues can thus be directly compared.

If a series of pregnant mice are studied, the variation with time of the maternal, placental, and fetal distribution pattern can be followed. Most of our data are from mice in a late state of gestation. The mice are injected, generally intravenously, each mouse receiving a single dose. After various predetermined times, the animals are rapidly frozen and sagittal sections are prepared at different levels through the whole frozen bodies. The sections are freeze-dried and pressed against a photographic film. After exposure the films are separated from the sections and are developed.

Quantitative data can be obtained by densitometry using an isotope staircase as a reference, or by pulse counting of pieces cut out from thick whole-body sections. Such pieces can also be used for radiochromatographic separation of possible drug metabolites.

Larger animals such as pregnant squirrel monkeys can also be sectioned. In experiments with large animals, the labeled compound may be injected in a cord vein to save isotopic costs or to avoid the metabolism by the maternal tissues. An experiment with autoradiography of perfused human fetuses has also been performed (Fig. 8).

Recently an attempt has been made to obtain improved autoradiographic resolution by permanently attaching 5- to 10-μ thick whole body sections on to fine-grain photographic emulsions, e.g., nuclear plates (Ullberg and Appelgren, 1969). This is, however, a rather tricky technique which cannot be applied on a large scale.

The results from an autoradiographic investigation may be complemented by radiochromatography to reveal the possible presence in the tissues of drug metabolites.

RESULTS

Relation between concentrations in mother, placenta, and fetus

Most drugs pass from the mother over to the fetus but to a different extent and at different rates. The pattern of transfer is also very variable. Most exogenous compounds seem to diffuse passively through the placenta without being specifically accumulated there, whereas some physiological substances accumulate first in the placenta and later in the fetuses apparently by an active placental transport mechanism.

Only the first, probably passive, type of transfer seems to be dependent on the physicochemical properties of the drug such as fat solubility and degree of ionization. Fat-soluble compounds generally pass both the placental barrier and the blood-brain barrier rather easily. This means that drugs which influence cerebral function, such as general anesthetics, also pass rapidly to the fetus and may influence the fetal brain, which is a particular problem in obstetric anesthesia.

Short-acting barbiturates and sedatives such as chlorpromazine pass very rapidly to the fetus (e.g., Sjöstrand, Cassano, and Hansson, 1965; Cassano, Ghetti, Gliozzi, and Hansson, 1967). They can be detected in the fetus within a couple of minutes after intravenous injection into the mother. All the fetuses are reached simultaneously by the drug. The fetal concentration soon reaches the level of that in the mother, but never seems to exceed it, not even during the phase of excretion, when the drug is in process of leaving the body. These drugs are accumulated in both maternal and fetal brains (Fig. 6), but the fetal brain concentration has always been found to be lower than the maternal.

For most drugs, the general fetal level is always lower than the maternal. Heavily ionized drugs pass especially slowly to the fetus; quaternary bases are frequently not found in detectable concentrations in the fetus (Allgén, Ekman, Reio, and Ullberg, 1960; Hanson and Schmiterlöw, 1961).

With respect to the relation between the ability of drugs to pass the blood-brain and placental barriers, it may be noted that many drugs such as the antibiotics penicillin and tetracycline are much more efficiently blocked by the blood-brain barrier than by the placental barrier (Ullberg, 1954; André, 1956). On the other hand, there are many drugs (among them many tertiary amines) which are accumulated rapidly and markedly in the adult brain but never reach maternal levels in the fetus. There thus seems to be a wider range of uptake in the brain than in the fetus with respect to drugs.

Active placental transfer

Some physiological substances such as vitamins, hormones, and microelements are accumulated in the fetus apparently by an active placental transport mechanism. The substance which leads this class is vitamin B_{12}, which can be accumulated more than a hundredfold if a low dose is given maternally. Two other water-soluble vitamins have also been investigated, namely vitamins B_1 (Hammarström, Neujahr, and Ullberg, 1966) and C (Hammar-

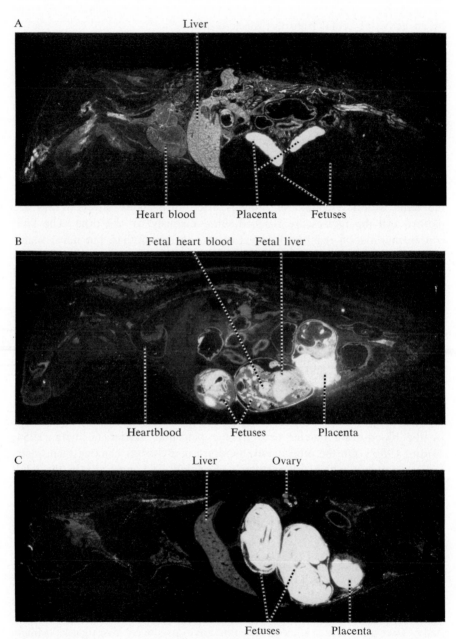

FIG. 1. Distribution of ⁵⁸Co-labeled vitamin B₁₂ in pregnant mice various times after intravenous injection.

ström, 1966), and these also were found to accumulate in the fetus, although to a much smaller extent. The placental transfer of the two fat-soluble vitamins A and E has, however, been found to be partially blocked (Ullberg, 1965). The behavior of these vitamins is thus in complete discord with the thesis that fat solubility favors the placental passage of drugs.

The physiological estrogen estradiol (Ullberg and Bengtsson, 1963) and the synthetic diethylstilbestrol (Bengtsson and Ullberg, 1963) are very similarly distributed in adult females. They are both accumulated in target organs such as the uterine wall and the vagina. However, the autoradiograms of estradiol showed a marked fetal accumulation, whereas the placental passage of stilbestrol was partially blocked.

With regard to microelements, both iron and iodide have been found to accumulate in the fetus. Iodine (Ullberg and Ewaldsson, 1964) is strongly accumulated in the fetal thyroid, which may be related to the somewhat surprising findings of congenital goiter after large iodide doses.

The pattern of active placental transport is illustrated in Fig. 1, which shows three stages in the fetal accumulation of ^{58}Co-labeled vitamin B_{12} (Ullberg, Kristoffersson, Flodh, and Hanngren, 1967; Flodh, 1968). Vitamin B_{12}, which is chemically very stable in the body, is first rapidly taken up by the placenta, which apparently has a very large receptor capacity, because the placental concentration soon reaches a level which may be several hundred times higher than the average concentration in maternal tissues.

The further transfer from the placenta to the fetus is slow. There is a delay before any activity shows up in the fetus, and the length of this period varies from fetus to fetus. [This variation between fetuses in rate of uptake is still more marked for iron (Ullberg, Sörbo, and Clemedsson, 1961).] The peak in the fetal concentration is not reached until after 2 to 4 days, when the vitamin is hardly detectable in the maternal tissues. After 4 hours, when the fetal concentration has just exceeded the maternal, the level is very low in the maternal but high in the fetal blood. The placental "pump" is dose-dependent, and it is also depressed by vitamin B_{12} analogs. The efficiency of the blocking effect seems to depend on the closeness of the resemblance of the analogs to B_{12} stereostructurally.

Vitamin B_{12} needs a carrier (the intrinsic factor) to be able to pass the intestinal mucosa, and this carrier mechanism is sometimes defective. It also seems possible that the active transport of vitamin B_{12} (and possibly some

A: After 15 min, a very high concentration is seen in the placenta but none in the fetuses. *B*: After 4 hr, transport has occurred to the fetuses. The fetal blood concentration is high, the maternal low. *C*: After 4 days, the maternal organs are nearly depleted while the fetal concentration is very high.

other essential nutrients such as iron) may sometimes be defective, and that such a deficiency may be responsible for some cases of fetal death or damage, which are presently not understood.

Distribution within the fetus

Vitamins

The fetal drug-distribution pattern shows many similarities with the adult, but is generally simpler and more even. Many sites of transport and accumulation which are found in the adult animal are lacking in the fetus. There is, however, a great difference between various substances; e.g., vitamin B_{12} shows a highly variant fetal distribution pattern, while the physiologically very indifferent compound benzyl penicillin is distributed very evenly.

When vitamin B_{12} reaches the fetal blood, it is not taken care of by any specific storage organ, but all fetal tissues reach higher concentrations than the corresponding maternal tissues. The highest concentrations in both the adult and fetal body are found in some endocrine organs.

In Fig. 2 it is shown that vitamin C accumulates in both the maternal and fetal brain and retina and that most, but not all, fetal tissues have reached higher concentrations than the corresponding maternal tissues. In spite of a very varied organ uptake, the fetal pattern is a simplified version of that of the mother, in that many maternal accumulation sites are lacking in the fetus (Hammarström, 1966).

Antibiotics

The most even fetal distribution pattern found in our material is that of the antibiotic benzyl penicillin. It is apparently a very indifferent substance in the body, and does not specifically bind to any tissue components. In the adult animal, it becomes concentrated in excretory sites, but in the fetus it seems to be distributed only in the extracellular space. The uniformity in the distribution picture is disturbed in the late-term fetus mainly due to the appearance of a functioning blood-brain barrier (Ullberg, 1954). This lack of a specific tissue uptake of penicillin can probably be regarded as an advantage with respect to the risks of fetal damage.

Another antibiotic, tetracycline (André, 1956; Blomquist and Hanngren, 1966), behaves rather differently. In the adult organism, it is firmly bound to the skeleton, where it is taken up in high concentration in the

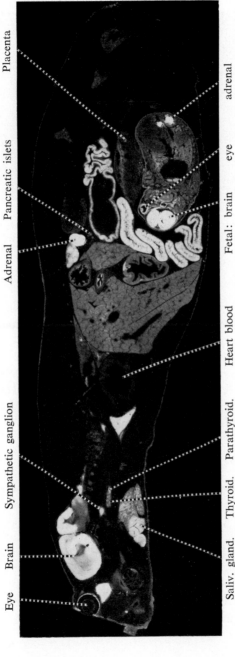

Eye　Brain　Sympathetic ganglion　Adrenal　Pancreatic islets　Placenta

Saliv. gland.　Thyroid.　Parathyroid.　Heart blood　Fetal: brain　eye　adrenal

FIG. 2. Autoradiogram of a pregnant mouse 3 days after intravenous injection of ascorbic acid-1-^{14}C. Note the accumulation (*light areas*) in both maternal and fetal brain, eye, and adrenal gland. There is also a marked uptake in the maternal sympathetic ganglia, thyroid, parathyroid, and pancreatic islets. No radioactivity is visible in the maternal or the fetal blood. (Hammarström, 1966.)

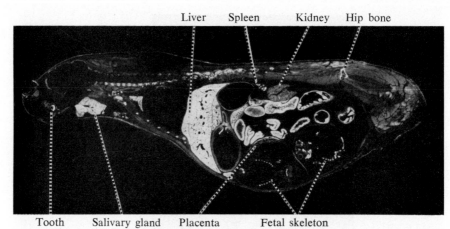

Liver   Spleen   Kidney   Hip bone

Tooth   Salivary gland   Placenta   Fetal skeleton

FIG. 3. Whole body fluorogram from a pregnant mouse 5 hr after intravenous injection of a tetracycline preparation (demethylchlortetracycline). In the fetuses, the drug is localized selectivity in the skeleton. In the mother, an accumulation can also be seen in many soft tissues. (Blomquist and Hanngren, 1966).

growth zones, but it is also temporarily accumulated in many soft tissues. In the fetus there is a very marked and persistent accumulation in the skeleton, but no soft-tissue uptake is seen (Fig. 3).

This hard-tissue affinity of tetracycline probably explains the brownish fluorescent enamel spots which may appear in the teeth of children after the mother has been treated with tetracycline during pregnancy. Higher doses of tetracycline given to pregnant experimental animals are known to cause arrest of bone growth and, occasionally, skeletal deformities.

Thyrostatics

In the case of thyrostatic drugs also, a well-known type of drug-induced congenital damage—fetal goiter—can be related to a selective uptake in the critical fetal organ.

When thiouracil is given to an adult animal, the autoradiograms show that the drug is accumulated at its main site of action, the thyroid; there is also accumulation in the lung and in excretory organs. In the fetus, however, the accumulation in the target organ is still more selective. There is a low and even concentration in the whole fetal body except for the thyroid, where there is a marked accumulation (Fig. 4) (P. Slanina, S. Ullberg, and L. Hammarström, *in preparation*).

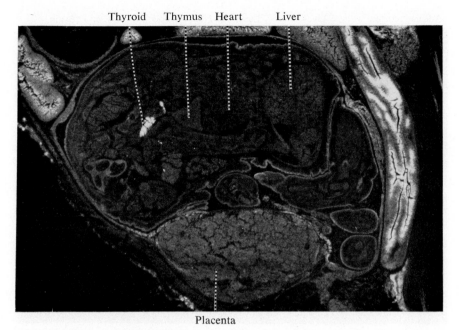

FIG. 4. Detail of autoradiogram of a pregnant mouse showing selective accumulation in the fetal thyroid 4 hr after maternal intravenous injection of ^{14}C-thiourea.

The blocking of the formation of iodinated hormones in the fetal thyroid may stimulate the fetal pituitary to an increased production of thyroid hormone, which in turn may cause an extensive growth of the fetal thyroid.

Enzyme affinity

A selective uptake in one type of fetal tissue is a rather frequent finding. Figure 5 is an autoradiogram showing that an agent with diphenylethene character is taken up selectively in the adrenal cortex. In the mother this substance is also accumulated at sites of steroid hormone formation. The most marked accumulation is seen in the corpora lutea, where it has been found to interfere with progesterone formation (Hanngren, Einer-Jensen, and Ullberg, 1965).

The accumulation of this substance at sites of steroid hormone formation is probably due to an enzyme affinity. Appelgren (1969) has found histochemically that it blocks the Δ5-3β-hydroxysteroid dehydrogenase activity.

Adrenal cortex   Liver   Lung   Heart blood   Brain

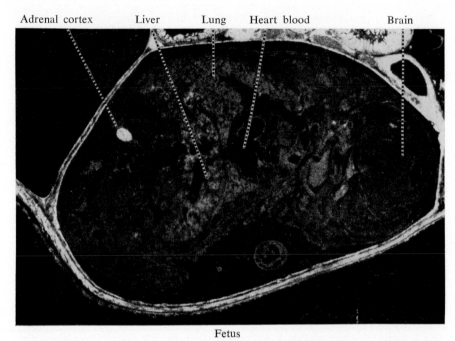

Fetus

FIG. 5. Detail of a whole body autoradiogram from a pregnant mouse showing a fetus 5 min (!) after injection of a nonsteroid compound, bis-(p-acetoxyphenyl)-2 methyl-cyclohexylidene-methane, which interferes with steroid hormone production. Selective accumulation in fetal adrenal cortex.

The accumulation of the diphenylethene substance is most marked a few minutes after injection and disappears rapidly.

Nicotine

Nicotine is excreted into the fetal intestinal lumen, but is also accumulated in the entire respiratory tract (lungs, trachea, and larynx). The pulmonary accumulation is more marked after birth (Tjälve, Hansson, and Schmiterlöw, 1968).

Eye melanin affinity

Many drugs, such as the phenothiazine tranquilizers, the tricyclic antidepressants, and also the antimalarial and antirheumatic compound chloroquine, show a strong and persistent affinity for the melanin-containing tissues of the body.

If chlorpromazine is given to a pregnant pigmented mouse, it passes the placenta and is accumulated in the uvea (not in albino mice) of the fetal eye (Ullberg, Lindquist, and Sjöstrand, 1970). The uptake in the fetal eye begins immediately after the drug has entered the fetal circulation, and the eye uptake is seen before the radioactive substance is observable elsewhere in the fetal body. After 1 hr, accumulation can be seen in the brain, but by far the highest uptake is present in the eye (Fig. 6). After 2 days, when the chlorpromazine has left the rest of the fetus, it is retained in the fetal eye; it can still be seen in the offspring 6 months after birth.

The fetal eye uptake can also be demonstrated *in vitro*. If a section through a non-injected pregnant mouse is just immersed in a water solution of the labeled drug, the drug is accumulated in the uvea (Fig. 7). The accumulation appears to be due simply to chemical affinity. Special physiological conditions such as body temperature and glucose in the medium are not needed.

With prolonged medication with one of these drugs, very high concentrations are built up, and these may cause secondary retinal damage in the fetus of a similar type to that which has been observed in adult humans and

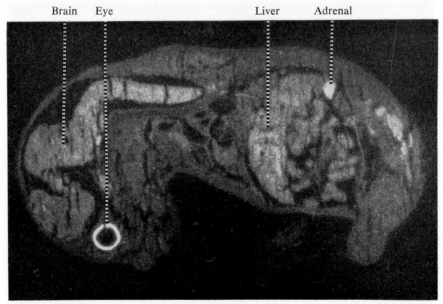

FIG. 6. Autoradiogram of a pigmented mouse fetus 1 hr after intravenous injection of ^{35}S-chlorpromazine to the mother. The fetus was removed surgically. Note slight accumulation in fetal brain and adrenal cortex and very marked accumulation in the uvea of the eye.

Placenta   Amniotic fluid   Uvea   Brain

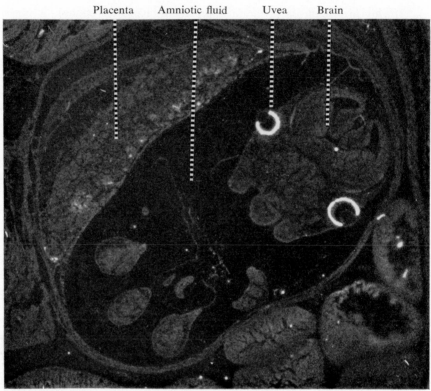

FIG. 7. Detail of an autoradiogram of a pregnant pigmented mouse showing the *in vitro* affinity of ^{14}C-chloroquine for fetal uveal melanin.

animals. I know of only one clinical report of congenital drug-induced retinal damage; this was observed in three children whose mother was treated with chloroquine during each pregnancy (Hart and Naunton, 1964). However, there may well be many undiscovered similar cases. If damage, which gives a slight reduction of vision, has occurred, this may not be observed until long after birth, and it may then be difficult to relate it to medication during pregnancy. There thus seems to be a need for carefully controlled studies of children whose mothers were taking these compounds during pregnancy.

Progesterone in the human fetus

Bengtsson, Ullberg, Wiqvist, and Diczfalusy (1964) studied the distribution of 4-^{14}C-progesterone in perfused previable human fetuses. The up-

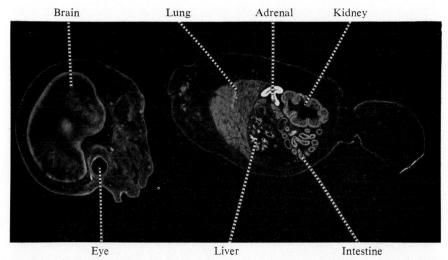

Brain   Lung   Adrenal   Kidney

Eye   Liver   Intestine

FIG. 8. Whole body autoradiogram of a human male fetus following administration to the fetus of progesterone-4-^{14}C. Note the marked uptake by the adrenal cortex.

take was highest in the adrenal cortex (Fig. 8). This accumulation may be related to the very rapid metabolism of progesterone by the fetal adrenal, which seems to use progesterone as a precursor in the formation of adrenal cortical steroids. A specific accumulation was also observed in the pituitary gland, testes, thyroid, and thymus.

SUMMARY

Whole-body autoradiography of pregnant mice has revealed a widely varying distribution pattern for different kinds of drugs.

The more "unphysiological" a compound is, the more its distribution is influenced by physicochemical properties such as high fat solubility, which facilitates the ability of a drug to pass to both the brain and the fetus. Short-acting barbiturates pass the placenta without being concentrated there; they are seen in the fetus within several minutes after intravenous injection into the mother. They rapidly reach a maternal level in the fetus but never seem to exceed it, not even during the phase of elimination.

Physiological substances, e.g., vitamins, hormones, and microelements, are apparently strongly influenced by specific mechanisms such as membrane pumps and blockage and selective binding to different proteins. Each substance has its characteristic distribution pattern. Some of them, e.g., vitamin

B_{12} and iron, are accumulated in the fetus apparently by an active placental transport mechanism, which probably involves a carrier. A deficient placental transport for an essential nutrient such as B_{12} may possibly cause fetal death or damage. The general pattern for such an active transfer is that the substance is first accumulated in the placenta. Then there is a delay, followed by a rather slow further transfer to the fetus. Vitamin B_{12} was accumulated more than a hundredfold in the fetus if a low dose was given.

The distribution pattern within a fetus generally shows certain similarities with the maternal pattern. However, the fetal distribution is generally more even than the maternal. The fetus seems to lack many of the transport and accumulation mechanisms, which are developed in adult animals. There is also, with exception for a few drugs, a lack of accumulation in fetal excretory pathways: kidney, urinary bladder, biliary ducts, intestine.

A rather frequent finding is a very strong and selective accumulation in one single type of fetal tissue, which may involve a risk for damage. Thus tetracycline accumulates selectively in the fetal skeleton, thiouracil in the fetal thyroid, and chloroquine and chlorpromazine in the pigment of the fetal eye. The affinity of many drugs to the fetal melanin-containing tissues seems to deserve more attention.

REFERENCES

Allgén, L.-G., Ekman, L., Reio, L., and Ullberg, S. (1960): Biological fate of S^{35}-labelled Secergan—a quaternary phenothiazine compound. *Archives Internationales de Pharmacodynamie et de Thérapie*, 126:1-16.

André, T. (1957): Studies on the distribution of tritium-labelled dihydrostreptomycin and tetracycline in the body. *Acta Radiologica*, suppl. 142.

Appelgren, L.-E. (1969): Histochemical demonstration of drug interference with progesterone synthesis. *Journal of Reproduction and Fertility*, 19:185-186.

Bengtsson, G., and Ullberg, S. (1963): The autoradiographic distribution pattern after administration of diethylstilboestrol compared with that of natural oestrogens. *Acta Endocrinologica*, 43:561-570.

Bengtsson, G., Ullberg, S., Wiqvist, N., and Diczfalusy, E. (1964): Autoradiographic studies on previable human foetuses perfused with radioactive steroids. *Acta Endocrinologica*, 46:544-551.

Blomquist, L., and Hanngren, Å. (1966): Fluorescence technique applied to whole body sections for distribution studies of tetracyclines. *Biochemical Pharmacology*, 15:215-219.

Cassano, G. B., Ghetti, B., Gliozzi, E., and Hansson, E. (1967): Autoradiographic distribution study of "short acting" and "long acting" barbiturates: ^{35}S-thiopentone and ^{14}C-phenobarbitone. *British Journal of Anaesthesia*, 39:11-20.

Flodh, H. (1968): Distribution and kinetics of labelled vitamin B_{12}. *Acta Radiologica*, suppl. 284.

Hammarström, L. (1966): Autoradiographic studies on the distribution of C^{14}-labelled ascorbic acid and dehydroascorbic acid. *Acta Physiologica Scandinavica,* 70, suppl. 289.

Hammarström, L., Neujahr, H., and Ullberg, S. (1966): Autoradiographic studies on ^{35}S-thiamine distribution in mice. *Acta Pharmacologica et Toxicologica,* 24:24-32.

Hanngren, Å. (1959): Studies on the distribution and fate of C^{14} and T-labelled *p*-aminosalicylic acid (PAS) in the body. *Acta Radiologica,* suppl. 175.

Hanngren, Å., Einer-Jensen, N., and Ullberg, S. (1965): Specific uptake in corpora lutea of a non-steroid substance with antigestagenic properties. *Nature,* 208:461-462.

Hansson, E., and Schmiterlöw, C. G. (1961): A comparison of the distribution, excretion and metabolism of a tertiary (promethazine) and a quaternary (Aprobit®) phenothiazine compound labelled with S^{35}. *Archives Internationales de Pharmacodynamie et de Thérapie,* 131:309-324.

Hart, C. W., and Naunton, R. F. (1964): The ototoxicity of chloroquine phosphate. *Archives of Otolaryngology,* 80:407-412.

Sjöstrand, S. E., Cassano, G. B., and Hansson, E. (1965): The distribution of ^{35}S-chlorpromazine in mice studied by whole body autoradiography. *Archives Internationales de Pharmacodynamie et de Thérapie,* 156:34-47.

Tjälve, H., Hansson, E., and Schmiterlöw, C. G. (1968): Passage of ^{14}C-nicotine and its metabolites into mice foetuses and placentae. *Acta Pharmacologica et Toxicologica,* 26:539-555.

Ullberg, S. (1954): Studies on the distribution and fate of S^{35}-labelled benzylpenicillin in the body. *Acta Radiologica,* suppl. 118.

Ullberg, S. (1965): Specific localization of labelled hormones and vitamins; whole-body autoradiographic observations. In: *Isotopes in Experimental Pharmacology,* edited by L. Roth. International Conference on the Use of Isotopically Labeled Drugs in Experimental Pharmacology, Chicago, 1964. University of Chicago Press, Chicago.

Ullberg, S., and Appelgren, L.-E. (1969): Experiences in locating drugs at different levels of resolution. In: *Autoradiography of Diffusible Substances,* edited by L. Roth. Academic Press, New York.

Ullberg, S., and Bengtsson, B. (1963): Autoradiographic distribution studies with natural oestrogens. *Acta Endocrinologica,* 43:75-86.

Ullberg, S., and Ewaldsson, B. (1964): Distribution of radio-iodine studied by whole-body autoradiography. *Acta Radiologica,* 2:24-32.

Ullberg, S., Kristoffersson, H., Flodh, H., and Hanngren, Å. (1967): Placental passage and fetal accumulation of labelled vitamin B_{12} in the mouse. *Archives Internationales de Pharmacodynamie et de Thérapie,* 167:431-449.

Ullberg, S., Lindquist, N. G., and Sjöstrand, S. E. (1970): Accumulation of chorioretinotoxic drugs in the foetal eye. *Nature,* 227:1257-1258.

Ullberg, S., Sörbo, B., and Clemedsson, C.-J. (1961): Distribution of radioactive iron in pregnant mice studied by whole-body autoradiography. *Acta Radiologica,* 55:145-155.

DISCUSSION

MCBRIDE: Your experiments with vitamin B_{12} are very interesting, in the high concentrations occurring in the fetus. Have you done similar experiments with folic acid? What were the results with folic acid? Was it found to be concentrated in the fetus?

ULLBERG: Yes, we have studied folic acid, but it was not accumulated in fetuses to an order of magnitude approaching that of vitamin B_{12}.

LUTWAK-MANN: As a brief comment on vitamin B_{12} in relation to placental passage of this compound into the mouse fetus, I would like to recall the spectacularly high level of vitamin B_{12} in the pre-implantation rabbit blastocyst as well as in the endometrial section. However, the concentration of vitamin B_{12} in rabbit blood is very high, too, many times higher than, for example, in man. It is therefore conceivable that both the high level of this vitamin in the young conceptus as well as its rapid placental transmission following maternal adminis-tration, are limited to and peculiar for the laboratory animal species. Perhaps before assigning to vitamin B_{12} a very special position in fetal-maternal exchange we should investigate the situation with respect to vitamin B_{12} also in human feto-placental relationships.

ULLBERG: Your observations on accumulation of vitamin B_{12} also at the blastocyst stage are very interesting. I believe that the high uptake of vitamin B_{12} is common for most species including man. In humans a high concentration has been observed in fetal cord blood compared to the maternal vein blood.

FABRO: Did you identify the radioactivity after administration of vitamin B_{12}? Is it possibly cobalt that accumulates?

ULLBERG: Vitamin B_{12} is chemically very stable in the body. In our separation studies the radioactivity in the tissues was practically totally unchanged vitamin B_{12}. In one experiment two minor metabolites were found in maternal organs. They were apparently closely related to vitamin B_{12}.

We have studied the distribution of inorganic cobalt ($^{58}CoCl_2$) and found its passage to the fetus to be partially blocked. Cobalt has no known physiological role except as part of vitamin B_{12}, and the placenta seems to be rather skillful in selecting substances which are transported actively to the fetus. The only unphysiological substances which in our material have been found to accumulate in the fetus are amino acid analogs, which probably are transferred by an amino acid transport mechanism.

KARCZMAR: Dr. Levy indicated earlier that cloxacillin does not but methicillin does penetrate into the fetus—particularly into fetal circulation. This indicates some similarity between the blood-brain barrier and the placental barrier, as in the adult methicillin penetrates better into body fluids, including cerebrospinal fluid than the other penicillins. On the other hand, you indicated relatively good penetration of benzyl penicillin into the fetus, which agrees well with Dr. Mirkin's concept that there is a difference between the blood-brain barrier and the placenta. Do you subscribe to the concept of a difference between the two barriers?

ULLBERG: Yes, some drugs—and among them benzyl penicillin and tetracycline—were found in our investigations to be more efficiently blocked from entering into the brain than into the fetus. However, there was a partial placental barrier. The fetal concentration was lower than the maternal.

FUCHS: Is it not true that your method is less useful with substances that are rapidly metabolized, such as ethanol?

ULLBERG: A rapid metabolism may complicate the situation. In the case of ethanol, preinjection of an enzyme blocker such as an alcohol dehydrogenase inhibitor seems to offer an interesting approach which may enable one to get round the problem and study the unmetabolized compound autoradiographically.

FUCHS: If the metabolizing enzyme systems are blocked by other compounds, one must be sure that such compounds reach the fetal organs rapidly enough and in adequate concentations.

ULLBERG: Yes. The distribution of the enzyme blocker in the body should preferably also be looked into. In the case when they do not reach the fetal tissues you may have only blocked the metabolism in the maternal organism, which may still be of sufficient interest to be studied.

In autoradiography with drugs, in general, a rapid metabolism does not create as great problems as might be suspected. Most drug metabolites are rapidly excreted. Many drugs are localized specifically in certain organs a few minutes after injection, when the metabolism has hardly started. A positive aspect is also that if autoradiography is combined with a microseparation method, such as thin layer chromatography, detailed drug metabolism studies can be carried out. The potentiality for autoradiography of rapidly metabolizing compounds is especially good if a substance is available in several labeled forms with each form labeled at a particular site of the molecule.

Another technical approach to obtain increased chemical information is to treat some sections with a solvent before the autoradiographic exposure, a method which is useful when either the unchanged drug or a metabolite is selectively soluble in a particular solvent.

RÄIHÄ: Regarding the experiments on ascorbic acid, I would like to ask whether there were any differences in the autoradiograms when using the oxidized or reduced form of ascorbic acid? I ask this because we showed some time ago that there is a marked difference at least in the guinea pig between the placental transfer of ascorbic acid and dehydroascorbic acid in favor of the latter form.

ULLBERG: Yes, you are right. Hammarström in our laboratory has studied the distribution of both ascorbic acid and dehydroascorbic acid (labeled with ^{14}C)

and there is a very marked initial difference in the distribution pattern of these two compounds. Thus dehydroascorbic acid accumulates in the brain of adult animals within 2 minutes after intravenous injection, while it takes ascorbic acid at least 24 hours to reach a significant concentration in the brain. But after 3 days the distribution pattern is about the same irrespective of whether ascorbic or dehydroascorbic acid was injected.

However, the fetal distribution pattern after injection of dehydroascorbic acid is almost identical with the ascorbic acid pattern, which probably means that dehydroascorbic acid is transformed into ascorbic acid in the placenta before being transferred to the fetus.

LIND: Dr. Ullberg mentioned the possibility of using human material for the drug distribution. Some experiences concerning the distribution of iodine organic compounds exist for human fetal angiocardiograms during cesarean section. If you have your X-ray equipment in the operation room, the injection of contrast medium into the umbilical vein can be carried out within 30 seconds after the cesarean section. Within less than a minute, the liver, the adrenal, and the kidneys are seen loaded with the contrast medium and even the ureters are visualized at the following X-ray exposure. In this way kidney capacity for excretion of contrast medium could be stated at an early fetal stage, in other words, 8 to 10 weeks of pregnancy.

HILL: Are there many areas of the brain in which chlorpromazine is deposited? I ask this question because we have seen a child with a Parkinson-like reaction in which the mother received chlorpromazine during her gestation. The infant had symptoms for 9 months post delivery. Mothers who receive other tranquilizers during pregnancy also have infants who manifest abnormal neurological symptoms for many months post delivery.

ULLBERG: Your observation is most interesting. Chlorpromazine is accumulated in all melanin-containing tissues including the neurons in the substantia nigra of the brain. The accumulation of chlorpromazine in these neurons is very likely to disturb the formation of dopamine, which might lead to parkinsonian symptoms.

There are many other sedatives, for example, all N-substituted phenothiazines, which behave similarly to chlorpromazine with respect to melanin affinity, and they are therefore likely to give the same side effects.

MIRKIN: Can you identify any specific characteristics of those drugs which tend to concentrate in discrete fetal tissues, for example, chlorpromazine in the retina?

ULLBERG: It is difficult to generalize. Many types of mechanisms seem to be involved. One is that a substance is taken up in a tissue, where it interferes with the metabolism. The tissue may, as in the case of thyrostatic compounds, be an endocrine gland. In many cases the drug has some kind of affinity to a certain structure. In the case of the diphenylethene compound, the drug apparently has an affinity to an enzyme and this affinity is likely to be due to a stereostructural relationship to the physiological substrate of the enzyme. The binding to the enzyme apparently leads to a temporary inhibition of the enzyme action. But drugs can also be bound to more indifferent structures. The affinity of tetracycline to growing bone may be related to the property of tetracycline to bind calcium by chelate formation.

In the case of accumulation of some drugs in melanin-containing tissues, the fact that it takes place *in vitro* under unphysiologic conditions indicates that it is simply due to chemical affinity. The drugs which show melanin affinity are polycyclic amines and they fluoresce in ultraviolet light.

JOST: Does your technique permit recognizing in which part of the placenta or in which placental cells a compound accumulates?

ULLBERG: The resolution of whole body autoradiograms is not very satisfactory for the purpose you mention if the photographic film is separated from the section before it is developed. But if, for example, a 10-μ thick whole body section has been permanently attached to a fine-grain photographic plate (such as a nuclear plate), observations may be made down to a cellular level.

HOLMSTEDT: With autoradiography it is possible to study the whole body of small animals and fetuses of all species. Is there a difference in the distribution pattern of one particular drug when several species are studied particularly with regard to drugs that have characteristic accumulation, for example, in the thyroid or the brain?

ULLBERG: Unfortunately our resources have not allowed us to do enough experiments of that kind to be able to draw any general conclusions. Based on the limited experience we have and by comparison with data from other laboratories, I am inclined to believe that there would be qualitatively similar findings between species for most compounds, with occasional exceptions.

Fetal Pharmacology, edited by L. Boréus
Raven Press, New York © 1973

Ontogeny of the Blood-Brain Barrier

Hugh Davson

Department of Physiology, University College, London, England

We are accustomed to think of the blood-brain barrier in terms of the restraint on the passage of material from blood to the extracellular fluid and cells of the brain and spinal cord; such a restraint has been well validated by recent work, in spite of earlier attempts to discredit the whole notion (e.g., Edström, 1958). It has also been shown that the blood-brain barrier, viewed in this way, is just a part of a complex homeostatic mechanism, involving, in addition to the nervous tissue, the cerebrospinal fluid (CSF) and meninges. This homeostatic mechanism serves to maintain the environment of central and peripheral neurons not only tolerably constant in the face of fluctuations in blood composition but also at a different composition from that of the blood plasma. Thus the study of the ontogenetic development of the blood-brain barrier cannot be restricted to the study of the restraint on passage of material from blood into brain, for example, by measuring the rate of uptake of a foreign solute such as sucrose, at different stages in development, since changes in this parameter may well be due to alterations in other features of the system, such as the total volume of the extracellular space, rather than to the impediment to passage across the capillaries of the brain.

Let us first consider briefly the general arrangement of the fluid compartments of the brain. These are illustrated schematically in Fig. 1 where the ventricles have been grouped together as a single cavity, into which projects a single schematic choroid plexus. The CSF is secreted by this plexus and flows out of the ventricles over the surface of the brain and cord, to be drained

75

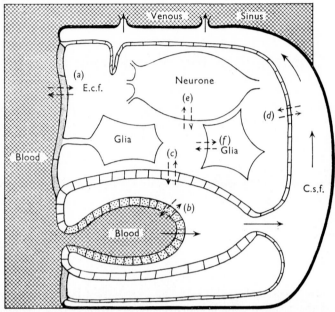

FIG. 1. Diagram of fluid compartments of the blood-brain CSF system. Continuous arrows represent proven directions of fluid flow. Interrupted arrows indicate where diffusion of water and solutes may occur between the different compartments, namely: (a) across the blood-brain barrier, between brain capillaries and extracellular fluid; (b) across the epithelia of the choroid plexuses; (c) across the ependyma; (d) across the pia-glial membranes; (e) and (f) across the cell membranes of neurons and glial cells. Thick line represents the arachnoid-dural enclosure of the system. (From Davson and Bradbury, 1965).

away through relatively large channels (i.e., large by comparison with the size of protein molecules) into the blood of the dural sinuses. Blood thus has access to the brain extracellular space by two main routes: the direct interchange across capillaries in the nervous tissue, indicated by the arrows in Fig. 1, and also less directly through the choroid plexuses and thence from the CSF into the adjacent tissue across the ependyma and pia-arachnoid. An additional site of interchange is through the dura, which is quite highly vascularized, and thence across the arachnoid membrane, which separates the dura from the subarachnoid fluid.

When considering the exchanges between blood and brain, therefore, it is important to appreciate that if a restraint is to be exercised, it is probably insufficient to exercise this solely at the capillary level of the brain parenchyma, since this restraint can be circumvented by passage through the choroid plexuses and thence from the CSF, or through the dura and across the arachnoid membrane. In fact, it is now well established, on the basis of both kinetic and morphological studies, that the passage of material from blood into the CSF, by way of the choroid plexuses, experiences similar restraints to those met by material passing across the brain capillaries; this results from the presence of an epithelial layer covering the choroid plexuses, the *choroidal epithelium,* the clefts between the individual cells being sealed by tight junctions (Brightman and Reese, 1969). Although the choroidal epithelium is embryologically similar to the ependyma lining the ventricles, with which it is continuous, the ependyma does not exhibit this restraint, so that if a substance that only penetrates across the choroid plexuses with difficulty, such as sucrose, is injected into the ventricular fluid, then it passes without serious restraint into the extracellular fluid of the brain. In fact, this is the basis for accurate determinations of the extracellular space of brain. Thus, when a steady level of sucrose was maintained for a long time in the blood, the measured volume of distribution was found to be very low, of the order of 5%. Yet, if the ventricular system was perfused with an artificial CSF containing a known and constant concentration of sucrose, the measured space after a long period was of the order of 15%, and this is a much closer approximation to the true extracellular space. With regard to the passage from dura to CSF, kinetic studies indicate that the substance of the dura comes into quite rapid equilibrium with the blood, exhibiting the absence of a significant barrier in the dural capillaries; however, morphological and some kinetic evidence indicates that the arachnoid membrane, immediately under the dura, exercises the restraint necessary to keep the blood-brain barrier intact.

The interchange between brain, on the one hand, and CSF on the other, is of more than academic interest. It has been demonstrated that, even when a steady level of, e.g., sucrose is maintained in the blood for very long periods (e.g., 24 hr), the volume of distribution is very much less than the extracellular space measured by ventriculo-cisternal perfusion; this means, in essence, that the CSF, because it is drained away continuously, can exert a "sink-action" on material diffusing into the brain from the blood. Thus, measurements of the concentration in the CSF during the maintenance of this steady level of sucrose in the blood indicate that the concentration is only a few percent of that in the plasma; hence, as sucrose passes into the extracellular space of the brain from the blood capillaries, the concentration tends to build up above that in the CSF, only to diffuse into this fluid and be carried away in the general stream back into the blood. It is precisely because the CSF is continuously being re-formed in the choroid plexuses, and drained away through the arachnoid villi, that such a sink-action is feasible; if it were stagnant, there would be nothing to prevent the concentration of sucrose from building up to that in the plasma, and the capacity for sink-action would be lost. Kinetically speaking, it is the presence of a strong restraint on passage into the newly secreted CSF—the *blood-CSF barrier*—and the absence of significant restraint on passage of the fluid out of the system in the arachnoid villi that permit the indefinite maintenance of a low concentration of the slowly penetrating solute in the CSF; this in turn permits the maintenance of a low volume of distribution in the brain. This low volume of distribution betokens, of course, a low concentration in the extracellular fluid of the brain by comparison with that in the plasma.

With these general principles clearly in mind, we may now pass to a consideration of the ontogenetic development of the various features that are involved in the concept of the blood-brain barrier.

Drainage

Weed's classical study (1917) on pig embryos was devoted to showing that the stage when the choroid plexuses develop, about the 14-mm embryo, corresponds to the stage when Prussian blue reagents are able to escape from the medullary tube into the adjacent mesenchyme. In other words, it seemed that some form of drainage mechanism developed at the point when bulk formation of fluid began, and Weed suggested that the specialized thinning of the roof of the wall of the IVth ventricle—the *area membranacea inferior*— was actually ruptured by the developing pressure resulting from secretion of CSF. More recent work on the human embryo by Brocklehurst (1969) has shown that the communication between internal and external CSF occurs between the 7th and 8th weeks. The lateral connections, corresponding to the foramina of Luschka, appear at 26 weeks.

Passage from blood to brain

The concept of a delayed development of the blood-brain barrier is largely based on the observations of Behnsen (1926, 1927), who reported that trypan blue, injected into young mice, was accumulated extensively in the nervous tissue, and he concluded that the blood-brain barrier was not fully developed in these immature animals. In very young animals, the staining of the central nervous system was extensive, and it was only by the 7th to 8th week that the staining picture became indistinguishable from that in the adult animal. Behnsen considered that the defects in the blood-brain barrier manifest in the young mouse were essentially exaggerations of those normally observed in the adult, in the sense that they were expansions of those localized areas, such as the area postrema, that normally permit the dyestuff to leave the blood stream. Stern and Peyrot (1927) arrived at an essentially similar conclusion as a result of their studies of the uptake of Prussian blue reagents by the brains of the rabbit, rat, mouse, cat, and dog; the uptake was extensive at birth and decreased until the eyes opened, at which time the adult picture was obtained. The guinea pig was an exception in that it showed adult features at birth, presumably because of its more advanced state of development; a study of fetal animals showed that only when their lids were still sealed and their hair was undeveloped would penetration from blood to CSF and nervous tissue occur.

The importance of this concept of a defective barrier in fetal life became manifest in the etiology of kernicterus, the jaundice of the brain nuclei that often accompanies jaundice in the newborn. Spatz (1934) emphasized that in the adult the dura is well stained in jaundice but not the substance of the brain, so that there is a definite blood-brain barrier to bilirubin. He attributed kernicterus to the poorly developed barrier in the fetus at the time of the maternal jaundice. Subsequent work, however, has shown that kernicterus is much more probably attributable to a defective conjugation of bilirubin by the liver, so that significant amounts of unconjugated bilirubin are present in the fetal circulation (Diamond and Schmid, 1966). Bilirubin is lipid-soluble, and, as such, would pass the blood-brain barrier with ease; this has been confirmed by experimental studies with the unconjugated form (Diamond and Schmid, 1966). The conjugated form, on the other hand, is water-soluble and meets considerable restraint at the blood-brain barrier.

If this is indeed the true explanation of kernicterus, the question as to whether the passage across the brain capillaries is really less restricted in immature animals and fetuses must be reexamined with care. At present, the position is not completely clear, and some of the recent quantitative studies carried out by my colleagues Bradbury, Saunders, and Segal, will be the subject of a following chapter. To recapitulate some of the earlier work, Bakay (1953) found a steady decrease in uptake of $^{32}PO_4$ by the brains of fetal and postnatal rabbits as they grew older; other and later studies on several species have agreed on greater uptakes of solutes in the fetal state, but the evidence that this represents a more *rapid* uptake rather than a more extensive uptake into a larger extracellular space has not been provided; in fact, the more probable interpretation is that the extracellular space in the immature animal is larger than in the adult. Thus, Vernadakis and Woodbury (1962, 1965) found a definite decrease in the chloride space of brain with development; however, they (1965) also found progressive changes in the kinetics of uptake of ions and inulin that suggested an increase in the height of the barrier with age.

In their most recent paper, Ferguson and Woodbury (1969) have followed uptake of ^{14}C inulin and ^{14}C sucrose into both brain and CSF of developing rats, and have discussed their results in terms of a steadily decreasing extracellular space, a variable sink-action of the CSF, and a variable blood-brain barrier to the solutes. There is little doubt that at the earliest stage studied (4 days before birth), the blood-CSF barrier is considerably reduced so that the concentration in the CSF nearly reaches the plasma concentration after about 24 hr. Such a situation might be expected were the CSF being formed as a simple filtrate of plasma at this early stage. In these animals the inulin space for brain was about 30%, and this doubtless corresponded with the extracellular space, which is high in the fetal animal (Brizzee and Jacobs, 1959). With increasing age, both rate of equilibration and absolute steady-state level decreased, and the results are consistent with an increasing barrier leading to more effective sink-action by the CSF, associated with a real decrease in extracellular space until the adult value of 13.5% is reached.

Changes in chemical composition of CSF

CSF is a secretion, and as such has a different composition from that which would be expected of a mere ultrafiltrate of blood plasma; characteristic deviations from an ultrafiltrate are given by the concentrations of Cl^- and Mg^{++} which are higher than in an ultrafiltrate, while the concentrations of K^+ and urea are definitely lower.

Flexner (1938) found that, in the pig, embryos 3 to 5 cm in length had values for the ratio R_{CSF} = concn. in CSF/concn. in plasma of about 1.04, corresponding to what would be expected of a plasma ultrafiltrate; at 6 to 7 cm, the value of R_{CSF} was 1.17, and at 10 to 15 cm, it had reached the adult value of 1.29. Figure 2 shows the progressive changes in R_{CSF} for Cl^-, Na^+, and K^+ in the growing rat as observed by Ferguson and Woodbury (1969). Here the most striking change is that for the K^+ distribution ratio, which falls from the dialysis value of about 0.94 in the fetal animal to about 0.6 in the adult.

Bito and Myers (1970) examined the changes in concentration of K^+, Ca^{++}, and Mg^{++} in the CSF of developing monkeys; they examined the fluid withdrawn not only from the cisterna magna, the usual site of withdrawal in

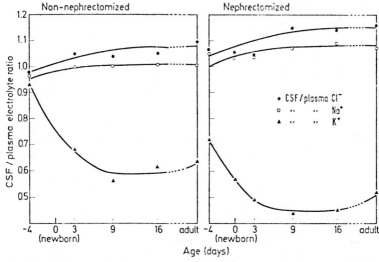

FIG. 2. Plot of CSF/plasma electrolyte concentration ratios for rats of various ages. (From Ferguson and Woodbury, 1969.)

animal studies, but also from the lateral ventricles and cortical and lumbar subarachnoid spaces. This was considered necessary since an earlier study (Bito and Davson, 1966) had shown that there were interesting gradients of concentration within the CSF; e.g., the concentration of K^+ in the cortical subarachnoid fluid was actually lower than that in the ventricular fluid, and this suggested that the extracellular fluid of the cortex had a low concentration of K^+, and was imposing this on that of the CSF. Thus, in general, there is reason to believe that the extracellular fluid of nervous tissue is formed by secretory processes across the capillaries or their astrocytic covering; only in this way can we conceive of the CSF maintaining concentrations of solutes such as K^+, Cl^-, Mg^{++}, and Na^+ that are considerably different from those in plasma or its ultrafiltrate. Mere secretion of a fluid by the choroid plexuses with these different concentrations would not be adequate, since exchanges between brain and CSF occur readily across the ependyma and pia-glia. The CSF and extracellular fluid of nervous tissue are, therefore, most probably of essentially similar composition, their compositions being maintained different from that of a plasma ultrafiltrate by secretory activity, on the part of the choroidal epithelium in the one case and the blood-brain barrier in the other. If the two fluids are not perfectly matched, we may expect some gradients of concentration as we proceed from the ventricles where the fluid is "newest" to the cortical subarachnoid space where it is older than the cisternal fluid; the lumbar fluid is probably old, too, since it constitutes a backwater, aside from the main flow of fluid.

The finding that the cortical subarachnoid has normally a lower concentration of K^+ than that in the cisternal and ventricular fluids suggests that the extracellular fluid of brain has an even lower concentration, and that it is influencing that in the CSF. The situation with Mg^{++} is essentially similar, in that the cortical subarachnoid fluid is different from the cisternal and ventricular fluids; in this case the concentration in all fluids is considerably higher than in a plasma ultrafiltrate, and the cortical fluid is the highest, i.e.,

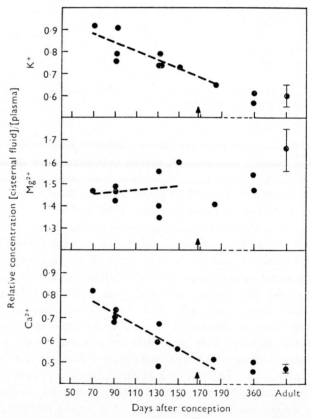

FIG. 3. The development of adult type of cisternal-CSF/plasma distribution ratio. The correlations between the distribution ratios and gestational age are significant for K and Ca ($p < 0.01$), but not for Mg. *Abscissa*: Days after conception linearly up to approximately 22 days of postnatal life. The normal time of delivery (168 days) is indicated by the arrow. The values for the 6-month-old (1 yr after conception) and adult monkeys are placed arbitrarily at the end of the scale. (From Bito and Myers, 1970).

the most discrepant from a plasma ultrafiltrate in the same way that the lowest concentration of K$^+$ in the cortical fluid shows it to be the most discrepant from a plasma ultrafiltrate.

Figure 3 shows that the cisternal R_{CSF} for K$^+$ decreases to reach its adult value of about 0.6 at some 360 days. The Mg^{++} ratio is already high at the earliest stage studied and increases less dramatically. The large changes in R_{CSF} for Ca^{++} may be related to the protein content of the fluid since a large fraction of the Ca^{++} is bound to protein. Of some interest is the development of the cortical/cisternal gradient of concentration, and this is shown in Fig. 4. During fetal life, this gradient does not exist, and the large

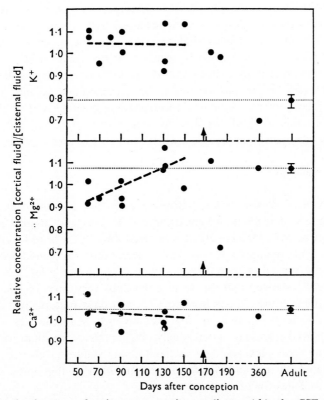

FIG. 4. The development of cation concentration gradients *within* the CSF system. The adult type of cortical-subarachnoid-fluid/cisternal-fluid ratios are indicated by the dotted lines. Only the Mg regression line is significant ($p < 0.01$). *Abscissa*: Days after conception linearly up to approximately 22 days of postnatal life. The normal time of delivery (168 days) is indicated by the arrow. The values for the 6-month-old (1 yr after conception) and adult monkeys are placed arbitrarily at the end of the scale. (From Bito and Myers, 1970.)

change occurs some time between 190 days (i.e., in the 3-week-old infant) and adulthood. By contrast, the cortical/cisternal gradient for Mg^{++} shows a significant increase during the second trimester of gestation, reaching the adult value by the 120th day of fetal life.

To return to the situation with K^+, we may note that the distribution ratio for the earliest fetuses studied, namely, 50 days after conception, is the same as for dialysis of adult plasma, and so at this stage there is no evidence for secretory activity. As shown in Fig. 3, the value of R_{CSF} for K^+ does not reach its adult value until after birth; however, if the *absolute concentration* in CSF is considered, rather than the R_{CSF}, it is found that the adult concentration is reached by about 130 days after conception, i.e., before birth. This is because the plasma K^+ decreases with age, and the finding that the adult concentration in CSF is achieved early means that the homeostatic mechanism that ensures that the CSF concentration is largely independent of plasma concentration is operative at this early stage.

In general, this study of Bito and Myers (1970) establishes the earliness with which secretory activity occurs in the cerebrospinal system. Since such activity is inconceivable without a corresponding development of the blood-brain barrier, this work shows that, in primates at any rate, "barrier activity" occurs at an early embryonic stage.

Active accumulation

The choroid plexus, besides secreting a fluid of characteristic composition, is capable of actively accumulating certain ions and organic molecules; in the intact animal, the actively accumulated ion is transferred to the blood, so that the CSF maintains a very low concentration compared with that in blood plasma; typical of these ions is iodide. Robinson, Cutler, Lorenzo, and Barlow (1968) showed that this feature develops very early in fetal cats and rabbits. In the earliest fetuses studied (7 to 10 days preterm in rabbits and 1 to 2 days preterm in cats), *in vitro* accumulation of iodide was as great as in adult choroid plexuses; interestingly, higher tissue/medium ratios were found in late fetal plexuses than in adult ones. Sulfate is also accumulated by the isolated plexus, and significant accumulation of this anion developed later, at 1 to 3 days after birth.

Secretory rate

Again, the rate of secretion may be expected to increase with development; Shaywitz, Katzman, and Escriva (1969) found that this increased from

3.3 μliters/min in 20-day kittens to 11.3 at 8 weeks of age, and to 17.1 in adults. Associated with this development there was a large drop in efflux of ^{24}Na from the ventricles, presumably associated with a decrease in passive permeability of the choroid plexuses and brain capillaries to sodium.

Morphology

Finally we may discuss the changing morphology of the developing choroid plexus; this has been reviewed by Tennyson and Pappas (1968). According to Kappers (1958), the development may be divided into three stages in man, and corresponding stages were described by Tennyson and Pappas in the rabbit. In the first phase, at about 6 weeks, the choroid plexus is represented by a simple fold into the lateral ventricle consisting of pseudo-stratified epithelium; the stroma is filled with developing blood cells and strands of angioblasts forming capillaries. The second phase appears at about 8 weeks when the plexus becomes lobular and occupies almost the entire ventricle; at this stage the epithelium consists of a single layer of low columnar cells containing glycogen. The third period occurs when the fetus is in its 4th month; the choroid plexus decreases in volume in relation to the ventricle; most of the epithelial cells still contain glycogen, but some cuboidal cells resembling the mature epithelium have appeared. According to the electron-microscopic study of Tennyson and Pappas (1968), Stage II is accompanied by an increase in the number of microvilli on the epithelial cells, as well as in the infoldings and interdigitations of the basal regions of adjacent cells. Stage III is associated with a reduction in the number of microvilli while the basal infoldings become less complex. Meller and Wechsler (1965), in their study of the chick, suggest that the early signs of development in the epithelial cells are related to the requirement for *absorption* from the primitive CSF. Only later does the secretion of fluid become important, and this is associated with the microvilli and lateral interdigitations. In this connection we may note that Smith, Streicher, Milkovic, and Klatzo (1964) observed that early chick embryonic plexuses actively absorbed labeled proteins.

To summarize this very brief review of the evidence relating to the ontogeny of the blood-brain-CSF relationships, we may say that the development of the special features that characterize them begins very early, so that to establish a significant difference between the newborn and the adult is extremely difficult; moreover, the complex interrelations that make up the blood-brain barrier concept so far preclude an unequivocal statement that the permeability of the brain capillaries is in any way different in, say, the late fetal animal than in the newborn or adult. The brain has not reached full development at term, however, so that changes in the complex interrelations must occur, and these may be reflected in altered parameters. It is the task of the experimenter to analyze these parameters so that ultimately the individual alterations, which may well include alterations in secretion rate of CSF, in permeability of the cerebral capillaries, in volume of extracellular space, and so on, may be demonstrated.

REFERENCES

Bakay, L. (1953): Studies on blood-brain barrier with radioactive phosphorus. III. Embryonic development of the barrier. *Archives of Neurology and Psychiatry,* 70:30-39.

Behnsen, G. (1926): Farbstoffversuche mit Trypanblau ar der Schranke zwischen Blut und Zentralnervensystem der wachsenden Maus. *Münchener medizinische Wochenschrift,* 73:1143.

Behnsen, G. (1927): U.d. Farbstoffspeicherung im Zentralnervensystem der weissen Maus in verschiedenen Alterszuständen. *Zeitschrift fur Zellforschung und mikroskopische Anatomie,* 4:515-572.

Bito, L. Z., and Davson, H. (1966): Local variations in cerebrospinal fluid composition and its relationship to the composition of the extracellular fluid of the cortex. *Experimental Neurology,* 14:264-280.

Bito, L. Z., and Myers, R. E. (1970): The ontogenesis of haematoencephalic cation transport processes in the rhesus monkey. *Journal of Physiology,* 208:153-170.

Brightman, M. W., and Reese, T. S. (1969): Junctions between intimately apposed cell membranes in the vertebrate brain. *Journal of Cell Biology,* 40:648-677.

Brizzee, K. R., and Jacobs, L. A. (1959): The glial-neuron index in the submolecular layers of the motor cortex in the cat. *Anatomical Record,* 134:97-105.

Brocklehurst, G. (1969): The development of the human cerebrospinal fluid pathway with particular reference to the roof of the fourth ventricle. *Journal of Anatomy,* 105:467-475.

Davson, H., and Bradbury, M. B. (1965): The fluid exchange of the central nervous system. *Symposium of the Society of Experimental Biology,* 19:349-364.

Diamond, I., and Schmid, R. (1966): Experimental bilirubin encephalopathy. The mode of entry of bilirubin-C into the central nervous system. *Journal of Clinical Investigation,* 45:678-689.

Edström, R. (1958): An explanation of the blood-brain barrier phenomenon. *Acta Psychiatrica et Neurologica,* 33:403-416.

Ferguson, R. K., and Woodbury, D. M. (1969): Penetration of ^{14}C-inulin and ^{14}C-sucrose into brain, cerebrospinal fluid, and skeletal muscle of developing rats. *Experimental Brain Research,* 7:181-194.

Kappers, J. A. (1958): Structural and functional changes in the telencephalic choroid plexus during human ontogenesis. In: *The Cerebrospinal Fluid.* Ciba Foundation Symposium. Churchill, London.

Meller, K., and Wechsler, W. (1965): Elektronenmikroskopische Untersuchung der Entwicklung der telencephalen Plexus chorioides des Huhnes. *Zeitschrift fur Zellforschung und mikroskopische Anatomie,* 65:420-444.

Robinson, R. J., Cutler, R. W. P., Lorenzo, A. V., and Barlow, C. F. (1968):

Development of transport mechanisms for sulphate and iodide in immature choroid plexus. *Journal of Neurochemistry,* 15:455-458.

Shaywitz, B. A., Katzman, R., and Escriva, A. (1969): CSF formation and ²⁴Na clearance in normal and hydrocephalic kittens during ventriculocisternal perfusion. *Neurology,* 19:1159-1168.

Smith, D. E., Streicher, E., Mikovic, K., and Klatzo, I. (1964): Observations on the transport of proteins by the isolated choroid plexus. *Acta Neuropathology,* 3:372-386.

Spatz, H. (1934): Die Bedeutung der vitalen Farbung für die Lehre vom Stoffaustausch zwischen dem Zentralnervensystem und dem übrigen Körper. *Archives fur Psychiatrie und Nervenheilkunde,* 101:267-358.

Stern, L., and Peyrot, R. (1927): Le fontionnement de la barrière hématoencéphalique aux divers stades de développement chez diverses espèces animales. *Comptes Rendus Hebdomadaires des Séances et Mémoires de la Société de Biologie,* 96:1124-1126.

Tennyson, V. M., and Pappas, G. D. (1968): The fine structure of the choroid plexus: Adult and developmental stages. *Progress in Brain Research,* 29:63-85.

Vernadakis, A., and Woodbury, D. M. (1962): Electrolyte and amino acid changes in rat brain during maturation. *American Journal of Physiology,* 203:748-752.

Vernadakis, A., and Woodbury, D. M. (1965): Cellular and extracellular spaces in developing rat brain. *Archives of Neurology,* 12:284-293.

Weed, L. H. (1914): The pathways of escape from the subarachnoid spaces with particular reference to the arachnoid villi. *Journal of Medical Research,* 31:51-91.

DISCUSSION

DEMPSEY: When the tonicity of blood is changed, the volume of extracellular space generally also is changed. In the brain, however, by electron microscopy, it is the glial cells which change in volume, not the extracellular space. Is it possible that in the brain we must consider a compartment not identical with either the extracellular or the intracellular space, identifiable perhaps as vacuolar extensions of the plasma membranes of the glial cells? If so, can the development of the blood-brain barrier be related to the development of glial cells?

DAVSON: The idea that the glial cells can act as an extracellular space is unsound; in brain edema, glial cells appear swollen in the electron microscope, but there is no reason to believe that neurons do not respond to osmotic changes by swelling and shrinking. So far as the development of the barrier is concerned, it is likely that the phase of proliferation of glia corresponds roughly in time with the manifestations of barrier activity but there need be no causal relation; in fact the low permeability of the cerebral capillaries is a function of the closing of intercellular clefts in the endothelium.

BRADBURY: I have no histological evidence on this, but amphibian central nervous system tissue may be incubated *in vitro* without swelling or electrolyte disturbance. Measurements of extracellular space enable cell volume to be estimated. The cellular component of the tissue behaves almost as a perfect osmometer in hypo- and hypertonic solutions; in other words, presumably both nervous and glial cells are responding equally and maximally to osmotic stress.

KARCZMAR: Most speakers so far seemed to describe the various barriers (blood-brain barrier, placental barrier) purely in terms of "passive" permeability barriers. Yet, active transport processes exist as well. Can not some of the brain protection which it exhibits in the adulthood depend on active extrusion of substances rather than on relative impermeability of its blood-brain barrier compared to the fetal state?

DAVSON: Yes, by all means. There is no doubt that active transport processes occur across the blood-brain and blood-CSF barriers.

MANN: I was greatly interested in the observation that in the sheep cerebrospinal fluid, the concentration of chloride changes so dramatically at about 50 days. Unless there is also a change in osmolality of that fluid, this must mean that the rise in chloride concentration must be compensated by a decrease in some other fluid constituents. Is it perhaps, that, for example, inositol or amino acids change their concentration?

DAVSON: Yes, to some extent the fall in bicarbonate helps to maintain osmolality; also the fall in urea concentration contributes materially.

DAWES: The period 40 to 60 days over which you have shown such rapid changes in CSF constitution corresponds exactly to that over which Bernhard and his group in Stockholm have shown, both anatomically and histologically, that there is a great development of the cerebral cortex. Can the ionic composition of the brain be regarded as homogenous at this time, as is implied for the adult, or is the cortex then in a different ionic environment?

DAVSON: Unfortunately we have no studies on different regions of the brain to answer that question adequately.

Fetal Pharmacology, edited by L. Boréus
Raven Press, New York © 1973

Uptake and Distribution of ³H-Ouabain in Brain and Other Tissues of Developing Rats

Hans E. Brøndsted and D. M. Woodbury

*Institute of Physiology, University of Aarhus, Aarhus, Denmark, and
Department of Pharmacology, University of Utah College of Medicine,
Salt Lake City, Utah 84112*

Among important enzyme systems which develop rapidly after birth in rat brain is the sodium-potassium-activated adenosine triphosphatase (Na^+-K^+-ATPase) which is closely related to the sodium pump. Pump activity, Na^+-K^+-ATPase, and electrical activity of the brain all develop rapidly after birth (Vernadakis and Woodbury, 1965; Abdel-Latif, Smith, and Ellington, 1970). It is well known that ouabain (g-strophantin) inhibits both the sodium pump and Na^+-K^+-ATPase. It also inhibits the transport of substances which are important for the brain, such as glucose (Brøndsted, 1970). It was therefore of interest to study the uptake and distribution of ³H-ouabain in the developing rat brain. Cerebrospinal fluid (CSF) was included in the studies because it probably has a composition similar to that of brain extracellular fluid (ECF). For comparison, plasma, muscle, heart, and liver were also included.

METHODS

Tritium-labeled ouabain of high specific activity was administered intraperitoneally to developing rats (3, 9, 16, and 35 days of age). At selected time intervals after the injection, tissues were taken during light ether anesthesia for determination of ^{3}H activity by means of scintillation counting. Chromatography studies showed no signs of metabolism of ^{3}H-ouabain within 8 hr after injection. Ultrafiltration studies on tissue homogenates (in water) permitted the determination of unbound ^{3}H-ouabain in the tissues. Electrolytes were determined by means of flame photometry (Na^+ and K^+) and electrometric titration (Cl^-).

RESULTS AND DISCUSSION

All tissues took up ^{3}H-ouabain rapidly. The concentrations of unbound ^{3}H-ouabain in muscle, heart, and liver from 3- and 9-day-old animals were about the same as or slightly higher than in plasma. In the 16- and 35-day-old animals, these tissue levels were several times higher than plasma levels, indicating maturation of a transport system for ^{3}H-ouabain (unbound) which accumulates the drug intracellularly. Liver slices from adult rats have similarly been found to accumulate the drug *in vitro* by a saturable mechanism (Kupferberg and Schanker, 1968).

The concentrations of unbound ^{3}H-ouabain in brain rapidly (within 5 min) reached near-maximal levels. These levels were much lower than in plasma, indicating the existence of a blood-brain barrier against ^{3}H-ouabain. The brain/plasma and CSF/plasma concentration ratios decreased with age (CSF/plasma ratios are shown in the Table). Although present shortly after birth, the blood-brain barrier against ^{3}H-ouabain thus still develops during the following weeks. A lipid-insoluble drug such as ouabain is not likely to pass the blood-brain barrier easily by simple diffusion. The rapid uptake and the constant levels in brain and CSF, which were seen in face of alterations in plasma concentrations, are, therefore, probably the result of a specific transport mechanism located at the blood-brain barrier.

Brain cells develop a transport mechanism which accumulates unbound ^{3}H-ouabain intracellularly. This was disclosed in the following way. The intracellular fluid (ICF)/ECF concentration ratios were derived from the water content of the brains and values for extracellular space (ECS) which had been determined previously (Ferguson and Woodbury, 1969). The ECF was assumed to be in equilibrium with CSF. This assumption is probably correct since it is valid for the much larger inulin molecule up to 16 days of age (Ferguson and Woodbury, 1969). The Table shows an increase in ICF/ECF ratios from zero in the young animals to 2.1 in the 35-day-old animals. The

TABLE 1. *Extracellular space and ³H-ouabain distribution ratios in developing rat brain.*

Age (days)	ECS	ICF/ECF	CSF/Plasma
3	41	0	0.076
9	33	0	0.067
16	30	1.0	0.034
35	15	2.1	0.013

ECS is extracellular space (% wet weight). Values were derived from previous determinations with ^{14}C-inulin (Ferguson and Woodbury, 1969). ICF, ECF, and CSF are concentrations of unbound ^{3}H-ouabain in intracellular fluid, extracellular fluid, and cerebrospinal fluid, respectively. Distribution ratios are based on values during steady state (about 1 hr after injection).

decrease with age of ECS largely caused by growth of glial elements is also shown in the Table.

Some of the animals received an LD_{50} dose of ouabain together with the ^{3}H-ouabain. The effect was a decrease almost to zero of intracellular unbound ^{3}H-ouabain in heart and muscle from the older animals; i.e., the transport mechanism was saturable. There was no effect in brain probably because the blood-brain barrier prevented the entry into or accelerated the exit from the brain of the drug.

Tissue electrolytes were determined after a LD_{50} dose of ouabain (intraperitoneally). Again the blood-brain barrier prevented clear effects from being seen in brain and CSF, but the sodium pump was clearly inhibited in muscle where K^+ was decreased and Na^+ and Cl^- were both increased. These effects only occurred in the older animals. No effects upon electrolytes were seen in the heart.

CONCLUSION

Unbound ^{3}H-ouabain is accumulated intracellularly in brain, muscle, heart, and liver of developing rats. The transport mechanism is saturable in muscle and heart as shown by the inhibitory effect of an LD_{50} dose of ouabain. Both the ability to accumulate ^{3}H-ouabain intracellularly and a blood-brain barrier against the drug mature after birth.

ACKNOWLEDGMENT

This work was supported in part by a U.S. Public Health Service International Postdoctoral Research Fellowship (1-F05-TW01677-01).

REFERENCES

Abdel-Latif, A. A., Smith, J. P., and Ellington, E. P. (1970): Subcellular distribution of sodium-potassium adenosine triphosphatase, acetylcholine and acetylcholinesterase in developing rat brain. *Brain Research,* 18:441-450.

Brøndsted, H. E. (1970): Ouabain-sensitive carrier-mediated transport of glucose from the cerebral ventricles to surrounding tissues in the cat. *Journal of Physiology,* 208:187-201.

Ferguson, R. K., and Woodbury, D. M. (1969): Penetration of ^{14}C-inulin and ^{14}C-sucrose into brain, cerebrospinal fluid and skeletal muscle of developing rats. *Experimental Brain Research,* 7:181-194.

Kupferberg, H. J., and Schanker, L. S. (1968): Biliary secretion of ouabain-H^3 and its uptake by liver slices in the rat. *American Journal of Physiology,* 214:1048-1053.

Vernadakis, A., and Woodbury, D. M. (1965): Cellular and extracellular spaces in developing rat brain. *Archives of Neurology,* 12:284-293.

Fetal Pharmacology, edited by L. Boréus
Raven Press, New York © 1973

The Development of the Internal Environment of the Brain

N. R. Saunders and M. W. B. Bradbury

Department of Physiology, University College and Sherrington School of Physiology, St. Thomas' Hospital, London, England

INTRODUCTION

It has long been suggested that the composition of the microenvironment of brain cells is maintained within closer limits than that of other tissues. This stability has been supposed to be important for the normal functioning of nervous tissue and to involve not only maintenance of a rather constant composition but also exclusion of harmful agents. This protection was supposed to reside in a morphological barrier between the blood and the brain (reviewed by Friedmann, 1942). The concept has been criticized, notably by Dobbing (1961), who argued that the composition of the extracellular fluid of the brain may be more a reflection of the activity of brain cells than directly due to the action of specific controlling mechanisms. However, there is now a substantial amount of evidence that the composition of cerebrospinal fluid (CSF) in adult animals is remarkably stable even when the external environment is severely perturbed (e.g., electrolyte composition; see below), but that a morphological barrier between blood and brain is only one of several factors which are involved in this stability. These factors are outlined below and are the same factors which may be involved in determining the steady-state or changing concentration of foreign solutes such as drugs introduced into the brain or CSF.

Experimental difficulty in separating the functions of different parts of the blood-brain-CSF system has hindered the development of models adequate to explain the behavior of different solutes in this system. In considering the distribution or movement of a solute, some or all of the following should be taken into account.

(1) The transport characteristics of the solute across at least five interphases: the blood-brain barrier between blood and interstitial fluid of brain (ECF); the choroid plexuses between blood and CSF; the plasma membranes of neurons and glial cells, between ECF and brain cells; the ependyma between ECF and ventricular CSF; and the pia-glial membrane between ECF and subarachnoid CSF. These characteristics of a single interphase may not be the same in all regions. Thus the blood-brain barrier is deficient in certain parts of the brain and the ependyma shows much structural specialization (e.g., Olsson, 1958).

(2) The volume and other dimensions of the different compartments within the system, i.e., the extracellular or interstitial fluid of brain, the CSF, and the intracellular fluids of neurons and glial cells. There may be compartments of the extracellular fluid which are not in free communication with the bulk of this fluid, e.g., the water associated with myelin sheaths. Similarly, intracellular organelles may not have the same composition as the rest of the cytoplasma.

(3) The density of capillaries within the brain and the blood flow through them. This may be different in different regions and may change with altered physiological conditions, e.g., arterial P_{CO_2}.

(4) The rate of flow of CSF and the possibility of bulk movement of fluid within the ECF spaces of the brain.

(5) The rate of diffusion of the solute within the cerebral ECF.

EXPERIMENTAL INVESTIGATION OF THE FETUS

It is of interest to know how the stable environment of the fetus develops, partly because this may help in understanding the mechanisms involved, and partly because of the possible clinical significance of inadequacies in the system which may be present during development, as a result either of immaturity or of damage imposed by adverse conditions. However, the variety of factors which may be involved in determining the stable environment of the adult brain make interpretation of the limited amount of information available about the developing brain even more difficult. Not only may transport characteristics of the interphases be quite different, but the different dimensions of the various compartments and the different rate of flow of CSF make comparisons with the adult very difficult. Thus greater uptake of a solute from blood by a young brain might be due to: (1) greater permeability of the blood-brain barrier; (2) greater permeability of the blood-CSF barrier; (3) less effective outward active transport at either of these sites; (4) less sink action of the CSF due to smaller production of CSF; (5) greater volume of ECF in the brain; and/or (6) greater metabolic incorporation.

Other factors might tend to mask an increased permeability of the blood-brain barrier: (1) a smaller capillary density and less blood flow; (2) a larger volume of ventricular CSF relative to brain size; or (3) greater weight of the choroid plexuses and perhaps secretion of CSF relative to brain size and distances within the brain for diffusion.

Ferguson and Woodbury (1969) have discussed the effect of some of these factors on the uptake of ^{14}C-inulin and ^{14}C-sucrose by the brain and CSF of fetal and postnatal rats.

An initial indirect approach to some of these problems would be a systematic study of electrolyte concentrations in fetal brain, CSF, and blood plasma at different ages. Since chloride and sodium occur in low concentration in intracellular fluid whereas potassium is largely an intracellular ion, the changing relative concentrations of these ions would suggest in which directions the volumes of the intra- and extracellular compartments were changing. Simultaneous comparison of fetal CSF and blood plasma would indicate at what stage the secretory processes for the individual ions and perhaps for the fluid as a whole were arising, although not necessarily indicating the site of these secretory processes. Several studies of this type have been made on fetuses of different species—and these will be discussed below—but brain, CSF, and fetal plasma all obtained simultaneously have not previously been compared at different ages in one species. We have compared five electrolytes (chloride, sodium, potassium, calcium, and magnesium) in the fetal sheep (Bradbury, Reynolds, Reynolds, Saunders, and Wilson, submitted for publication). The sheep was chosen not only because it is a readily available species for which techniques of exteriorizing the fetus have been developed (Dawes, 1968), but because the fetus even at 40 to 45 days is large enough to yield volumes of fetal plasma and CSF suitable for precise analysis. The arterial pH, P_{CO_2} and P_{O_2} of the mother could be controlled within defined physiological limits (pH 7.40 $\pm$ SE 0.02;

TABLE 1. *Potassium contents of plasma, CSF, skeletal muscle, and brain from rabbits dieted 3 weeks.*

Level of potassium	Plasma (mequiv/liter)	CSF (mequiv/liter)	Muscle (mequiv/kg wet wt)	Brain (mequiv/kg wet wt)	Arterial pH
Control [6]	4.15 ± 0.27	2.83 ± 0.08	111.0 ± 2.7 (75.1)	95.4 ± 1.3 (78.5)	7.41 ± 0.03
Low K [5]	1.58 ± 0.09	2.72 ± 0.06	72.2 ± 2.6 (76.3)	94.5 ± 1.3 (79.1)	7.41 ± 0.02
Low K [5] + KCl infusion	4.45 ± 0.18	2.84 ± 0.05	93.5 ± 4.2 (77.8)	95.5 ± 1.7 (78.9)	7.39 ± 0.02
High K [7]	7.09 ± 0.59	3.02 ± 0.12	109.8 ± 0.9 (77.2)	94.9 ± 0.8 (78.5)	7.29 ± 0.05

No. of animals given in brackets. Water, percent wet weight, given in parentheses. Values are ± S.E. (Bradbury and Kleeman, 1967).

P_{CO_2} 38 mm Hg $\pm$ 2.1; P_{O_2} 111 mm Hg $\pm$ 10) by altering the composition of the ewe's inspired air. Checks of these variables in the fetuses showed them to be within physiological limits in most cases, although in the youngest age group there was insufficient blood volume for these measurements to be made.

ELECTROLYTES IN FETAL CSF

An extremely important aspect of any internal environment is its electrolyte composition. Because substances, even of large molecular weight, such as inulin, penetrate relatively easily from CSF to brain extracellular space, and because introduction of active solutes, including ions into CSF (Leusen, 1949), produces marked effects on the adjacent neurons, it is likely that the CSF represents a useful indicator of the brain-cell microenvironment. The electrolyte composition of CSF in the normal adult is relatively constant under normal conditions and rather similar in different species (Davson, 1967). Also, the composition of CSF remains stable even in the face of gross and prolonged changes in plasma electrolytes. This homeostasis of CSF electrolytes applies to hydrogen, potassium, calcium, and magnesium ions. An example of the excellent control of the potassium concentration in the cisternal CSF of rabbits rendered hypokalemic and hyperkalemic by dietary means is shown in Table 1. Since the potassium content of brain is also quite constant whereas muscle becomes depleted in chronic hypokalemia, the potassium concentration in the ECF of brain must also presumably be controlled.

However, there is relatively little information about the composition of CSF in the fetus at different ages and still less about its stability in the face of changes in the fetal and maternal blood. In the classical study in this field, Flexner (1938) obtained CSF from the fetal pig and analyzed it for chloride, urea, and sodium. For fetuses of crown-rump length of 5.0 cm and less, the ratio of the concentration of the solute in CSF water to the concentration in plasma water (R_{csf}) was for each of these solutes close to 1.00. For lengths of 6.5 cm and longer, R_{csf} for chloride and sodium rose rapidly, reaching 1.25 and 1.16 at 20 cm, whereas R_{csf} for urea fell, reaching 0.80 at this time. Flexner correlates this change with development of secretory activity by the choroid plexuses. There is no proof that the choroid epithelium is the site of this secretory activity although histochemical studies may support such a view (Flexner, 1951-1952). Rather similar changes in chloride and sodium were noted in the rat by Ferguson and Woodbury

(1969). In this species the crucial change occurs during the period between 4 days before and 3 days after birth. The apparent lateness of the change in the rat is no doubt due to the fact that this species is born at an early stage of general development compared to the pig and the sheep (see below).

Bito and Myers (1970) studied potassium, calcium, and magnesium in cisternal and cortical subarachnoid CSF in the rhesus monkey. Magnesium was higher in concentration in cisternal and cortical CSF than in plasma at all ages, R_{csf} being at least 1.4 from a fetus 70 days after conception. Since the ratio of concentration in a dialyzate to that in plasma is 0.75, Bito and Myers argue that there must be active transport of magnesium into CSF from an early age. Potassium and calcium in CSF showed rather different behavior in that their concentrations in CSF were close to that expected of a dialyzate of plasma at 70 days and fell thereafter to reach the lower value typical of the adult at or shortly after birth at 170 days. Similarly in the rat (Ferguson and Woodbury, 1969), potassium in CSF, initially high, only reached the adult value at 9 days. Thus the active processes

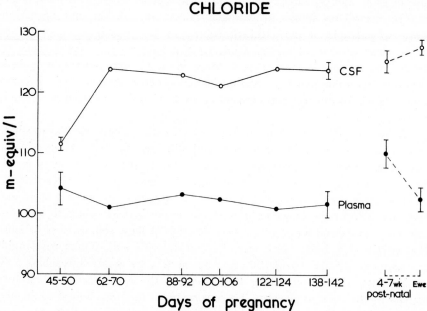

FIG. 1. The chloride concentration in CSF and blood plasma from fetal, postnatal, and adult sheep. Points are means from (generally) three to six fetuses, and limits are standard errors.

SODIUM

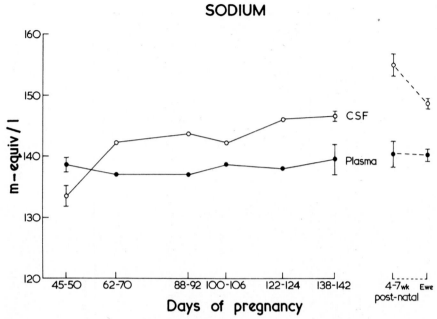

FIG. 2. The sodium concentration in CSF and blood plasma from fetal, postnatal, and adult sheep. Points are means from (generally) three to six fetuses, and limits are standard errors.

concerned in maintaining ionic concentrations in the CSF develop at quite different times for individual ions.

Our findings in the sheep confirm and complement the above observations. At most ages, chloride in CSF is substantially higher than in plasma, R_{csf} being 1.18 at 90 days and 1.22 at 139 days (Fig. 1). These values are close to R_{csf} in the ewe—1.24—but have not been corrected for water content. At 45 to 50 days, R_{csf} is significantly less—1.05. R_{csf} for sodium is also reduced at this stage, 0.98 instead of 1.045 at later ages (Fig. 2). Magnesium in CSF was higher than in plasma at all fetal ages (Table 2). This gradient was established in the earliest fetuses, CSF magnesium being 1.96 mequiv/liter and plasma magnesium 1.63 mequiv/liter at 45 to 50 days. Reliable figures for potassium and calcium were only available from 90 days. At this stage, both potassium and calcium were present at substantially higher concentrations than in adult CSF, 3.53 and 3.41 mequiv/liter as against 3.14 and 2.45 mequiv/liter, respectively, in the adult. Parity with the adult was not reached for either of these ions in CSF by 140 days.

TABLE 2. *Potassium, calcium, and magnesium concentrations in fetal and maternal CSF and blood plasma of the sheep.*

Age of fetuses (days)	Potassium		Calcium		Magnesium	
	CSF	Plasma	CSF	Plasma	CSF	Plasma
45-50	—	—	—	—	1.96 ± 0.11 (5)	1.63 ± 0.16 (5)
58-70	—	—	—	—	2.32 ± 0.56 (4)	1.96 ± 0.09 (6)
85-92	3.53 ± 0.04 (3)	3.81 ± 0.08 (6)	3.41 ± 0.06 (3)	6.05 ± 0.11 (6)	1.87 ± 0.05 (3)	1.77 ± 0.08 (6)
100-106	3.56 ± 0.08 (6)	3.71 ± 0.08 (5)	3.12 ± 0.07 (3)	6.18 ± 0.04 (2)	1.99 ± 0.03 (8)	1.91 ± 0.09 (7)
122-124	3.53 ± 0.10 (5)	4.46 ± 0.21 (5)	—	—	—	—
138-142	3.26 ± 0.13 (4)	4.20 ± 0.10 (5)	2.85 ± 0.08 (3)	6.45 ± 0.35 (3)	1.91 ± 0.07 (7)	1.78 ± 0.05 (8)
Lambs 4-7 weeks	3.02 ± 0.05 (7)	3.99 ± 0.27 (7)	—	—	1.95 ± 0.05 (7)	1.52 ± 0.05 (7)
Ewes (maternal)	3.14 ± 0.05 (8)	3.41 ± 0.16 (8)	2.45 ± 0.05 (5)	3.37 ± 0.17 (5)	1.83 ± 0.04 (9)	1.42 ± 0.06 (10)

Values given are mequiv/liter ± S.E. No. of experiments in parentheses.

Potassium had reached the adult concentration at 5 to 8 days postnatal; figures are not available for calcium.

Thus there is no discrepancy in the order in which the concentration of each ion reaches its adult value in different species. This order in which active ion secretion matures in the sheep is magnesium first (before 48 days), sodium and chloride next (by 65 days), and potassium and calcium last (after birth). The active processes concerned are presumably sited at either the choroid plexuses or the blood-brain barrier or both; it is not yet possible to relate the sites to transport of individual ions.

ELECTROLYTES IN BRAIN

Flexner and Flexner (1949) estimated the extracellular space of the developing brain of the guinea pig from the distribution of total chloride and from that of ^{22}Na. The chloride space was high, 48% at 40 days, and fell to reach the adult value of 29% shortly after birth. The ^{22}Na space was slightly higher than that of chloride at most ages, but followed the same pattern. One fetus at 33 days had spaces which were smaller than the optimum at 40 days. The water in brain fell progressively over the above period.

Vernadakis and Woodbury (1962) analyzed the brains of young rats; sodium and chloride were high, 57 and 48 mequiv/kg, respectively, at 1 day postnatal. Potassium was low at 78 mequiv/kg. Sodium and chloride began falling rapidly and potassium rising at 12 days, adult concentrations being approximately reached by 21 days. Brøndsted and Woodbury (1971) have obtained similar results in the developing rat.

Our results on brain extend the picture available from other species. Fetal cerebral hemispheres contained more water than maternal brain, 89.1% as compared to 77.7%. The water content of brain was fairly constant to about 105 days after which there was a progressive fall to the adult value. The chloride content was low at 45 days, 47 mequiv/kg, increased progressively to 62 mequiv/kg at 105 days and then fell steeply to 48 mequiv/kg at term, still rather greater than the adult value of 40 mequiv/kg (Fig. 3). The sodium content behaved in a precisely similar fashion to chloride but at each age was about 16 mequiv/kg greater than the chloride content. The potassium content varied in the opposite direction to that of chloride and sodium in such a way that the sum of potassium and sodium was approximately constant at 146 mequiv/kg. At 89 and 105 days, the equivalent concentration of potassium was less than that of sodium. These

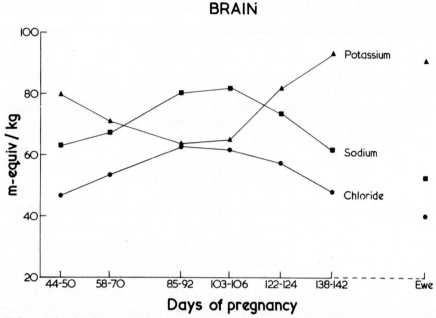

FIG. 3. The chloride, sodium, and potassium content of wet brain from fetal and adult sheep. Points are from (generally) six fetuses. Standard errors were small, less than 2.5 mequiv/liter in every case.

results therefore show unequivocally what has only been a suggestion before—that there is a well-defined maximum in sodium and chloride content during the development of brain and an equivalent minimum in potassium content.

The calcium content of the fetal brain averaged 3.0 mequiv/kg, a value not very different from the adult value of 3.2 mequiv/kg. It remained fairly steady throughout pregnancy except that the average value at 65 days was rather lower than at other times.

BEARING ON DEVELOPMENT OF BLOOD-BRAIN BARRIER AND EXTRACELLULAR FLUID

Ionic gradients between CSF and blood plasma could not, of course, be maintained unless there was a restriction on free diffusion between these fluids. The same argument naturally applies to the net production of CSF.

The findings above suggest that the blood-brain barrier is developed early. In the sheep, sucrose uptake into fetal brain and CSF from fetal blood is rather greater than into these compartments in the adult. However, a marked increase in uptake is only seen at ages before 60 days (Evans, Reynolds, Reynolds, Saunders, and Segal, *in preparation*) (Fig. 4). A similar situation appears to exist in developing rat brain where high uptake of sucrose occurs at 4 days before term and presumably earlier (Ferguson and Woodbury, 1969). In both species, there thus appears to be an association between the age at which sucrose penetrates more readily and the age at which R_{csf} for chloride and sodium diverges markedly, at least in the case of chloride, from unity. It is tempting to suppose that development of a barrier enables the results of secretory activity to become more manifest.

The maximum values for chloride and sodium content of brain observed between 85 and 105 days could have two possible causes. They might be due to a greatly enlarged extracellular space or to increased amounts of sodium and chloride in the brain cells. It is impossible at present to distinguish definitively between these two causes.

Indirect evidence favors the first possibility. A large extracellular space is a feature of many developing tissues (Friis-Hansen, 1957). Opinion is returning toward the view that the chloride space of brain is in the adult vertebrate not much greater than the extracellular space (Bradbury, Villa-

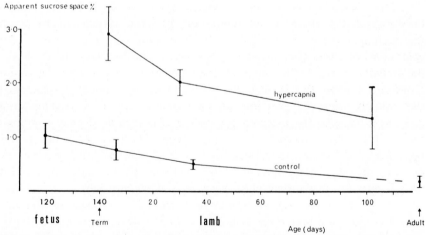

FIG. 4. Entry of ^{14}C-sucrose into brain of fetal and adult sheep from blood plasma. Sucrose was maintained effectively constant in fetal plasma by intermittent intravenous injection. The apparent space is c.p.m. brain/c.p.m. plasma $\times$ 100, and has been corrected for blood content of brain. Points are means $\pm$ S.E.M. (n = 4 or 5).

mil, and Kleeman, 1967; Levin, Fenstermacher, and Patlak, 1970). Ferguson and Woodbury (1969) have argued from the nature of the uptake of ^{14}C-inulin into developing brain and CSF from blood that there must be a high extracellular space as well as differences in the permeability of the barrier or in the rate of secretion of CSF. Any hypothesis as to the function of a high extracellular space must be speculative; it could provide a space suitable for the growth, branching, and connection of dendrites and the terminal fibers of axons.

If the above interpretations are correct, might there be a causal relation between the onset of secretory activity for chloride and sodium and the peak in extracellular space which follows it in time? Davson (this volume) has argued that the increase in sodium and chloride ratios in CSF might well be due to secretory activity at the blood-brain barrier rather than at the choroid plexuses. If sodium and chloride ions are being secreted at this interphase directly into the extracellular fluid, what could be a more likely result than that its volume would increase due to water following under the influence of osmotic forces? This explanation begs the question as to why the extracellular space reduces in size at a later stage in growth.

THE STABILITY OF THE FETAL BRAIN INTERNAL ENVIRONMENT

The relatively constant electrolyte composition of adult CSF and the resistance of CSF electrolyte concentrations to severe changes in the plasma has been mentioned above. The early development of rather steady concentrations of electrolytes in fetal CSF suggests that mechanisms involved in the stability of the brain's internal environment develop early in gestation. However, it is worth stressing that the fetal brain is doubly protected, in that not only does its own internal environment appear to develop at an early age, but also the placenta provides a considerable degree of stability for the internal environment of the whole fetus. Thus marked gradients have been found for some electrolytes between fetal and maternal plasma. For example, in our sheep experiments the maternal plasma calcium was 3.38 mequiv/liter but in the fetal plasma it was 6.31 mequiv/liter.

However, as soon as an animal is born, this additional protection is lost; it is therefore important to know to what extent the internal environment of the fetal and newborn brain can resist external change. An indication that a high degree of stability of the brain's internal environment develops *in utero* comes from experiments in which ewes and newborn lambs were subjected to gross disturbances of blood gas and pH homeostasis. Neither severe hypercapnia (arterial P_{CO_2} over 100 mm Hg) nor hypoxia (fetal arterial P_{O_2} intermittently reduced to 1 to 2 mm Hg by cord occlusion) had any marked effect upon concentrations of CSF electrolytes. Only the potassium showed a significant increase (Evans et al., *in preparation*). A similar effect has been described by Cameron (1971) in the adult dog in response to hypercapnia. Olsen and Sørensen (1971) found that the CSF magnesium concentration was not affected by prolonged severe hypercapnia in either young or adult rats. Low magnesium diets were also without effect upon the CSF magnesium.

DEFICIENCIES IN STABILITY

Deficiencies in stability could be due to immaturity or maldevelopment of the system or, alternatively, to damage induced by some external cause. From the evidence presented above, immaturity only seems likely to be a possible cause of instability in the very early stages of gestation or in animals which are very immature when born, e.g., the rat. Nevertheless, it is a rather common (e.g., Brown, 1962; Bakay, 1968) but poorly substantiated assertion that immaturity and/or damage to the blood-brain barrier of the fetus or newborn allows penetration into the brain of substances which would be kept out of the adult brain. Further, it has been said that such a deficiency is important in the pathogenesis of some clinical conditions, e.g., kernicterus. Confusion seems to have arisen because kernicterus commonly occurs in newborn infants when the serum bilirubin rises above 15 to 20 mg/100 ml; at similar levels of serum bilirubin in the adult, kernicterus is exceedingly rare. The difference is that in the newborn the bilirubin is almost all unconjugated and lipid-soluble (because of immaturity of the liver glucuronyl transferase system) and bound to serum albumin, whereas in the adult it is largely conjugated and in solution in the plasma (Diamond, 1968). Neither form would be expected to cross cell membranes with ease, but should any of the lipid-soluble unconjugated bilirubin become unbound, it would cross cell membranes freely.

The critical factor appears to be the binding capacity of albumin for bilirubin, since this can be affected by a number of factors such as albumin concentration and competition by other substances for binding sites on the albumin molecule. Thus several drugs (e.g., salicylates and sulfonamides) displace bilirubin from albumin and are associated clinically with the occurrence of kernicterus at lower serum bilirubin concentrations than in their absence (Stern, 1970). In animal studies, Diamond and Schmid (1966) have shown that salicylates increase the uptake of unconjugated bilirubin into brain and that this can be partly reversed by increasing the plasma albumin concentration. This is not due to immaturity of the blood-brain barrier since in the very rare instances in which high levels of unconjugated bilirubin do occur in the adult, kernicterus also occurs (Arias, 1962). Several authors (e.g., McKay, 1969; Stern, 1970) have listed clinical conditions which apparently predispose to the occurrence of kernicterus, e.g., asphyxia, hypoxia, hypercapnia, and acidosis. Others have shown experimentally that such conditions will cause unconjugated bilirubin to be deposited in the brain and may give the clinical and histological picture of kernicterus in animals (Lucey, Hibbard, Behrman, Esquiral de Gallardo, and Windle, 1964; Chen, Lien, and Lu, 1965). The usual explanation has been that these adverse conditions damage the supposedly immature blood-brain barrier and allow bilirubin to penetrate the brain. However, the binding of bilirubin to albumin is pH-dependent (Odell, 1965; Bratlid and Fog, 1970). It seems more likely that these adverse effects predispose to kernicterus because the low blood pH, which they all cause, produces unbinding of bilirubin.

The binding of dyes to plasma proteins is also pH-dependent; hence, studies involving their use are subject to similar considerations (e.g., Clemedson, Hartelius, and Holmberg, 1958). It should be emphasized that the factors which affect bilirubin binding to albumin (i.e., pH and competition from drugs) may also affect the immature liver glucuronyl transferase systems and thereby cause a rise in plasma unconjugated bilirubin. Thus the factors which produce kernicterus are several and interrelated, but immaturity and/ or damage to the blood-brain barrier seem most unlikely to be involved.

Other evidence suggests that neither hypercapnia nor hypoxia has any marked effect upon blood-brain barrier permeability. For example, severe hypercapnia (arterial $P_{CO_2} > 100$ mm Hg) increases the penetration of sucrose from blood into brain both in the adult rabbit (Cameron, Davson, and Segal, 1970) and in the newborn lamb (Evans et al., in preparation). But sucrose penetration is extremely slow under normocapnic conditions, and although it may increase three or four times in the newborn lambs in hypercapnia (Fig. 4), there is still an appreciable barrier to sucrose penetration. Furthermore, the effect is reversible, which would not be expected if damage had occurred. It may well be related to the marked increase in cerebral blood flow which occurs in hypercapnia, although presumably as a result of the increased volume of vascular bed, and therefore of surface area for exchange, rather than directly as a result of the flow increase itself. The very slow penetration of sucrose into brain makes it unlikely that it is flow-limited. We have indeed found a striking correlation between the cerebral blood flow response to hypercapnia and the amount of sucrose penetration into the brain.

SUMMARY AND CONCLUSIONS

A review has been made of significant information available concerning changes in electrolyte concentrations in brain and CSF during early growth in different species. These results have been compared with a recent systematic study of five electrolytes in brain and CSF from the fetal sheep. Good agreement between results in different species has allowed a composite picture to be built up. Concentrations of the various ions in CSF, the same or similar to those in the adult, are established at very different ages for different ions. It appears that specific transport processes for the ions mature in this order: magnesium first (before 48 days in the sheep), sodium and chloride next (by 65 days), and potassium and calcium last (after birth). The ionic gradients observed between CSF and plasma at early stages would suggest that the blood-brain and blood-CSF barriers also develop early. Studies on the uptake of sucrose from blood into brain support such a concept. Changes in the chloride, sodium, and potassium content of brain during early growth strongly suggest that at early ages the extracellular space is small, that it increases enormously to a maximum between 90 and 105 days in the sheep, and thereafter decreases towards the adult value. The magnesium content of brain is fairly steady and similar to that in the adult. These studies provide the basis for a more kinetic approach to a study of the origin of mechanisms producing homeostasis of cations in CSF and the interstitial fluid of brain. They also provide normal values, useful in any investigation into the effect of abnormal conditions such as hypoxia or asphyxia on the brain of the fetus or the newborn. However, preliminary studies indicate that neither moderate hypoxia nor severe hypercapnia has any marked effect on the CSF electrolytes apart from a rise in potassium concentration. These factors have been supposed to affect the brain's internal environment by exerting a damaging effect upon the blood-brain barrier. But it seems likely that the results of many of the experiments which purport to show this may, in fact, be caused by changes in the physicochemical properties of the marker substance, notably its protein binding.

REFERENCES

Arias, I. M. (1962): Chronic unconjugated hyperbilirubinaemia without overt signs of kernicterus in adolescents and adults. *Journal of Clinical Investigation*, 41:2233.

Backay, L. (1968): Changes in barrier effect in pathological states. *Progress in Brain Research*, 29:333-339.

Bito, L. Z. (1969): Blood-brain barrier: Evidence for active cation transport between blood and the extracellular fluid of brain. *Science*, 165:81-83.

Bito, L. Z., and Myers, R. E. (1970): The ontogenesis of haematoencephalic cation transport processes in the rhesus monkey. *Journal of Physiology*, 208:153-170.

Bradbury, M. W. B., and Kleeman, C. R. (1967): Stability of the potassium content of cerebrospinal fluid and brain. *American Journal of Physiology*, 213:519-528.

Bradbury, M. W. B., Villamil, M., and Kleeman, C. R. (1968): Extracellular fluid, ionic distribution and exchange in isolated frog brain. *American Journal of Physiology*, 214:643-651.

Bradbury, M. W. B., Reynolds, J. M., Reynolds, M., Saunders, N. R., and Wilson, J.: Electrolytes and water in the brain and cerebrospinal fluid of the foetal sheep. (*submitted*)

Bratlid, D., and Fog, J. (1970): The binding capacity of human albumin for bilirubin and its significance in the pathogenesis of kernicterus. *Scandinavian Journal of Clinical and Laboratory Investigations*, 25:257-261.

Brøndsted, H., and Woodbury, D. M.: Uptake, distribution, and intracellular accumulation of tritiated ouabain in brain, cerebrospinal fluid, heart and other tissues of maturing rats. (*submitted*)

Brown, A. K. (1962): Bilirubin metabolism with special reference to neonatal jaundice. *Advances in Pediatrics*, 12:121-187.

Cameron, I. R. (1971): The effect of acid-base changes on K^+ homeostasis in CSF. In: *Ion Homeostasis of the Brain*, edited by B. K. Siesjö and S. C. Sørensen. Münksgaard, Copenhagen.

Cameron, I. R., Davson, H., and Segal, M. B. (1969-70): The effect of hypercapnia on the blood-brain barrier to sucrose in the rabbit. *Yale Journal of Biology and Medicine*, 42:241-247.

Chen, H. C., Lien, I. N., and Liu, T. C. (1965): Kernicterus in newborn rabbits. *American Journal of Pathology*, 46:331

Clemedson, C. J., Hartelius, H., and Holmberg, G. (1958): The influence of carbon dioxide inhalation on the cerebral vascular permeability to trypan blue ("the blood-brain barrier"). *Acta Pathologica Scandinavica*, 42:137-149.

Davson, H. (1967): *Physiology of the Cerebrospinal Fluid*. Churchill, London.

Dawes, G. S. (1968): *Fetal and Neonatal Physiology*. Year Book Medical Publishers, Chicago.

Diamond, I. (1969): Bilirubin binding and kernicterus. *Advances in Pediatrics*, XVI: 99-119.

Diamond, I., and Schmid, R. (1966): Experimental bilirubin encephalopathy. The mode of entry of bilirubin-^{14}C into the central nervous system. *Journal of Clinical and Laboratory Investigations*, 45:678-689.

Dobbing, J. (1961): The blood-brain barrier, *Physiological Reviews*, 41:130-188.

Ferguson, R. K., and Woodbury, D. M. (1969): Penetration of ^{11}C-inulin and ^{14}C-sucrose into brain, cerebrospinal fluid, and skeletal muscle of developing rats. *Experimental Brain Research,* 7:181-194.

Flexner, L. B. (1938): Changes in the chemistry and nature of the cerebrospinal fluid during fetal life in the pig. *American Journal of Physiology,* 124:131 135.

Flexner, L. B. (1951-1952): The development of the cerebral cortex: A cytological, functional and biochemical approach. *Harvey Lectures,* 47:156-179.

Flexner, L. B., and Flexner, J. B. (1949): Biochemical and physiological differentiation during morphogenesis. IX. The extracellular and intracellular phases of the liver and cerebral cortex of the fetal guinea-pig as estimated from distribution of chloride and radio-sodium. *Journal of Cellular and Comparative Physiology,* 34:115.

Friedmann, U. (1942): Blood-brain barrier. *Physiological Reviews,* 22:125-245.

Friis-Hansen, B. (1957): Changes in body-water compartments during growth. *Acta Paediatrica.* 46:suppl. 110.

Levin, V. A., Fenstermacher, J. D., and Patlak, C. S. (1970): Sucrose and inulin space measurements of the cerebral cortex in four mammalian species. *American Journal of Physiology,* 219:1528.

Leusen, I. (1949): The influence of calcium, potassium and magnesium ions in cerebrospinal fluid on vasomotor system. *Journal of Physiology,* 110:319-329.

Lucey, J. F., Hibbard, E., Behrman, R. E., De Gallardo, E. F. O., and Windle, W. F. (1964): Kernicterus in asphyxiated newborn rhesus monkeys. *Experimental Neurology,* 9:43-58.

McKay, R. J. (1969): The fetus and the newborn infant. In: *Pediatrics,* edited by W. E. Nelson. Saunders, Philadelphia, pp. 346-410.

Odell, G. B. (1965): Influence of pH on the distribution of bilirubin between albumin and mitochondria. *Proceedings of the Society for Experimental Biology and Medicine,* 120:352-354.

Olsen, O. M., and Sørensen, S. C. (1971): Stability of Mg^{++} in cerebrospinal fluid during plasma changes and during hypercapnia in young and in adult rats. *Acta Physiologica Scandinavica,* 82:466-469.

Olsson, R. (1958): Studies on the subcommissional organ. *Acta Zoologica,* 39:71-102.

Stern, L. (1970): Temperature control, hydration and feeding, bilirubin and calcium metabolism. *Biology of the Neonate,* 16:92-100.

Vernadakis, A., and Woodbury, D. M. (1962): Electrolyte and amino-acid changes in rat brain during maturation. *American Journal of Physiology,* 203:748-752.

Fetal Pharmacology, edited by L. Boréus
Raven Press, New York © 1973

Drug-Receptor Interactions in the Human Fetus

Lars O. Boréus

Department of Clinical Pharmacology, Karolinska Hospital, Stockholm, Sweden

The interaction between drugs and living cells is usually very specific: a minor change in the chemical structure of the drug molecule may lead to a drastic change in the pharmacological effect. It is natural, therefore, to postulate the existence of selective "active sites" on or in the cells with which the drug molecules must interact in order to produce the effect. These sites are usually called *receptors*. The drug-receptor interaction is of fundamental importance for the final result of the pharmacological stimulation.

Since the influence of growth and development upon the pharmacological response can be fully understood only if the various part-processes of the total drug action are considered separately, we started a study on drug-receptor interactions during ontogenesis in man. This area of developmental pharmacology had not been subjected to systematic investigation but could be explored since the principal experimental approach involves studies on isolated tissues *in vitro*. Human fetal tissues from the middle trimester of pregnancy could be obtained without ethical difficulties from legal abortions. Such tissues behaved technically very well under various experimental conditions in the laboratory, and the data obtained from the studies are summarized in this chapter.

THE CONCEPT OF DRUG RECEPTORS

The term "drug receptor" is functional rather than structural since chemical isolation of receptor substance has not yet been accomplished. The main reason for this is that any procedure for chemical extraction of the receptor from the tissue may destroy it and will exclude the possibility of measuring the pharmacological effect since the integrity of the tissue is broken. Furthermore, it is likely that receptors are part of membrane structures, and thus their behavior after extraction might be very different from that observed in solution (Ariens, 1964; Ehrenpreis, Fleisch, and Mittag, 1969). The main experimental approach to analysis of receptor function is, therefore, to expose isolated tissues to graded concentrations of active drugs (agonists and antagonists) and to record the degree of response. The tissue is preferably some kind of muscle-cell preparation because contraction or relaxation are easily recorded effects. If the response is reproducible for a sufficient time period, repeated concentration-effect curves can be obtained.

The drug-receptor interaction results in the formation of a drug-receptor complex (Fig. 1) which, in turn, may stimulate the effector system so that a certain degree of effect is produced. The stimulus is supposed to be proportional to the quantity of drug-receptor complex present at a certain moment. The relation between drug concentration and final effect may thus give information about the nature of the drug-receptor interaction in the given experimental situation, provided the effector system itself is intact during the experiment. In the present studies, the concentration-effect relationship has been examined in various human fetal tissues where both the drug-receptor interaction and the effector systems may be expected to be subjected to ontogenetic changes.

METHODS

The studies described in this chapter were performed *in vitro* on fresh muscle-containing tissues from human fetuses. The specimens were mount-

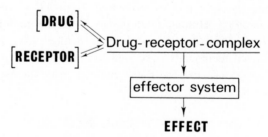

FIG. 1. The drug-receptor interaction is thought to lead to the formation of a more or less transient drug-receptor complex which may stimulate a specific effector system. Species or age differences in effect may be due to either differences in the receptor itself or in the effector system.

ed in 20-ml overflow baths with constant temperature (37°C) in Tyrode solution, which was bubbled with a $O_2 + CO_2$ mixture to keep the pH at 7.4. *Ileum* and *esophagus* were cut in segments, about 1 cm in length, and mounted in the bath. The isometric tension of the longitudinal muscles was recorded. *Trachea* was cut in three or four rings and a chain prepared which was mounted in the bath. *Aorta* was removed in its entire length, and a spiral strip was made with a fine pair of scissors before mounting in the bath. The *heart* was cut out and immediately placed in oxygenated Tyrode solution. Even if the circulation of the fetus had stopped, it was possible to restore spontaneous beating of the heart muscle. Usually the whole right auricle was used in the experiment. In very small fetuses, the heart was cut in a transverse section and both auricles mounted in one piece in the bath. In some cases a small amount of isoprenaline was added to the bath in order to start spontaneous beating. Regular mechanical activity of the heart without fatigue usually lasted for several hours. In some experiments, the heart muscle was driven electrically with a needle electrode. *Ductus arteriosus* was perfused with Tyrode solution at constant speed with continuous monitoring of pH, P_{CO_2}, and P_{O_2}. Any contraction of the ductus, due to drugs in the perfusion fluid, resulted in an increase in the perfusion pressure.

The isometric tension of the various specimens as well as the perfusion pressure of the ductus was measured with strain gauge or pressure transducers and recorded on a polygraph. Drugs were added directly to the bath or to the perfusion fluid.

Human fetuses were obtained at legal abortions performed for sociomedical reasons. The gestational ages were 12 to 24 weeks, corresponding to crown-rump lengths (CRL) of 5.5 to 20 cm. The operation was performed by abdominal hysterotomy under ether-nitrous oxide anesthesia after premedication with morphine-scopolamine or meperidine-scopolamine. The whole fetus, usually with the membranes intact, was immediately brought from the operation room to the laboratory and the tissues removed and immersed in Tyrode solution. The methods have been described in detail earlier (Boréus, 1967, 1971; McMurphy and Boréus, 1968, 1971).

RESULTS AND DISCUSSION

Sensitivity of human fetal smooth muscles to drugs

All tissues examined, except the aorta, reacted with prompt contractions or relaxations upon exposure to a variety of drugs. Strong responses were

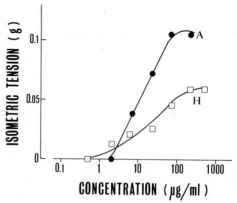

FIG. 2. Contractile response induced by acetylcholine iodide (A) and histamine hydrochloride (H) in the tracheal muscle from a human fetus (CRL = 13.5 cm).

noted for the physiological transmitters acetylcholine and adrenaline-noradrenaline, and the cholinergic and adrenergic responses will therefore be discussed in some detail below. Histamine (Fig. 2) and 5-hydroxytryptamine also contracted the fetal smooth muscles but in a more sluggish and irregular fashion. For both these drugs, there was a tendency of tachyphylaxis upon repeated stimulation; reliable and reproducible concentration-effect curves were therefore sometimes difficult to obtain. Bradykinin strongly contracted the ileum but not the trachea, aorta, or ductus arteriosus.

The cholinergic receptor function

It appeared logical to consider first the response of the human fetal smooth muscle to acetylcholine. The only information that could be found on this point in the literature was a study by Hughes (1957) which demonstrated that preparations of the esophagus from fetuses of 20 to 26 weeks responded with immediate isotonic concentrations when exposed to acetylcholine *in vitro*. It was also shown that this reaction could be inhibited by atropine. However, no attempts were made to determine the relationship between drug concentration and effect or to relate the response to the age of the fetus.

In our studies, a cholinergic contraction could easily be produced in all smooth-muscle tissues examined, including the aorta. The response in ileum (Fig. 8), esophagus, trachea, and ductus arteriosus was rapid and

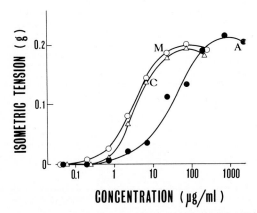

FIG. 3. Contractile response induced by acetylcholine iodide (A), methacholine bromide (M), and carbacholine chloride (C) in the tracheal muscle from a human fetus (CRL = 15 cm).

usually well sustained. The cholinergic contraction of the aorta was slower but equally reproducible. Removal of the drug from the bath resulted in return of the tension to the previous baseline, allowing reliable determination of the concentration-effect curve for each specimen. The most convenient tissue for systematic studies was the ileum since it was possible to obtain two to four consecutive segments from one fetus which made more extensive experiments possible, for instance, a study on the "spare receptor" phenomenon (see below).

The cholinergic response in the fetal tissues was similar to that described in laboratory animals. The log concentration-effect curves for acetylcholine, metacholine, and carbacholine have the classical S-formed shape and reach the same maximum in the same preparation (Fig. 3). The contractile response was potentiated by physostigmine (Table 1).

The tissues from even the smallest fetuses (12 weeks) reacted as well and with similar speed to acetylcholine as did those from the larger individuals (24 weeks), although the strength of the response increased with gestational age. The degree of maximal response cannot, therefore, form a meaningful basis for evaluation of ontogenetic changes in receptor function. If the concentration-effect curves from many fetuses of various gestational ages are compared, it is more interesting to consider the position of the curve on the concentration axis rather than the maximum values (Fig. 4). The pD_2 values do not differ significantly when the fetus increases its CRL from 6.5

TABLE I. *Potentiation of acetylcholine-induced contraction of ileum from a human fetus (CRL = 13.5 cm) by means of simultaneous addition of physostigmine salicylate to the bath.*

Physostigmine (μg/ml)	Increase of contraction	
	mg	%
0.05	64	11
0.15	164	26
0.5	173	28
1.5	273	43
5	145	22
15	55	8
50	—127	—19
150	—300	—46

Concentration of acetylcholine iodide 0.5 μg/ml. Note that high concentrations of physostigmine inhibit the response.

to 20.5 cm, a period which covers essentially the entire second trimester of pregnancy when the body weight increases about 40-fold. In other words, relative to the maximum values, the dose-effect relationship does not change during this phase of ontogenesis in man. An extension of this study to later fetal ages, to the newborn period, and to adults cannot be done in man but has been performed in experimental animals. Thus, the cholinergic response in guinea pig ileum (Fig. 5) has been followed in the same manner from fetal to adult ages, and the same phenomenon was observed: the pD$_2$ values

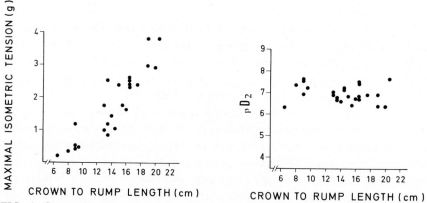

FIG. 4. Contractile response induced by acetylcholine iodide in the longitudinal muscle of the ileum from 25 human fetuses of various gestational ages. *Left*: The maxima of the concentration-effect curves plotted against CRL. *Right*: The pD$_2$ values (the log molar concentration for half-maximal response) for the same fetuses plotted against CRL. (Courtesy of *Biologia Neonatorum*.)

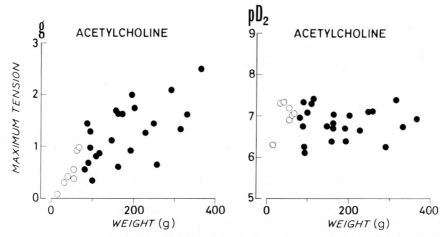

FIG. 5. A similar plot as in Fig. 4 for acetylcholine-induced contractions in ileum from 30 guinea pigs. *Left*: Maximum isometric tension. *Right*: pD₂ values. Open circles represent fetuses and closed circles represent newborns and adults. The age of the animals is expressed as body weight. (Courtesy of *Acta Physiologica Scandinavica.*)

are essentially the same both in the pre- and postnatal life of the animal (Boréus and McMurphy, 1971).

If the quantitative relation between agonist molecules and receptors, which is assumed to follow the law of mass action, stays the same during fetal development, then a similar unchanged relationship should be expected with a pure competitive antagonist in the same system. Experiments were therefore done (Boréus, 1967) with atropine acording to the technique suggested by Schild (1947). This involves determination of the pA_2 value, i.e., the negative logarithm of the molar concentration of the antagonist that is required to reduce the effect of a double dose of a stimulant drug to that of a single dose. As seen in Fig. 6, such a determination could be made without difficulties in human fetal ileum. The conclusion of these experiments was that the pA_2 values for atropine do not change significantly during fetal growth in the second trimester of pregnancy.

It is not possible to determine the total number of receptors in a given test preparation. This might have been of some interest in a developing tissue. However, the size of the receptor population does not seem to be of relevance for the position or shape of the concentration-effect curve since only a small part of the total number of receptors needs to be activated for even a maximal response. This phenomenon of "spare receptors" or

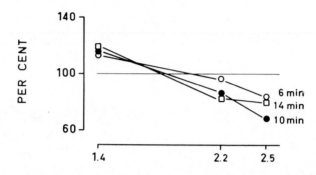

CONCENTRATION OF ATROPINE (moles × 10^{-9}/liter)

FIG. 6. Inhibition by atropine of response in human fetal ileum to a doubling of the standard dose of acetylcholine, determined according to Schild (1947). The response to the standard dose before addition of antagonist is equal to 100%. Atropine was present in the bath for 6, 10, or 14 min. (Courtesy of *Biologia Neonatorum*.)

"receptor reserve" (Nickerson, 1956; Stephenson, 1956) may be demonstrated in a tissue if a "nonequilibrium antagonist" (Nickerson, 1957) such as phenoxybenzamine is added to the bath in such a concentration and for such a time period that only a part of the receptors are blocked. By means of a step-wise increase of this blockade, which is essentially irreversible, the relative size of the receptor reserve can be estimated. This approach was used on fetal ileum (Boréus, 1968), and a considerable "surplus" of cholinergic receptors could be demonstrated even in the smallest fetuses examined (12 weeks). Furthermore, the proportion of receptors "in excess" did not change during growth from 12 to 24 weeks of gestational age.

Thus, various experimental approaches all seem to show that the cholinergic receptor is fully developed early during human fetal life. Smooth muscles probably play important roles in the fetus even if the organ does not have the same function as in postnatal life. For instance, the tiny smooth muscle of the fetal trachea has well-developed acetylcholine receptors which may play some role for the resistance to movement of fluid in the tracheobronchial tree.

The adrenergic receptor function

The effects of adrenaline and noradrenaline on the fetal cardiovascular system have been studied in animals by many authors (for review, see Dawes, 1968). A fetal tachycardia following injection of an adrenergic drug to the mother may be difficult to interpret, since both a direct drug effect

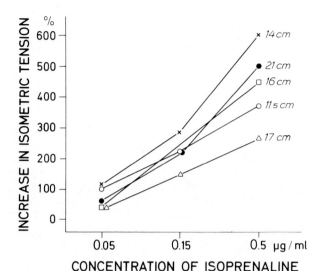

CONCENTRATION OF ISOPRENALINE

FIG. 7. Effect of isoprenaline on the maximal isometric tension of each beat in spontaneously beating preparations of right atrium from human fetuses. There is no apparent correlation between the effect and the CRL of the fetuses.

on the fetal myocardium and a secondary effect due to vasoconstriction of uterine vessels may contribute. Again, the best quantitative approach to the adrenergic receptor function must be to use isolated tissues. This was considered to be of great interest from the clinical point of view, since drug therapy in human pregnancy often involves interaction with the adrenergic system (hypertensive drugs, tricyclic antidepressants, uterine-relaxing agents, etc.). Experiments *in vitro* were therefore performed on myocardium, ileum, ductus arteriosus, and aorta from human fetuses.

It was found (Boréus, *unpublished results*) that the isolated myocardium

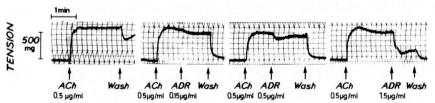

FIG. 8. Actual recording of an experiment with human fetal ileum. Repeated contractions were produced by addition of a constant dose of acetylcholine (ACh) to the bath. Relaxations were produced by additions of adrenaline (ADR) when the isometric tension was stable. Return to the original baseline was allowed between determinations. As the concentration of adrenaline was increased, the percentage of relaxation from the plateau also increased. (Courtesy of *Biologia Neonatorum*.)

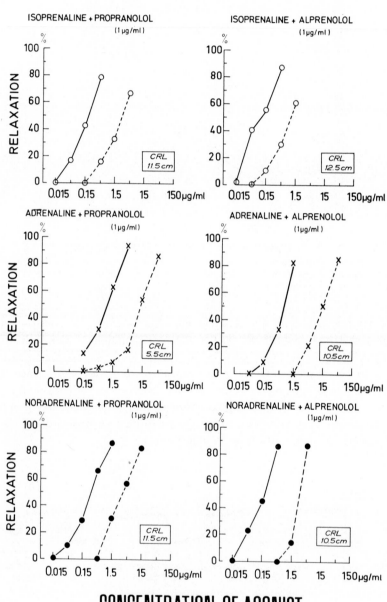

CONCENTRATION OF AGONIST

from the human fetus was very sensitive to the action of beta-adrenergic drugs (Fig. 7). Spontaneously beating atrial preparations responded in a dose-dependent fashion to isoprenaline in concentrations as low as 0.05 μg/ml with a drastic increase in peak tension and contraction rate. In electrically driven specimens, it was found that the isometric tension of each beat was inversely related to the stimulation frequency. This complicates the analysis for drugs that have both positive inotropic and chronotropic effects (Koch-Weser and Blinks, 1963). The point of maximum of the concentration-effect curve is also difficult to define because of the tendency toward arrythmias at higher concentrations of the drug. A complete concentration-effect curve for each specimen was therefore not attempted, and no pD_2 values were calculated. However, the relative increase in isometric tension and in frequency was similar in all fetuses, and it was not possible to demonstrate any correlation between degree of response and fetal age. The interindividual variations in this tissue, however, were relatively large; the resting spontaneous heart rate varied between 100 and 140 beats per minute. This is slightly lower than the basal fetal heart rate in man *in vivo* for this age as reported by Caldeyro-Barcia and Schifferli (1972). In our experiments, the spontaneous heart rate was found to be very sensitive to temperature; if the bath temperature was decreased only by 1°C, the rate decreased about 10 beats per minute. This reaction was accompanied with an increase in isometric tension of the myocardium. The reverse reaction could be obtained by increasing the bath temperature up to about 45°C when failure occurred. This phenomenon is well known from studies in adult animal preparations (Blinks and Koch-Weser, 1963).

In a study on four fetal atrial preparations, the effect of isoprenaline was compared to that of orciprenaline and terbutaline. Both these drugs have been used as uterine-relaxing agents in the treatment of threatened premature labor. Both were found to have similar effects on tensions and frequency of the fetal myocardium as had isoprenaline; however, between 10 and 100 times higher concentrations were needed to produce the same effect as isoprenaline. Propranolol effectively and reversibly blocked the

---

FIG. 9. Log concentration-effect curves for the relaxing effect of adrenergic drugs in human fetal ileum. Total relaxation = 100%. Contractions were produced with acetylcholine and the relaxing effects of isoprenaline, adrenaline, and noradrenaline were determined in the absence (solid lines) and in the presence (dashed lines) of the beta-antagonists propranolol and alprenolol. The inhibitors caused a shift to the right of all three agonist curves. No correlation to CRL was found. (Courtesy of *Biologia Neonatorum.*)

action of isoprenaline. These studies are in agreement with the *in vivo* observation of Caldeyro-Barcia and Schifferli (1972) that injection of orciprenaline into the peritoneal cavity of a human anencephalic fetus caused an immediate increase in fetal heart rate, which could be inhibited by subsequent injection of a beta-adrenergic blocking drug.

The fetal adrenergic receptor function was further explored in the longitudinal muscle of the ileum (McMurphy and Boréus, 1968). Acetylcholine-contracted strips were found to be very useful for such an analysis, since a dose-dependent relaxation was produced with catecholamines (Fig. 8). No changes in pD_2 values were observed for isoprenaline, adrenaline, or noradrenaline relaxation during the middle trimester of pregnancy. Extensive studies on the specificity of this relaxation were made, since it has been reported from experiments on laboratory animals that both alpha- and beta-adrenergic receptors may be involved. It was found that beta-adrenergic blocking drugs inhibited the relaxation competitively (Fig. 9) and that a complete blockade could easily be obtained. On the other hand, alpha-adrenergic drugs could not relax the muscle unless extremely high concentrations were used, and alpha-adrenergic blocking compounds were not able to antagonize the relaxation. It was concluded that only beta-adrenergic receptors are involved in the relaxation of the contracted smooth muscle of the fetal ileum. In a recent short communication, Hart and Mir (1971) reported that alpha-adrenergic receptors were also operating for relaxation in some of their preparations of human fetal ileum. However, no concentration-effect curve was presented, and in some cases a contraction rather than a relaxation was noted for the alpha-stimulating drug phenylephrine.

In the search for a suitable tissue to test the alpha-adrenergic response, the ductus arteriosus and the aorta from human fetuses were studied (Boréus, Malmfors, McMurphy, and Olson, 1969). It was found that the perfused ductus responded to noradrenaline and that this contraction could be reversibly blocked by the alpha-adrenergic inhibitor phentolamine. The effect of noradrenaline was associated with a marked degree of tachyphylaxis, and it was difficult to determine reliable concentration-effect curves. It was easier to do so when spiral-strip preparations of the ductus were tested, but this could not be done with the younger fetuses because of the small size of the vessel. From the quantitative point of view, it was more profitable to analyze the cholinergic response of the perfused ductus arteriosus than the adrenergic response (Fig. 10). It was interesting to note that strips of human fetal aorta did not react to noradrenaline stimulation but were sensitive to acetylcholine. This is in contrast to aortic strips from fetal guinea pigs which contracted with alpha-adrenergic stimulation. The difference in sensitivity to noradrenaline between the ductus arteriosus and the aorta was correlated to a difference in appearance of adrenergic nerve terminals, demonstrated by the histochemical fluorescence technique. Such terminals were abundant in the ductus but absent in the aorta of human fetuses. These results on the ductus arteriosus have been confirmed and extended by Aronson, Gennser, Owman, and Sjöberg (1970). Both studies indicate that adrenergic as well as cholinergic receptor function is present in the human ductus arteriosus. It is therefore possible that they play a functional role in the

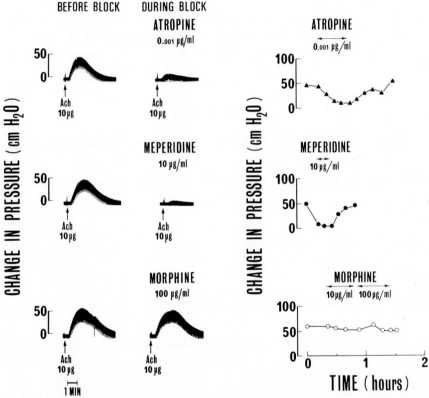

FIG. 10. Antagonism of acetylcholine contraction in ductus arteriosus from human fetuses by atropine, meperidine, and morphine. Left panel shows actual pressure recordings before and during presence of antagonists. Right panel demonstrates the time course before, during, and after the presence of antagonists in the perfusion fluid. Each symbol represents the maximum pressure obtained by injection of a standard acetylcholine dose (10 μg) into the perfusion system. CRL = 13.5 cm. Both atropine and meperidine give an effective reversible blockade. Recovery from blockade is much faster for meperidine than for atropine. Morphine has no antagonistic action. (Courtesy of *American Journal of Obstetrics and Gynecology*.)

closure of the vessel at birth.

It may be concluded that adrenergic receptors are operating early in the fetus and that they can be readily separated into alpha- and beta-functions according to the concept of Ahlquist (1948). For beta-adrenergic receptors, there is no quantitative change in the concentration-effect relationship during the middle trimester of human pregnancy. The alpha-adrenergic receptor has, for technical reasons, been more difficult to evaluate quantitatively in the human fetus, but animal experiments (McMurphy and Boréus, *unpublished*) have shown that fetal guinea pig aorta strips contract when exposed to noradrenaline in the same concentration as the aortic strip from its mother, although the strength of the response is weaker in the fetus. It is probable, therefore, that the alpha-adrenergic as well as the beta-adrenergic receptors have the same affinity to the specific agonist during growth in the same way as described above for the cholinergic receptor.

CONCLUSIONS

Specific drug-receptor interactions have been demonstrated in various tissues from human fetuses of 12 to 24 weeks gestational age. Quantitative analyses show that the relation between concentration of the stimulus and resulting effect, relative to the maximum obtainable response, stays the same during ontogenesis. Intricate characteristics, such as the "spare receptor" phenomenon, can be demonstrated even in the smallest fetuses, and it is likely that the typical drug-receptor interaction may occur as soon as organogenesis is completed. However, the strength of the response increases with age when the efficiency of the effector system increases. Parallel animal experiments show that species differences in receptor pharmacology are discernible early in prenatal life. Autonomic receptor mechanisms probably play important functional roles in the fetus. Consequently, maternal drug therapy may strongly interfere with the function of the fetus if autonomically active drugs or metabolites can reach the fetal circulation. If drug distribution to the fetus can be controlled, the existence of active drug receptor function in the tissues is a basis for future development of therapeutic measures directed toward the human fetus.

ACKNOWLEDGMENTS

This work was supported by the Association for the Aid of Crippled

Children, New York, the Swedish Medical Research Council, and Prenatal-forskningsnämnden, Stockholm.

REFERENCES

Ahlquist, R. P. (1948): A study of the adrenotropic receptors. *American Journal of Physiology*, 153:586-600.

Ariëns, E. J. (1964): *Molecular Pharmacology*, Vol. 1. Academic Press, New York.

Aronson, S., Gennser, G., Owman, C., and Sjöberg, N. O. (1970): Innervation and contractile response of the human ductus arteriosus. *European Journal of Pharmacology*, 11:178-186.

Blinks, J. R., and Koch-Weser, J. (1963): Physical factors in the analysis of the actions of drugs on myocardial contractility. *Pharmacological Reviews*, 15:531-599.

Boréus, L. O. (1967): Pharmacology of the human fetus: Dose-effect relationships for acetylcholine during ontogenesis. *Biologia Neonatorum* (Basel), 11:328-337.

Boréus, L. O. (1968): Demonstration of a receptor reserve for acetylcholine in the human fetus. *Acta Physiologica Scandinavica*, 72:194-199.

Boréus, L. O. (1971): Use of human fetal ileum for evaluation of smooth muscle effects of narcotic analgesics. *European Journal of Pharmacology*, 15:127-131.

Boréus, L. O., Malmfors, T., McMurphy, D. M., and Olson, L. (1969): Demonstration of adrenergic receptor function and innervation in the ductus arteriosus of the human fetus. *Acta Physiologica Scandinavica*, 77:316-321.

Boréus, L. O., and McMurphy, D. M. (1971): Ontogenetic development of cholinergic receptor function in guinea pig ileum. *Acta Physiologica Scandinavica*, 81:143-144.

Caldeyro-Barcia, R., and Schifferli, P.-Y. (1972): Effects of atropine and beta-adrenergic drugs on the heart rate of the human fetus. *This volume*.

Dawes, G. S. (1968): *Foetal and Neonatal Physiology*. Year Book Medical Publishers, Chicago.

Ehrenpreis, S., Fleisch, J. H., and Mittag, T. W. (1969): Approaches to the molecular nature of pharmacological receptors. *Pharmacological Reviews*, 21:131-181.

Hart, S. L., and Mir, M. S. (1971): Adrenoreceptors in the human foetal small intestine. *British Journal of Pharmacology*, 41:567-569.

Hughes, F. B. (1957): Drug responses of human fetal esophagus. *American Journal of Physiology*, 191:37-39.

Koch-Weser, J., and Blinks, J. R. (1963): The influence of the interval between beats on myocardial contractility. *Pharmacological Reviews*, 15:601-652.

McMurphy, D. M., and Boréus, L. O. (1968): Pharmacology of the human fetus: Adrenergic receptor function in the small intestine. *Biologia Neonatorum* (Basel), 13:325-339.

McMurphy, D. M., and Boréus, L. O. (1971): Studies on the pharmacology of the perfused human fetal ductus arteriosus. *American Journal of Obstetrics and Gynecology*, 109:937-942.

Nickerson, M. (1956): Receptor occupancy and tissue response. *Nature*, 178:697-698.

Nickerson, M. (1957): Nonequilibrium drug antagonism. *Pharmacological Reviews*, 9:246-259.

Schild, H. O. (1947): pA, a new scale for the measurement of drug antagonism. *British Journal of Pharmacology*, 2:189-206.

Stephenson, R. P. (1956): A modification of receptor theory. *British Journal of Pharmacology*, 11:379-393.

DISCUSSION

KARCZMAR: What is the time of innervation of the tissues in reference to the dose-effect relationships which you obtained? In other words, did your receptors respond, and how did they respond, prior to innervation? Second question: do your pD_2 values express the affinity of the tissues, or better still, of the receptor, to the drug equally as well as the affinity constants developed on the basis of reaction rates such as those used by Paton and others?

BORÉUS: In all human fetal tissues that responded to adrenergic stimulation, we found varicose fluorescence nerve terminals. Younger fetuses than 12 weeks could not be used since their tissues are too undifferentiated and small to be tested with this technique. In the tissues that did not respond (human fetal aorta), no adrenergic fluorescence was observed. From our experiments we therefore cannot decide if a receptor response can be elicited prior to innervation. "Affinity" is dependent upon the probability that drug molecules and receptors approach each other in such a way that they interact with each other (Ariens). It should be emphasized that the reaction rate in a living tissue is hard to define on the receptor level. It depends not only on the drug-receptor interaction itself (like the situation with enzymes in solution) but also on other factors such as diffusion barriers which may influence the access of the drug molecules to the "biophase." The concentration-effect curves are based on individual equilibrium values.

DAWES: It has been shown that stimulation in the rabbit of the peripheral vagus caused intense bradycardia a day or two after birth. The effect was much less 7 to 10 days later, attributed to the appearance of cholinesterase. Have you looked for such an effect in your preparations during innervation?

BORÉUS: We have found that the isolated human fetal myocardium responds to acetylcholine with a dose-dependent bradycardia which can be abolished by atropine. It has not been investigated if these reactions are changing with age.

OWMAN: With regard to the question by Dr. Karczmar, there appears to be a discrepancy between innervation and responsiveness. In Burnstock's laboratory it has been shown on vas deferens of mouse that excitatory junction potentials do not appear until 18 days post partum, although structurally the adrenergic innervation is fully developed before that stage.

ARONSON: I should like to comment on the question of affinity. We have shown that the receptivity to acetylcholine and especially to noradrenaline declines in anoxia in the isolated guinea pig ductus. In the human fetal ductus, a similar lowering of sensitivity has been found for noradrenaline but not yet for acetylcholine. This finding may be of importance for the postnatal closure of the ductus.

Fetal Pharmacology, edited by L. Boréus
Raven Press, New York © 1973

Cholinergic Function in the Developing Fetus

A. G. Karczmar, R. Srinivasan, and J. Bernsohn

The Institute for Mind, Drugs and Behavior, and the Department of Pharmacology of Loyola University Medical Center, Maywood, Illinois; and the Neuropsychiatric Research Laboratory, Veterans Administration Hospital, Hines, Illinois

INTRODUCTION

In the thirties, Nachmansohn (1938*a*) proposed that cholinesterase (ChE) is related to the emergence of nerve function and to motility during development. This was a heuristic concept, and it generated numerous studies which still continue. In the context of his hypothesis, Nachmansohn spoke of ChE because at that time it was the readily measurable component of the cholinergic system, and also because of his particular view of its role in nerve function and conduction. However, the pertinent studies that ensued were concerned with, in addition to ChE's and particularly acetylcholinesterase (AChE; EC 3.1.1.7), other components of the cholinergic system such as acetylcholine (ACh) and choline acetylase (ChAc; EC 2.3.1.6). Even more particularly, although sometimes only by implication, the investigators were concerned with the ontogenesis of the cholinergic synapses. It must be emphasized that, while Nachmansohn might now consider the ontogenesis of ACh rather than that of ChE as being related to the functional development of the nervous system, he may not be willing to consider the former in terms of the synapses, since his concept of the role of ACh in the nervous system is "unitarian," and since he does not wish to consider conduction and synaptic transmission in separate categories (*cf.* Nachmansohn, 1963 and 1970).

Notwithstanding Nachmansohn's position, the term "cholinergic system" will be employed here in its strict sense, i.e., with reference to synapses activated by ACh liberated from the presynaptic nerve terminals. In a more general sense, the term "ACh system" will be used. Indeed, to identify and to prove the presence of cholinergic synapses is difficult enough in the adult; the term ACh system may therefore be particularly appropriate in the context of this review chapter, especially since it will be shown that the ontogenetic presence of ACh or of ChE's may have other than transmissive or synaptic function.

Nine years ago, I (Karczmar, 1963*a,b*) felt that there were many exceptions to and inconsistencies within Nachmansohn's hypothesis, because the ontogenetic appearance of the components of the cholinergic system (ChAc, AChE, and ACh) frequently did not coincide with that of nervous or related function.

Today, since the development of the microtechniques for the determination of ACh, various ChE's, and ChAc, and because the microneurochemical data can be correlated with equally precise neurophysiological and neuropharmacological results, certain inconsistencies noted in 1963 seem resolved and certain exceptions may be looked at in a new light. These new aspects of the problem are concerned with the possibility that ACh, ChAc, and AChE may exert morphogenetic and trophic influences as well as be concerned with transport and metabolic phenomena. The new explorations and a brief review of the field constitute the major context of this chapter. Moreover, the problem of fetal responses to cholinergic agents and particularly that of the possible changes in adult behavior following an early cholinergic effect on the fetus should not be neglected.

An interesting, related problem is that of the phylogenetic appearance of the ACh system. In 1935 Bacq proposed a phylogenetic hypothesis of ChE analogous to Nachmansohn's ontogenetic hypothesis. Again, many inconsistencies are apparent (cf. Karczmar, 1963*a,b*). For instance, exceptions may be found to Bacq's (1935) prediction that ChE's (and ACh) should be present in motile but not in non-motile invertebrates (Karczmar, 1963*a,b*; Willmer, 1970). Although it may be expected that the ACh system should be present throughout the chordate phylum—it is indeed present already in *Amphioxus*—it seems absent in the urochordate *Cyona* (Durante, 1956, 1957; Scudder, Akers, and Karczmar, 1963, 1966; Scudder and Karczmar, 1966); in fact, the ganglion of *Cyona* does not respond to ACh (Scudder et al., 1963, 1966). The new technical advances and the conclusions reached in this chapter may elucidate not only the problems concerned with ontogenesis but also those related to phylogenesis of the ACh system.

AChE AND ACh IN DEVELOPMENT AND THEIR POSSIBLE RELATION TO FUNCTION

Following his proposal about the parallelism between ontogenesis, particularly of the nervous system, and AChE, Nachmansohn (1938a,b, 1940) and also Sawyer (1943a,b, 1944) provided data in support of this hypothesis. Sawyer showed, in the fish *Fundulus* and the amphibian *Amblystoma*, striking increases of the enzyme localized presumably in the nervous tissue at the time of intense neurogenesis and development of function. Recently, Filogamo and Marchisio (1971) referred to this synchrony as "striking" and as being "closely correlated with synaptic transmission." Actually (cf. Table I in Karczmar, 1963a), this synchrony is rather tenuous, and it is optimistic to suggest a strict correlation of AChE and ACh with synaptic transmission. This is particularly true since both AChE and ACh were found present in many forms long before the onset of neurogenesis, in fact, in the fertilized or even unfertilized egg and/or early blastula (see below). Yet, certain progress has been made in this area, and this will be reviewed with regard to the development of the central nervous system, of the skeletal and cardiac neuromyal junctions, and of the sensory systems. Because the data differ from form to form (Karczmar, 1963a), systematic description for each of these forms is impossible at present, and only summaries and generalizations will be presented here.

Certain tissues will not be considered because of the paucity of the data available, as in the case of blood and hypophysis (Cohn and Richter, 1956; Ferrand and Le Douarin, 1971). The data, however, particularly with regard to blood, are of interest as they relate to non-neural organs in which AChE and butyrylcholinesterase (BUChE) appear early in development (for earlier references, see Karczmar, 1963a). As in the case of neurogenesis, the changes in blood ChE's seem to continue postnatally (Muslin, 1968; Ozand, Artuinis, and Yarimigan, 1970; Zsigmond and Downs, 1971).

Sensitivity of the ACh system during development

Another aspect of ontogenesis of the ACh system should be stressed, namely, its plasticity and sensitivity during development. Prenatal handling, X-radiation, drugs, stimulation, and nutritional state of the mother (Nair, 1966; Kling, Finer, and Nair, 1965; Kling, Finer, and Gilmour, 1969; Adlard and Dobbing, 1971; Karczmar, Srinivasan, and Bernsohn, 1972b,c; Srinivasan, Karczmar, and Bernsohn, 1972; Richardson, Karczmar, and Scudder, 1972) all seem to affect brain ChE's during pre- and postnatal development; these changes may or may not be related to the changes in the brain weight (Adlard and Dobbing, 1971). It is of interest in this context that both anti-cholinergics and anti-ChE's given to mothers in single doses during gestation affected postnatally mouse brain isozymes of AChE and ChE (Karczmar, et al., 1972b,c). The brain enzymes (not only ChE's) and ACh of young animals may be also susceptible to various forms of experiential or other stimulation (Rosenzweig, Bennett, and Diamond, 1967; Kling et al., 1969; for the criticism of Rosenzweig et al., see Karczmar, 1969, and Bennett and Rosenzweig, 1969). It is impossible at this time to ascertain if these changes reflect the sensitivity of synaptization processes and the development of memory patterns (Eccles, 1972), the increase in cell number, or nonspecific growth phenomena.

Preneural appearance of the ACh system

In my earlier review (Karczmar, 1963a), I cited many animal forms (insects, tunicates, amphibia, birds, and many mammals) which exhibited AChE and/or ChE prior to neurogenesis and, in fact, in the unfertilized egg. These data may not be as pertinent to the ACh system and to its significance as the data concerning ChAc or ACh (Karczmar, 1969). Unfortunately, the ChAc and ACh data are incomplete. Yet, presence of ACh in unfertilized sea urchin and amphibian eggs as well as during their early, preneuronal development are well documented (Numanoi, 1953; Buznikov, Chudakova, Berchysheva, and Vyazmina, 1968; Reshetnikova, 1970). Very low but measurable amounts of ACh, ChAc, and ChE seem to be present during the early development of many insects (Smith and Salkeld, 1966; Karczmar, 1963a) including *Drosophila* (Dewhurst, McCaman, and Kaplan, 1970). In view of the presence of ACh in adult and ephemeral aneural tissues (see Karczmar, 1963a; Hebb, 1957, 1963), this is not an unexpected finding; it simply cautions us to look at other than transmittive functions of ACh (see sections on Morphogenesis and General Discussion, below) as pertinent for the significance of its presence.

Neurogenesis

The development of the chick. In the chick, AChE is present already in the Hensen's node and in the neural folds by the 1st and 2nd days of development and ACh by the end of the 2nd day (Tables 1 and 2; Karczmar, 1963a). This early appearance of AChE has been confirmed more recently by micrometric (Rizzoli, 1964) and by histochemical electron-microscopy (Brzin and Tennyson, 1967; Tennyson, 1970) methods, as well as on the basis of the electrophoretic separation and measurement of this enzyme (Maynard, 1966; also section on Isozymes, below).

The presence of ChAc and/or ACh was recorded at the time of the early differentiation of the primitive brain (Table 2; Karczmar, 1963a), by 3½ days in the brachial spinal cord (Burt, 1968) and by the 6th day in a number of regions such as cervical cord, cerebral hemispheres, motor column, and optic lobes (Filogamo, 1963; Marchisio and Giacobini, 1969; Giacobini, 1970a,b).

AChE subsequently increases gradually in the neuroblasts of ventral horn, of the dorsal root ganglion, and in the axolemma of the fibers of the Lissauer tract (subsequent to the entry of these fibers into the spinal cord on the 11th day). Thus, AChE formation in the spinal ganglion preceded that in the Lissauer tract; ChAc also may have been present earlier in the spinal ganglion than in the tract (Giacobini, Marchisio, Giacobini, and Koslow, 1970). However, at least as far as AChE is concerned, the trend was reversed by the 13th day, and the enzyme activity of the Lissauer tract continued increasing subsequently relative to the ganglion (Tennyson, 1970). Tennyson suggested that this distal-proximal gradient of activity is contrary to the concept of the formation of various substances—including AChE —in the perikaryon and their proximo-distal migration via the axonal flow (Weiss and Hiscoe, 1948). Tennyson prefers the concept of Koenig and Koelle (1961; Koenig, 1965, 1967) of the axonal formation of AChE. The precocious proximal appearance of AChE in the spinal ganglion must, however, be emphasized (see below). The antero-posterior sequence of ChAc appearance (earlier in the optic lobes and in the cerebral hemispheres and later in the midbrain and cerebellum; Filogamo and Marchisio, 1971) seemed contrary to the ontogenetic sequence of AChE (Karczmar, 1963a); however, the methods used were probably not sensitive enough to demonstrate the actual time of the first appearance of ChAc, as suggested by the much earlier presence of ACh (already in the 2-day-old brain).

Drastic increases of the components of the ACh system occur during the differentiation of the central nervous system and particularly at the onset of reflexes (see Karczmar, 1963a, for references). More recent data confirm this notion, indicating, for instance, a considerable increase in ChAc and AChE during chick neurogenesis, the latter occurring earlier, and the former later, both continuing generally quite steadily (Rogers, deVries, Kepler, Kepler, and Speidel, 1960; Rizzoli, 1964; Burdick and Strittmatter, 1965) and in parallel with cytological physiological maturation of the nervous system (Burdick and Strittmatter, 1965; Burt, 1968; Marchisio and Giacobini, 1969; Burt and Narayan, 1970). For instance, the 14-to-18-day peak in ChAc seemed to coincide with the establishment of early hatching movement and of polysynaptic reflexes (Burt and Narayan, 1970; Corner and Bot, 1967; Corner, Schadé, Sedlacek, Stoeckart, and Bot, 1967). The establishment of new connections seemed of importance, as the deafferented ventral spinal cord showed lesser gain in ChAc (Burt and Narayan, 1970). This is supported by the data obtained in tissue culture, as the brain cells of 7-day-old chick embryo showed increases of ChAc corresponding to those observed *in situ,* concomitantly with cell proliferation and differentiation (Werner, Peterson, and Shuster, 1971). If one may extrapolate from the data derived from tissue culture of the chick neuroblastoma cells, this period may also characterize the development and differentiation of synaptic contacts, concomitant with cholinoceptivity and the generation in at least some cells of the electric potential in response to electrophoretically applied ACh (Nelson, Peacock, Amano, and Minna, 1971a; Nelson, Peacock, and Amano, 1971b).

Thus, the ontogenetic appearance of AChE or even of ChAc does not suffice as an indicator of the functionability of the ACh system and of the cholinergic connections. In agreement with this concept, Marchisio and Giacobini (1969) were unable to show any correlation between changes in ChAc and the onset of electrical activity in several areas of chick embryo brain. In further agreement with this concept, whereas the electron-microscopy studies (Duffy, Tennyson, and Brzin, 1967; Tennyson and Brzin, 1972) demonstrate that initially AChE appears in the nuclear envelope of the neuroblast (4-day-old chick) and somewhat later at the—possibly cholinergic—synapse, a "primitive" synapse is present in the chick spinal cord after 5 days of development (Glees and Sheppard, 1964), and it matures only at 16 days. Thus, both ChAc and AChE appear precociously relative to the functional cholinergic transmission.

How do the data regarding AChE, ACh, and ChAc relate to brain function and motility? Head movements appear in the chick at 66 hours and the motility progresses caudadally, the trunk and tail movement appearing at 85 and 88 hours, respectively (Table 2; Karczmar, 1963a). The electric activity of the brain appears at 90 hours (Sharma, Dua, Singh, and Anand, 1964), but the mature activity of the EEG can be demonstrated only postnatally. Obviously, the presence of all the components of the cholinergic system antedates these phenomena. In fact, the earlier statement of

Rogers et al. (1960) about the relationship between the appearance of the electric activity which these authors assigned to the 15th day of development, and the increase in ChE activity, is not true today. Iqbal and Talwar (1971) suggested that the appearance of an AChE isozyme at day 9 "coincides" with the functional activity. This statement is obviously not precise; in any event, the functional role of the various AChE isozymes is completely unknown at present (see section on Isozymes, below).

Finally, it should be emphasized that the patterns of electric activity and, particularly pertinent in the current context, the effects of ACh and eserine differed as late as in the neonate chick compared to the adult (Corner et al., 1967). Altogether, although there is no reason to doubt the role of the ACh system in functional maturation of the chick brain, its appearance alone cannot be synonymized with either that of function or of cytological maturation of the latter.

Mammalian development. Data on mammalian development are sparse, and particularly the values for the components of the ACh system early in gestation are lacking. Generally, ChE's were found in the various forms prior to gestation, but no measurements were carried out during the earliest stages (Karczmar, 1963*b*). For instance, AChE was first measured in the whole embryo and in the spinal cord of the rat on the 8th and 11th days (Maletta, Vernadakis, and Timiras, 1966).

New findings were reported on several brain parts of the human fetuses, ranging in age from 8 to 32 weeks (Bull, Hebb, and Ratkovic, 1970). ChAc was present and rising "very steeply" throughout this period in most brain parts. This was naturally expected, and presumably ChAc, ACh, and AChE would be found in the human fetus considerably earlier (the central nervous system of the 8-week-old human fetus contained significant levels of AChE, as had been reported in 1941 by Youngstrom). Perhaps less expected was the finding that the distribution of ChAc in the fetal brain differed from that of the adult (Bull, Hebb, and Ratkovic, 1956). The most important exception was the cerebellum which showed at the 8th week the highest activity among the parts studied; its low ACh, AChE and ChAc activity in the adult mammals is well known. Relatively low levels of ChAc activity were found in the caudate nucleus, again contrary to the findings in the adult. The spinal cord and medulla seemed to catch up with the cerebellum as the development progressed.

Apparently, even weeks after birth, the brain of mammals such as the rat and dog is functionally immature not only insofar as the EEG patterns are concerned, but also as indicated by the postnatal changes in the potential evoked by the application of ACh or of anti-ChE's and by the relatively late postnatal appearance of the EEG activation by these substances (Sobotka, Myslivecek, and Springer, 1964; Myslivecek, Hassmannova, Rokyta, Sobotka, and Zahlava, 1965; Zahlava, 1965; Rozanova, 1967). This agrees with the fact that the components of the cholinergic system continue increasing postnatally in most forms (Karczmar, 1963a; Maletta et al., 1965; Maletta and Timiras, 1966), although they may decrease in some animals (the chick; Rizzoli, 1964). This may be true also in man where the levels of these components may increase postnatally and begin decreasing after 9 to 10 days of life (McGeer and McGeer, 1971). It should be added that AChE is present in what appears to be motoneurons in the tissue culture of rat neonate spinal cord, and, in fact, an AChE-rich Renshaw cell may also be present in such cultures (Hösli and Hösli, 1971). AChE seemed to be located in the soma and in the dendrites, but perhaps was not present to any extent in the nerve endings (Hösli and Hösli, 1971). This distribution may then be still immature. In the case of the tissue culture of the adult neurons, AChE is present in the perikaryon, fibers, and presynaptic nerve endings in cultures of human and rabbit brain cortex (Geiger, 1962); the presynaptic localization is teleologically important (Koelle, 1969). Altogether, as in the case of the chick, mammalian CNS function depends on many more factors of maturation than the presence of the components of the cholinergic system. Such maturation as well as the presence of synaptic vesicles (presumably containing ACh) were shown to coincide with electric activity in explanted spinal cord of the rat fetus at the period corresponding to that of similar occurrences in the course of the postnatal development (Bunge and Bunge, 1965). In fact, the cholinergic system cannot be considered as isomorphic throughout the development. The patterns of isozymes, which differ at various stages of development, are pertinent here (see below, section on isozymes and arylesterases). Similarly, the ratio of bound to free ACh differs in development, and Mann, Pleul, and Kewitz (1971) suggested that free ACh predominates at the time when the synapses are still poorly developed.

The neuromyal junction

As reviewed earlier (Karczmar, 1963a; Koelle, 1963), there is no doubt that, whether in terms of the estimations of the whole embryonic muscle or in those of cytochemical studies, AChE is present already in the myoblast, prior to the maturation of the muscle and of its innervation (see particularly Kupfer and Koelle, 1951; Gerebtzoff, 1954, 1959; Goodwin and Sizer, 1965); this seems true in many vertebrate (chick, *Amblystoma*) and mammalian (from rat to human) forms. In fact, chick embryo skeletal muscle grown in tissue culture has been shown to be capable of developing AChE aneuronally (Engel, 1961; Mumenthaler and Engel, 1961).

Altogether, the time of the appearance of the components of the cholinergic system in the muscle embryogenesis approximates that of their appearance in the neuroblasts, particularly of the future motoneurons. There was equally no doubt at the time of the writing of the earlier review (Karczmar, 1963a) that the early appearance of the enzyme was diffuse, while its localization in the end plates was concomitant with the arrival of nerves. In fact, aneuronal myoblast could not develop AChE-rich end plates in the tissue culture (Engel, 1961). This possibly morphogenetic role of the innervation is described and emphasized below.

Recently, Filogamo and Marchisio (1971) argued that "in every class of vertebrates" there is "a close temporal correlation . . . between the earliest arrival of nerve fibers and the appearance of AChE in the myoblasts." To support this conclusion, they refer to the data of Begliomini and Moriconi (1960) and Filogamo (1963) which indicate that AChE is present in the chick at 70 hours, while myotome of the chick is reached by the nerves between 60 and 70 hours (see Filogamo and Marchisio, 1971, for additional references). Additionally, Giacobini (1970b) described a ChAc peak in the chick embryo axial myotome at the time of its innervation. Yet, while the Italian authors are, of course, correct with regard to the *arrival* of the nerves at the chick myotome at the Hamburger stage 14 (53rd hour of development), the actual formation of the primitive junctions occurs considerably later, as does muscle movement (see Karczmar, 1963a; Table 2). Moreover, the histochemical method employed following formalin fixation does not reveal full enzyme activity, and it is very likely that even the early stain reported by the Italian workers and by Gerebtzoff (1959) does not reveal the first appearance of the enzyme (Koelle, 1963; Karczmar, 1963a; Holmstedt and Sjöqvist, 1961). When Kupfer and Koelle (1951) employed fresh-frozen sections in their determination of ACh activity in the embryogenesis of the rat neuromyal junction, they indubitably demonstrated the presence of AChE in aneural myoblast.

This is not to be construed as denying the role of nerves either in the increase of the muscle AChE activity upon innervation, or, as already stated, in the neuromyal morphological, biochemical, and pharmacological differentiation. Moreover, while the Italian investigators described lack of AChE stain in myotomes grown in culture following the explanation at stages 11-13, or in the case of older explants obtained from despinalized embryos (Filogamo and Mussa, 1967), these data are not in agreement with those of Engel (1961) and Mumenthaler and Engel (1961). It seems that in this case the positive result—the presence of AChE stain—may be more significant than the negative datum—the absence of the stain.

It is of interest that the activity of AChE seems to decrease postnatally (Nachmansohn, 1938b; Karczmar, 1963a); it is possible that this is simply due to the concentration of AChE in the end plate and concomitant decrease in the reading of AChE of the whole muscle. However, there may also be a change in the characteristics of AChE as well as a loss of certain isozymes postnatally (see section on Isozymes and Arylesterases).

The heart

In my earliest review (Karczmar, 1963a), the ontogenesis of ChE in relationship to the morphogenesis and to the functional development of the amphibian (*Amblystoma*), the chick, and the mammalian (several species) heart was discussed at length. In most forms, ChE's seemed to appear some time *after* the onset of cardiac contractility, but *prior* to the cardiac neurogenesis. For instance, in *Amblystoma,* while AChE may be demonstrated at Harrison stage 37 (Sippel, 1955), the heart beat is present at Harrison stage 34, the cross-striations occur at stage 37, the vagal nerve penetrates the sinus at stage 44, and the heart can be inhibited reflexly by stage 45 (Table 4; Karczmar, 1963a). A similar situation occurs in the chick heart, where ACh was found to be present at 3 days (Lissak, Toro, and Pasztor, 1942), and it could be released at that time by direct stimulation (Coraboeuf, LeDouarin, and Obrecht-Coutris, 1970); yet, the nerve penetration occurs in this form on day 4. Finally, vesicular bodies resembling ACh-containing synaptic vesicles were found in several vertebrate, embryonic non-innervated hearts (Page, 1967; Staley and Benson, 1968).

These data, as well as those on the precocious responsiveness of the fetal heart to autonomic drugs (see section of morphogenesis), strongly suggest that the ontogenetic appearance of the components of the ACh system relate better to the emergence of contractility or perhaps to the pacemaker functions than to that of the nervous control of the heart. Moreover, in the case of the heart just as in that of the skeletal neuromyal junction, the neurogenic control seems to depend on the maturation of the system as a whole rather than on the mere presence of the components of the

ACh system. This point is well illustrated by the recent electron-microscopy studies of Hagopian, Tennyson, and Spiro (1969) and Tennyson (1971). While they showed clearly that ChE was present in non-innervated embryonic rabbit hearts, which they interpreted as being "in favor of an ACh-ChE system of myogenic origin," they found important differences between the fetus and the adult as to the type of enzyme involved and its distribution. For instance, embryo heart contained predominantly AChE, while BuChE was also present in adult heart (although not as the "only" enzyme, as stated by Hagopian et al., 1969); there was ChE activity in the Golgi complex but not in the sarcolemma of the embryo heart, whereas the converse was true for the adult tissue. Finally, the adult tissue exhibited the enzyme in the T system and in the M bands, which were not as yet differentiated in the embryos studied by Hagopian et al. (1969) and Tennyson (1971). Indubitably, more studies of this particular type are needed before the question of the functional role of ACh system in the control of cardiac function and rhythmicity can be resolved.

It would be of interest to attack the problem of the ontogenetic role of ACh system in contractility and related phenomena by investigating the development of the smooth muscle, its innervation, and its contractility. The pertinent studies are few. It is of interest that the fetal ductus arteriosus, pulmonary trunk, and aorta of the lamb exhibited, shortly before birth, AChE-positive nerve fibers and ganglia; synaptic vesicles, possibly containing ACh, were also present (Silva and Ikeda, 1971). Also in this case there was a possibility that these nerves terminate differently than, and that their relationship to the adrenergic nerves differs from, those of the adult. Thus, this study affords an explanation for the apparent change in the response of the ductus arteriosus after birth (Boréus, Malmfors, McMurphy, and Olson, 1969; Smith, Morris, and Assuli, 1964; see also section on Morphogenesis, below, for ontogenetic change in pharmacological response of smooth muscle), and it accentuates the concept of the complex nature of the functional maturation of the nerve-effector response.

Sensory systems

It is well known that in the adult vertebrates AChE activity is very low (as compared, for instance, to motoneurons) in the primary afferent neurons as represented by the dorsal roots, their ganglion cells, and their terminations in the spinal cord; however, in the case of the secondary and tertiary sensory relay neurons, AChE activity increases peripherally (Koelle,

1963). It is of interest to follow the ontogenesis of these systems and relate them to the appearance of the sensory function.

There is a puzzling difference between the *olfactory* and *auditory* systems on the one hand, and the *visual* system on the other. In the olfactory and auditory systems, AChE appears early in the elements which are not considered as cholinergic, and its activity may diminish in subsequent development (Filogamo and Marchisio, 1971). AChE appeared in the neuroblasts of the olfactory placode of the chick on the 3rd day and in those of the rabbit and rat on the 13th or 14th day (Filogamo, 1963; Filogamo and Robecchi, 1969). Subsequently, the AChE stain appeared in the central processes of the neuroblasts which constitute the rudiment of the olfactory nerves. Filogamo and Marchisio (1971) found no correlation between AChE of the olfactory neuroblasts, the future olfactory neurons, and the development of their synaptic contacts; the stain disappeared before birth. Somewhat similarly, those cells of the acoustic ganglion of the guinea pig embryo which give rise to the propioceptive neurons of the vestibular ganglion showed marked AChE activity, which diminished postnatally; the ganglion cells of the future cochlear ganglion showed weak activity which disappeared prenatally. It should be stressed that in the adult the efferent olivocochlear bundle shows AChE activity which, on the basis of electron-microscopy data may be particularly localized at the synapses with the hair cells (Lehrer, Maliner, and Gioia, 1966; see Koelle, 1963, for other references) and that this part of the acoustic system may be cholinergic in nature (Koelle, 1969).

More extensive data are available with regard to the *optic pathways*. In the two extensively studied forms, the urodele *Amblystoma* and the chick, AChE appears almost simultaneously in the central midbrain rudiments of the optic pathways and in the peripheral optic-cup rudiments of the future retina (for references, see Karczmar, 1963a); in mammals, the former appears postnatally (Siou, 1958).

It has been demonstrated histochemically (Shen, Greenfield, and Boell, 1956) for the neuroretina of these two forms that the AChE stain appears earliest in the bodies of the ganglion and amacrine cells, forming subsequently several bands localized apparently at the time of the arborization and synaptization of these cells. Although several light bands appeared subsequently in the chick horizontal cells and at the future site of the rods and cones, the bodies of bipolar cells never stained, and at hatching the enzyme distribution resembled that of the adult vertebrate forms (Koelle, Wolfand, Friedenwald, and Allen, 1952; Francis, 1953; Leplat and Gerebtzoff, 1956; see Koelle, 1963, and Karczmar, 1963a, for additional references); moreover, the bands corresponded to the several layers of synaptic contacts between the ganglion and amacrine cells. The early appearance of an intense AChE stain in the amacrine cells is of interest, since Koelle (Nichols and Koelle, 1968) proposed that these cells activate cholinergically the ganglion cell as well as inhibit the bipolar neurons; this last action depends on a "percussive" mechanism, the terminals of the amacrine cells releasing ACh which in turn releases from the terminals an inhibitory transmitter capable of blocking the ganglion cell (Koelle, 1969; Karczmar, 1969). It should be added that ACh can be found in the chick retina (Lindeman, 1947) at the time of the appearance of the AChE stain in the regions of the synaptizations.

Centrally, AChE in the optic tectum of the chick (Filogamo, 1960a,b) appeared quite early and increased subsequently; in the superior colliculus of the mouse, it seemed to appear postnatally (Siou, 1962). Altogether, it seems that the appearance of both AChE and ChAc (Marchisio and Giacobini, 1969) in the tectal neurons is independent of the arrival of the afferent retinal fibers. However, the denucleation experiments indicate that the afferent fibers are responsible for maintenance of the collicular neurons and for the further production of their AChE (Hess, 1960, 1961) and ChAc (Marchisio, 1969), although afferent fibers from other than retinal origin may play this role; this is Hess' explanation for the fact that denucleation of the adult mice, rabbits, and guinea pigs did not cause a decrease of collicular AChE, since the adult contrary to the fetal neurons may be maintained by nonretinal afferents. In fact, Hess (1960) states that "there may be a quantitative relationship between the capacity of the neuron to produce cholinesterase and the number of synapses that it receives . . . at the time of initial production of cholinesterase."

It should be stressed that Boell, Greenfield, and Shen (1955) found a reduced content of AChE in the optic tectum of denucleated adult frog, contrary to the findings in the chick and the rodents. They believed that ChE was located in the nerve fibers and ascribed this result to the reduction in neuropil rather than to that of cell body enzyme or of the number of neurons. These results were not confirmed by Hess (1961) or Filogamo (1960a,b). Hess (1961) discounted hypoplasia and reduction of neuronal number as the cause of the diminution of AChE following enucleation of the embryo chick or frog. While Filogamo in 1960 emphasized hypoplasia as involved in the loss of AChE content in the tectal layer, more recently he came nearer to Hess' new point as he states (Filogamo and Marchisio,

1971) that "the rapid loss of synaptization alters the trophic equilibrium of tectal neurons and . . . prevents the critical increase of AChE at this stage" (for trophic effects, see below).

It is of interest that, in spite of the obvious role of afferent innervations in AChE synthesis of the tectal pathways, this synthesis is not synonymous with function. Indeed, tectal electric activity (Sedlacek, 1967) occurs subsequent to the rapid increase in tectal AChE and ACh. Similarly, the light reflex in the chick is established on the 19th day of the development (Lindeman, 1947), long after the appearance of retinal ACh and the establishment of the retinal, AChE-rich synapses (both on the 12th day). Thus, we are confronted with still another instance of the degree of complexity of the neurochemical-morphogenetic differentiation which is sufficient and necessary for function, while no single component of this differentiation may play this role by itself.

Spinal and sympathetic ganglion of the chick

In the rudiments of the *spinal* ganglion and related structures, AChE activity was noticed as early as at the 52nd hour of incubation in the case of the cells of the mesencephalic root of the fifth nerve and a day later in spinal ganglia, including their small and large neuron populations (Filogamo and Strumia, 1958; Filogamo, 1960b; Strumia and Baima-Bollone, 1964).

Early appearance of AChE in the spinal ganglia of the rabbit was confirmed by Tennyson and Brzin (1970). ChAc could not be demonstrated till the 6th day (Marchisio and Consolo, 1968; Giacobini, 1971).

In the *sympathetic* ganglion of the chick, AChE and ChAc were found by the 6th day (Marchisio and Consolo, 1968; Giacobini et al., 1970; Giacobini, 1971). In the related Remak's ganglion, AChE was found to be present at the same time (Cantino, 1969). In the case of the spinal ganglion, AChE increased to a peak at 12 days and subsequently declined, whereas ChAc exhibited a two-peak pattern, first declining from its early (6th day) level peaking again on the 18th day, and declining subsequently. The ultimate decline of both ChAc and AChE in the spinal ganglia relates obviously to their ultimately noncholinergic nature. To the contrary, AChE and ChAc of the sympathetic ganglia increased—somewhat irregularly— from the 6th day into the post-hatching period, and Cantino (1969) remarked that the increase of AChE in the Remak's ganglion coincides on day 13 with distinct synaptizations (see also Giacobini, 1971). Altogether, AChE and ChAc of the spinal ganglion are obviously not related to the final synaptic function, and Filogamo and Marchisio (1971) relate them to the "maturational events"; they comment further that even in the case of the sympathetic ganglion the ups and downs of ChAc activity resemble those of RNA and protein synthesis in these structures (Larrabee, Partlow, and Brown, 1969); this similarity is, at best, superficial.

MORPHOGENESIS, ONTOGENETIC PHARMACOLOGY, AND TROPHISM

There are new data which suggest that the ACh system may be involved in morphogenesis and differentiation and in the related phenomena of growth. Relatively complete data have been reported on the role of ACh—and other transmitters or transmitter-like substances—in echinoderm development and on the differentiation of the vertebrate skeletal end plate. In a related context, the cholinergic nerves may be concerned with trophic influences upon the muscle and limbs, and may be needed for regeneration in the case of the forms capable of the latter; the evidence is not all in, however. In view of this, the effects of cholinergics and anti-cholinergics on development, known since the turn of the century, may be not surprising.

The role of ACh and serotonin in echinoderm development

The early appearance of AChE and of ACh in the echinoderm development has been already stressed. On the basis of the pattern of their development as well as that of serotonin, and particularly on the basis of the pharmacological data, Gustafson and Toneby (1971) put forth a hypothesis which relates these substances to various phases of sea urchin morphogenesis. They relate serotonin to the early gastrulation and to the formation of mesenchyme. After a low in serotonin level, it increases in the cells of the primitive gut which are subsequently related to the pigmented rudiment of the pluteus ciliated bands and, ultimately, to the nerve cells of the ganglion of the adult sea urchin. Serotonin precursors and antagonists exerted expected action on gastrulation and the formation of the nervous system. ACh, on the other hand, may be involved in the late gastrulation as well as in mesenchyme-ectoderm association. Altogether, Gustafson and Toneby (1971; see also Gustafson, 1963, 1969; Gustafson and Wolpert, 1967; Gustafson and Toneby, 1970; and Buznikov, Chudakova, and Zvezdina, 1964) stress the fact that sea urchin development consists of phases dependent on intense cellular pulsatory activity and on movement and contraction of the cellular pseudopods. The effectiveness of ACh and serotonin with regard to such processes is well known; this is seen particularly clearly in the tissue cultures (Geiger, 1960). In fact, this type of event and active aggregation of all layers of different origins—such as mesenchyme and ectoderm—and transfer of materials from one to another may have been unduly disregarded as a mechanism of morphogenesis. Moreover, Gustafson and Toneby (1971) point out that pharmacology of the early organs and of the muscle elements of the sea urchin larva agrees with the pharmacology of the sea urchin ontogenesis.

Several cautionary statements should be made. First of all, Gustafson and Toneby employed relatively high concentrations of the various agents in their pharmacological analyses. Second, many of these agents have more than one pharmacological action, and it is faulty to consider the results obtained with quinidine, for instance, as due solely to its anti-cholinergic action (Gustafson and Toneby, 1971). Finally, Buznikov, Kost, Kucherova, Mndzhoyan, Suvorov, and Berchysheva (1970) showed that frequently both cholinomimetics *and* cholinolytics showed similar blocking effects during echinoderm development; these effects were obtained at various stages, in addition to those which Gustafson found to be sensitive in his studies.

The effects of cholinergics and anti-cholinergics on development

Since the early reports of Mathews (1902) and Sollman (1904) on the developmental effects of cholinergics in the sea urchin, reports on morphogenetic action of these substances are available but are certainly not systematic. The data of Mathews and of Sollman are somewhat unusual, in that they show that low concentrations of pilocarpine (10^{-6} M) accelerated echinoderm growth and morphogenesis as early as during gastrulation; atropine blocked this effect and at higher (and yet relatively low, 10^{-7} M) concentrations had an opposite effect. Much later, this block of gastrulation by atropinics was confirmed by Gustafson and Toneby (1970, 1971). Yet, as described subsequently, cholinergics generally caused malformation and/or growth inhibition during the development of the chick, fish (Sawyer, 1944; Whiting, 1955), amphibia, and insects (for references, see Karczmar, 1963*b*).

Amphibia. In the case of *urodeles,* exogastrulation was induced by very low (10^{-10} M) concentrations of diisopropyl phosphofluoridate (DFP; Karczmar and Koppanyi, 1953) and by higher concentrations of physostigmine and neostigmine (Sawyer, 1947). Death of the early blastulae and older embryos was also noticed. Interestingly, some resistance to DFP seemed to occur with the progress of development. The rate of the lethality of the motile, stage 26-

34 *Amblystoma* larvae seemed proportional to the concentration of DFP rather than to the rate of inhibition of AChE which is present in these larvae at these stages and earlier (see preceding section; Karczmar and Koppanyi, 1953; Karczmar, 1955). Nontoxic concentrations of anti-ChE's affected morphogenesis of larval fins, the head skeleton (Sawyer, 1943a, 1947; Koppanyi and Karczmar, 1947; Karczmar and Koppanyi, 1953), and gills. The latter effect may have been mediated via pituitary or peripheral vascular effects (Sawyer, 1943a).

Altogether, the earliest morphogenetic and toxic effects of anti-ChE's occurred in amphibia prior to the ontogenesis of organ systems and to the neurogenesis or development of function. Subsequent to initiation of neurogenesis, anti-ChE's affected the overt, motor behavior of urodeles and fish (see Karczmar, 1963b for references), the type of the effects being seemingly related to reflexogeny and to the ontogenesis of ChE's (see Table 2 in Karczmar, 1963b). In fact, in the case of *Fundulus* (Sawyer, 1944), the early somatic, independent of innervation (Coghill, 1933; also Karczmar 1963a, b), motility was not, while the subsequent neurogenic swimming and reflex activity were, affected by anti-ChE's. An interesting speculation was that of Boell (1948); he suggested that the motor malfunction induced by the anti-ChE agents at any particular stage of neurogenesis resembled the motor activity of an earlier stage, since the amount of ChE left after the DFP treatment at a later stage resembled that characteristic for an earlier stage of development.

The chick. In the chick development, the effects both of anti-ChE agents and of the cholinergic stimulants such as pilocarpine (see Karczmar, 1963b), eserine (Agarval and Monga, 1958), and nicotine or nicotine analogs (Ancel, 1945; Landauer, 1960; for further references, see Karczmar, 1963b) resembled those described for amphibian or fish development. These agents could induce, at relatively high concentrations, arrest of the chick development and death even during the 1st day of development, i.e., prior to neurogenesis or onset of cardiac function (Ancel, 1945; Landauer, 1949; for further references, see Karczmar, 1963b). Somewhat in contrast to these data, Torre (1970) reported that DFP was relatively nontoxic until the 7th day of incubation.

When anti-ChE and related agents were employed after 4 days of incubation, serious defects of skeletal development were induced, resulting in "wry neck," "rumplessness," micromelia, and syndactilism (see Table 1 in Karczmar, 1963b). Somewhat similar teratologies were induced by the treatment of the duck egg (Khera, LaHam, Ellis, Zawidzka, and Grice, 1966). As these effects required relatively larger concentrations of the cholinergic or anti-ChE agents, and as the effects somewhat resembled (see, however, Karczmar, 1963*b*) those induced by the drugs interfering with carbohydrate metabolism, Landauer (1954) suggested that carbohydrate metabolism was involved. Subsequently, however, Landauer (1960), upon demonstrating the effectiveness of lysine and proline in antagonizing nicotine-induced malformations suggested interference with the protein synthesis, or with a more specific step in somatogenesis as the mechanism of the action of nicotine. He also pointed out that this action results in a phenocopy paralleling the "crooked-neck dwarf" mutation; in fact, nicotine was particularly teratogenic in embryos heterozygous for the gene in question.

It is of further interest that the early (days 0–14 of development) administration into the yolk sac of the chick egg of hemicholinium, an agent which as a blocker of ACh synthesis could be expected to produce opposite or at least different effects compared to those induced by the cholinergic stimulants, did indeed exhibit its own teratogenic action (Becker, Linder, and Gibson, 1967; Gibson and Becker, 1969). A larger dose (10 mg per egg) caused 100% mortality at hatching, independently of the time of administration. Teratologic and related effects of this and a much smaller dose (1 μg per egg) included shortening of long bones, necrosis of the brain, and exencephaly, liver, muscle, and kidney pathology, and ankylosis with foot dorsoflexion. Additionally, temporary ataxia, reversed by neostigmine (a myasthenia-like syndrome), was noticed after hatching; this effect and the dorsoflexion resembled that induced by *d*-tubocurarine by Drachman and Coulombre (1962). It is of interest that transient myasthenia was noticed recently in human neonates (Wise and McQuiller, 1970).

Insects. The effect of carbamate and organophosphorus anti-ChE's on insect development is widely known (O'Brien, 1960; Chadwick, 1963; Karczmar, 1963*b*; Smith and Salkeld, 1966); the insecticidal action may depend on this developmental, ovicidal effect as well as on the effect on the mature insect. Yet, many investigators claimed that the effect on the egg is delayed and does not occur until the initiation of the neurogenesis, or that it may even depend on the storage of the poison till the maturation of the insect. On the whole, it does not seem doubtful that high concentrations of anti-ChE's are ovicidal for a number of insect forms (Smith and Salkeld, 1966), but it is less certain if this effect depends on the ontogenetic appearance of ACh and of ChE's even though ChE inhibition and ACh accumulation was demonstrated during early stages of development (see Karczmar, 1963*b*, and Smith and Salkeld, 1966). The matter is complicated by two more facts. First, the appearance of ChE's and perhaps also that of ACh may antedate that of neuroblasts (Poulson and Boell, 1946; Chino and Yushima,

1953; for other references, see Karczmar, 1963a, and Chadwick, 1963); thus, the ovicidal effect of the anti-ChE's may be related to the ACh system but not to neurogenesis. The fact that with few exceptions, the eggs were more resistant to organophosphorus agents than the larvae or adults (Kerr and Brazzel, 1960) does not necessarily militate against this conclusion. Second, ali-esterases and related enzymes also appear early in the insect egg (see Fig. 2 in Karczmar, 1963a) as well as in the insect nervous system, although, unlike AChE, they abound outside of the nervous system (Chadwick, 1963). It is well known that aliesterases split esters other than those of choline, and, although inhibited by organophosphorus agents, they are generally not inhibited by eserine (Usdinn, 1970). It is, however, of interest that some nontypical insect esterases may be sensitive to carbamate but not to organophosphorus anti-ChE's (Salkeld, 1965). Many such esterases appear early in development and are sensitive to anti-ChE's (Smith and Salkeld, 1966). Thus, these enzymes may be also involved in ovicidal or insecticidal action of anti-ChE's. Recently, Krysan and Guss (1971) pointed out that insect lipases are very sensitive to organophosphorus agents, and that those insect embryos which use only a small part of their fat for embryogenesis (*Oncopeltus fasciatus*) are insensitive to those drugs at least until hatching (Zschintzsch et al., 1965). In fact, ChE is present early in the development of *Oncopeltus,* and anti-ChE agents did penetrate into its egg (Zschintzsch et al., 1965; Bracha and O'Brien, 1966); thus, Krysan and Guss (1971) on the whole favored the concept of the involvement of a non-cholinesterasic factor in the ovicidal action of several organophosphorus agents.

It should be added finally in this context that anti-ChE's also exerted other actions on the insect development, preventing hatching and prolonging the diapause. The cycle of ACh and AChE has been described for insect diapause (Van der Kloot, 1955, 1960), and the termination of diapause and reinitiation of growth may depend on the re-emergence of ChE; Van der Kloot postulated that the latter and the concomitant brain activity lead to brain neurosecretion which in turn causes the release of the growth hormone from the prothoracic gland. The inhibition of this mechanism may be then responsible for the anti-ChE effect on diapause (Chadwick, 1963; Karczmar, 1963b).

The above data dealing with generalized effects of anti-ChE's and cholinergics on development indicate sufficiently the difficulty in resolving two questions: do these compounds, so closely related in our mind to both nervous transmission and to the ACh system, act concomitantly with the onset of neurogenesis and synaptic, particularly cholinergic transmission? Or do they exhibit earlier actions, either related to non-neuronal ACh, AChE, and ChAc, or even non-cholinesterasic in nature? On the whole, the precocity and preneuronal character of their actions seems well documented; on the other hand, in view of the early appearance of all or of some components of the ACh system (see preceding section), these early actions may be at least dependent on the latter. However, further evidence is necessary, namely that pertaining to the action or inaction of the cholinergic agents during late neurogenesis and development of function, such as that related to the somatic and cardiovascular system.

Pharmacologic responses of the neuromyal junction and of the heart

In the case of the development of the *skeletal neuromyal junction,* it seems certain that ACh response is present prior to penetration of nerve endings into the young muscle. In fact, as soon as the myoblasts fuse into myotubules (chick embryo)—prior to the development or striation—ACh response is present, although relatively high concentrations are needed (de Lustig, 1942, 1943). However, ACh sensitivity increases with the development of cross-striations which is also the time of the increased membrane potential (Fischback, Nameroff, and Nelson, 1970) and of increased sensitivity to electrical stimulation (Szepsenwol, 1947). Moreover, in the case of the tissue culture of the skeletal embryonic cells, similar phenomena were observed. In the chick these cells responded to relatively high concentrations of ACh upon their differentiation into myotubes; the sensitivity increased and a more mature pattern of response occurred later (Dryden, 1970). Both these and more mature muscle cells (Kano, Shimada, and Ishikawa, 1971) responded along all their length similarly to the fetal muscle investigated *in situ* (Diamond and Miledi, 1962; Redfern, 1970). These phenomena should be related to the precocious presence of AChE and of ChAc (see preceding section) in the muscle rudiment.

However, the significance of this early response cannot be construed as indicating the muscle response is to a great extent myogenic and independent of innervation. In fact, the adult response pattern to ACh and to nerve stimulation has to await the arrival of the nerve endings at the muscle. While the myogenic fetal response to ACh resembles that of the denervated muscle (Axelsson and Thesleff, 1959; Miledi, 1960a,b) in that it covers the entire fiber surface, the adult response is confined to the end plate region, and this effect is accompanied by the appropriate organization of AChE, which becomes concentrated at the end plate (see Karczmar, 1963a, and Filogamo and Marchisio, 1971; also preceding section) coincidentally with the nerve release of the transmitter (Diamond and Miledi, 1962). Analogously, the rat and chick muscle cultivated *in vitro* showed, upon innervation, brief excitatory junctional potentials restricted to innervated cells (James and Tresman, 1969; Robbins and Yonezawa, 1971). A similar relationship between the cytological maturation on the one hand and the development of the neuromyal transmission on the other was found *in situ,* and in fact it resembled the relationship characteristic for the reinnervation of the denervated muscle (Koenig and Pecot-Dechavassine, 1971).

The pharmacological analysis indicated that, in the rat at least, the junctional potentials were due to ACh, and that the response, like that of the adult neuromyal junction, was quantal in nature (Robbins and Yonezawa, 1971). Altogether, a myogenic ACh response, not dependent on innervation, is replaced subsequently in development by the adult neurogenic response. For instance, there is a postnatal change in the response to succinylcholine, and the pattern of this response may ultimately relate to the differentiation of the slow and fast muscle (Mann and Salafsky, 1970). The question remains whether the earlier response to exogenous ACh indicates the presence of, and response to, endogenous ACh; in turn, the existence of the latter may explain the spontaneous activity of the non-innerval muscle frequently observed both in tissue culture and *in situ* (Hirano, 1967; Dryden, 1970). This endogenous ACh could be either myogenic (see Giacobini, 1970a,b) or due to the neurogenic ACh diffusing to the muscle from the still distant nerve (Kupfer and Koelle, 1951).

Interestingly, although only sporadic data are available for the fetal smooth muscle, Boréus (1967, 1968, 1971) found that the fetal ileum is responsive to ACh in the case of human embryo from the beginning of the second trimester of pregnancy, and in the guinea pig during the last week of gestation. On the basis of the pD_2 values, Boréus felt that the affinity of the cholinergic receptor to ACh did not change during prenatal and early postnatal development, although the contractility did increase. Since the first responses were recorded by Boréus (1971) relatively late in development, his data may bear out the contention of Filogamo and Marchisio (1971), based on the ontogenetic appearance of AChE (Cantino, 1970) and ChAc in the alimentary canal of the chick, that the "acquisition of the cholinergic system" in the smooth muscle depends first of all on the presence of neuroblasts.

The responses of *the heart* to ACh and to cholinergic and related drugs generally follow the pattern described above for the skeletal neuromyal junction. In reviewing earlier literature (Karczmar, 1963b), I had concluded that in both the chicken and rat hearts ACh responses may be found considerably prior to the innervation of the heart; in fact, the ACh sensitivity did not seem to change upon innervation. Although the response to the anti-ChE agents seemed to occur later than that to ACh, it also preceded innervation; ChE appears in these hearts also prior to innervation although possibly after the appearance of myogenic ACh (see below, and Karczmar, 1963a). It should be added that adrenergic responses also antedated, in these forms, the appearance of the cardiac innervation. Recent investigations seem to support these conclusions. (Roberts, Gimeno, and Webb, 1965; Obrecht-Coutris and Coraboeuf, 1967; Coraboeuf et al., 1970; Gennser and Nilsson, 1970). Interesting data were obtained with regard to the human 9- and 10-week-old hearts, prior to its innervation; in this preparation, ACh caused negative chronotropic and conduction effects (Gennser and Nilsson, 1970). Similar negative chronotropic action of ACh was described for the non-innervated chick heart. Related evidence was found in the case of the chick heart by Coraboeuf et al. (1970); prior to the onset of innervation, the heart, upon direct stimulation, exhibited slowing and decreased diastolic depolarization which were blocked by atropine. These data are consistent with the presence of myogenic ACh and ChAc as known from earlier work (see Karczmar, 1963a); in fact, Coraboeuf et al. (1970) confirmed the presence of ACh in the non-innervated heart by bioassay.

Trophic and regenerative effects of cholinergic nerves

The above data indicate the presence of organ and tissue function prior to innervation or independently of the latter, as well as the presence under these conditions of ACh and/or anti-ChE sensitivity; however, they indicate also that the *adult* type of response and function is neurogenic and that it depends on the arrival of the nerves at the receptor site. This then may suggest that the innervation has a morphogenetic effect, inducing functional and morphological differentiation of the synapses and/or junctions. The pertinent data will be adduced; moreover, evidence is available which indicates that the cholinergic nerves may exert a trophic influence as well as be important in regenerative processes.

Some of the data indicating the morphogenetic effect of the cholinergic motor nerves upon the neuromyal junction and particularly the end plate were already cited. It appears that the distribution of AChE (see above; Mumenthaler and Engel, 1961; Kovács, Kover, and Balogh, 1961) and perhaps also of ChAc (Giacobini, 1970a,b) and the mature organization of the end plate depends on the innervation of the fetal muscle (see also Zelena, 1962; Teravainen, 1968; Kelly and Zacks, 1969; Lentz, 1969a,b). Not only do the distribution and the end plate localization of AChE depend on the presence of nerves, but also the amount of the enzyme activity seems to be regulated by the innervation; for instance, after administration of DFP, the rate of AChE resynthesis was greater in the innervated than in the denervated muscle (Rose and Glow, 1967). Finally, the important recent contribution to our understanding of the role of innervation is the evidence that the innervation of the muscle may, in the process of ontogenesis, regulate the pattern of the isozymes of both AChE and BuChE and control the appearance—generally postnatal—of the adult pattern of the molecular forms of ChE's (Maynard, 1966; Barron et al., 1967; Karczmar et al., 1972b,c; see section on Isozymes and Arylesterases).

The problem here is that it is not necessarily the presence or release of ACh which regulates the synthesis of the enzyme, as the botulinum toxin did not produce the loss of AChE (Strömblad, 1960; also Guth, 1969). However, the release of ACh from the nerve endings seems to add to the maturity and integrity of the end plate. For instance, differential sensitivity of the latter versus the insensitivity of the rest of the muscle membrane was ascribed to ACh by Thesleff (1960); the prevention of ACh release by botulinum toxin (Thesleff, 1960) or by the chronic application of local anesthetics to the motor axon, as done in these laboratories (Robert and Oester, 1970a,b), induced the spread of ACh sensitivity to the whole muscle membrane without causing the degeneration of the nerve. Further examples of the dependence of the functional maturity of the muscle on its denervation—such as the role of the latter in preventing the hyper- (or multiple) innervation and its role in the differentiation of the white and red muscle —were thoroughly described in a recent review by Guth (1969).

Additional support for the concept of the role of nerves in the morphogenesis of the neuromyal junction comes from the data obtained following amputation of the urodele limbs. In fact, under those circumstances the muscle changes observed are converse (Lentz, 1969a) to those observed during ontogeny of the muscle and of its innervation. For instance, the junctional folds disappear, persisting as long as the nerve remains in contact with the muscle (Lentz, 1970), and the muscle loses its specialization— including the end plate—and dedifferentiates into mesenchyme. Additionally, AChE ceases to be localized in the sarcoplasmic end plate (Lentz, 1969a,b, 1970). These changes become reversed upon the regeneration of the distal axon and nerve ending. When the nerve is transected jointly with amputation, the end plates degenerate speedily (Reger, 1959; Nickel and Waser, 1968) and can be only reformed upon nerve regeneration and their growth into the amputation area, i.e., depending on the presence of the vesicle-filled axon terminals (Lentz, 1969b). It should be stressed, however, that both dedifferentiation and subsequent differentiation of the muscle upon amputation are not entirely dependent upon the innervation, as the nerve section without amputation produces lesser and slower, although related, changes (Couteaux, 1955; Guth et al., 1964; Nickel and Waser, 1968; for further references, see Guth, 1969); particularly slower are the changes in activity and pattern of AChE (see Lentz, 1970). On the other hand, new neuromyal junctions could be induced by causing motor nerve regeneration and escape from the glial cells by crushing; this induction occurred readily in younger rats at the sites of undifferentiated plasma membranes, and both infoldings and typical ACh distribution were observed (Juntunen and Teravainen, 1970).

It has already been indicated that certain problems arise when the differentiation of the end plate is ascribed *solely* to the cholinergic innervation and the concomitant appearance of the activity of ACh; particularly doubtful is this interpretation of the neural control of ChE activity (see above and Guth, 1969). Particularly important may be that changes in ChE do not seem to be related to various surgical and pharmacological maneuvers which affect the release of ACh (Guth, 1969). Similarly, the data from this laboratory (Robert and Oester, 1970a,b) indicated that "excitatory . . . functions of the motor nerve" are not strictly related to trophic influences, and a similar position was taken by Guttman (1963). On the other hand, particularly on the basis of his pharmacological analysis of the situation, Drachman (1964, 1967; Drachman and Romand, 1970; see, however, below, and Drachman and Singer, 1971) stated that the blockade of ACh transmission was responsible for "denervation atrophy" produced by drugs, and that this transmission is "essential for the maintenance of enzymatic differences between 'red' and 'white' muscle fibers." Even he, however, is not sure if "ACh alone is capable of mediating the nerve's trophic influence"; altogether, Drachman feels that the trophic effect of nerves—not necessarily coupled with cholinergic terminals—seems concerned not so much with morphogenesis of the cholinergic junctions, the development of their AChE pattern, and their functional maturation, but with general trophic phenomena such as protein synthesis and maintenance of muscle structure (Guth, 1969). It is true that the definition of the trophic action and of its mechanism appears vague; Guth (1969), for instance, states that "this is the basic question of trophic nerve function—the influence of the nerve over the genetic activity of the cell."

Perhaps the clearest indication of the trophic role of the nerves as well as of its noncholinergic character emerges from the investigations on amphibian limb and tail regeneration, which have continued unabated since the turn of the century (Rubin, 1903). Upon amputation of the limbs of such forms as urodele larvae, the regeneration can occur only in the presence of the nerves (the brachial plexus is generally the resected site; see Schotté, 1922, and Karczmar, 1946, 1963a). Without their presence, not only cannot regeneration occur, but dedifferentiation of, particularly, the muscle occurs and the stump is resorbed ("regression," Schotté and Butler, 1941; Schotté and Karczmar, 1944, 1945); these events thus resemble ontogenesis in reverse, as described above in the case of the blocked motor innervation. It appears clear, however, that in regeneration the role of nerves is not type dependent since regeneration was shown to be related to the amount rather than to the type of nerves transected (Karczmar, 1946); additionally, there is a continuous relationship between the amount of innervation left and the frequency of the occurrence of regeneration (at least in the case of *Amblystoma*; Karczmar, 1946).

Upon investigation of ACh and AChE changes during regeneration, Singer (Singer, Davis, and Arkovitz, 1960a; Singer, Davis, and Sheuing, 1960b; Singer, 1960) emphasized the possible role of ACh in regeneration since ACh peaked at the time of rapid onset of regeneration; at that time the latter was particularly sensitive to denervation. Pharmacological analysis seemed to support this notion; atropine and inhibitors of ACh synthesis were shown to inhibit regeneration not only in urodeles (Singer et al., 1960a,b; Hui and Smith, 1970) but also in *Hydra* (Lentz and Barnett, 1963). Yet, Singer (1960) pointed out certain inconsistencies of the situation, and recently Drachman and Singer (1971) demonstrated that botulinum toxin did not induce the regression of amputated limbs of *Triturus viridescens* and, in fact, did not prevent or slow the regeneration.

In summary, a trophic factor not identical with the cholinergic system may be involved in regeneration, as suggested by Karczmar (1946). In fact, besides AChE, other enzymes also decline in activity upon denervation (Karczmar and Berg, 1951), and the process thus resembles other nerve-dependent phenomena in which protein synthesis and other metabolic activities are affected (Guth, 1969), and which Guth therefore considers as dependent on a trophic factor. It even may be argued that after denervation the tissues return biochemically to the embryonic state, in keeping with the concept of not only the trophic but also the maturation role of the nervous system (Karczmar and Berg, 1952; Karczmar, 1955). The presence of a trophic factor is also indicated by experiments suggesting a systemic diffusion of the factor from the contralateral innervation (Tweedle, 1971). Furthermore, homogenates or supernatants of the brachial plexus and other nerves could restore denervation-induced inhibition of protein synthesis, and increase AChE activity of *Triturus* muscle in organ culture (Lebowitz and Singer, 1970; Lentz, 1971); however, AChE stimulation was also induced by the liver homogenate (Lentz, 1971). The nerve growth factor (NGF), a protein isolated from certain tumors (Levi-Montalcini and Hamburger, 1953) and other tissues, also accelerated early stages of regeneration, although it was not tested in the case of amputated *and* denervated limbs (Weis and Weis, 1970). Finally, the puzzling phenomenon discovered by Yntema (1959) may be explained by trophism. Yntema (1959) demonstrated that "aneurogenic" *Amblystoma* larvae produced by removal of appropriate portions of the spinal cord at an early developmental stage can regenerate their amputated limbs. Tweedle (1971) points out that in this case the trophic factor may persist in the non-neural tissues, provided certain other conditions also exist. It must be added, however, at least in the case of regeneration, that the trophic effect of nerves cannot be synonymized with an effect on growth. Indeed, provided the nerves are present, the growth of the amputated limb may be blocked by certain agents without inducing regression (Karczmar and Berg, 1951, 1952). Certain lytic agents, such as colchicine, or irradiation, which obviously do more than arrest growth, will cause regression under these conditions.

Altogether, the data indicate clearly a morphogenetic effect of cholinergic nerves in the neuromyal development. Whether ACh is the carrier of this effect is more doubtful, as is the role of ACh and its components in the trophic and in the regeneration phenomena. The trophic factor of the cholinergic nerves may depend on, without being identical with, ACh or ChAc; it may be related to that present in other nerves, but it is not a "growth factor."

ISOZYMES AND ARYLESTERASES

ChE's constitute a family of enzymes; the two sub-groups of this eserine- and organophosphorus-sensitive family are BuChE (pseudocholinesterase; EC 3.1.1.8), which has as its optimal substrates butyryl, benzoyl, and propionylcholine, and AChE (EC 3.1.1.7), the ACh-preferring enzyme. These two sub-groups contain a number of variants and isozymes; while both are genetically determined (Liddell, Newman, and Brown, 1963; for other references, see Goedde, Doenicke, and Altland, 1967; Usdin, 1970; Holmes and White, 1970), the variant is a wider term since the variants presumably exhibit isozymes. Furthermore, variants differ conspicuously in substrate activity, whereas isozymes differ physically and in their chemistry but not, at least conspicuously, in their activity (Massoulie, Rieger, and Bon, 1971).

ChE's in turn belong to the wider family of B-esterases, organophosphorus-sensitive enzymes; B-esterases include, in addition to eserine-sensitive choline hydrolases, the *ali-esterases* which are generally insensitive to eserine and which hydrolyze non-choline esters such as those of carboxylic acid. On the other hand, A-esterases differ from B-esterases in that they are insensitive to organophosphorus compounds and to eserine; while they hydrolyze, similarly to ali-esterases, non-choline carboxylic esters, they are particularly effective against aromatic esters of naphthol and phenol and hence are commonly called arylesterases.

In the present context, these related enzymic types present certain opportunities and certain difficulties. Teleologically, it may be more revealing to look at the ontogenetic appearance of all these forms rather than only at that of AChE or BuChE; on the other hand, the role in the nervous system of most of these forms, including ali- and arylesterases, and of the isozymes of BuChE and AChE, is unknown. In fact, the organophosphorus-insensitive hydroxylases of carboxylic and aromatic esters (A-esterases) were not known until recently to characterize the mammalian brain (Barron and Bernsohn, 1968) and neuromyal junctions (Barron et al., 1967), and naturally occurring substrates of these compounds are not known.

Isozymes

There is a general agreement as to the ontogenetic change in the isozymes of aryl-, ali-, Bu-, and AChE. Most of the studies involved the development of the muscle and/or neuromyal junction and of the brain; blood and several other tissues were studied more sporadically (Pantelouris and Arnason, 1966; Maynard, 1966; Szafran and McCarty, 1968).

With regard to the muscle, increased activity (quantitative change) and qualitative change in isozyme pattern were found to occur during ontogenesis. In the chick, mouse, and guinea pig, there was generally an increase in the number of bands (isozymes) of aryl- and ali-esterases (Barron and Bernsohn, 1965, 1968; Barron, Ordinario, Bernsohn, Hess, and Heduck, 1968; Pakhomov, Aronshtam, and Margulis, 1970).

The isozymes of AChE differentiated less during ontogenesis (Maynard, 1966; Wilson, Montgomery, and Asmundson, 1968; Barron et al., 1968; Szafran and McCarty, 1968; Wilson, Mettler, and Asmundson, 1969). It is, in fact, of interest that the postnatal decrease in AChE activity reported first by Nachmansohn (1938b) corresponded to the disappearance of certain AChE isozymes (Maynard, 1966; Barron, Bernsohn, and Hess, 1966; Barron et al., 1967; Wilson et al., 1968, 1969). This disappearance coincided with the localization and acquisition of the mature pattern of AChE at the end plate and at the myotendon junctions (Wilson et al., 1969). In fact, as in the case of the total activity of AChE and of its pattern during ontogenesis, the nerves may be responsible for a repressing activity, which controls the enzymic types in question (Wilson et al., 1969). It was suggested that these mechanisms may be deficient in dystrophic chicken (Wilson et al., 1968, 1969), and that there are similarities between dystrophic and denervated mouse muscle (McCaman, 1966).

The brain seems to be particularly rich in various molecular forms of esterases; 25 or more forms were reported for the adult human brain (Barron, Bernsohn, and Hess, 1963; Estrugo, Bernsohn, Barron, and Hess, 1969). Generally, a pre- and/or postnatal increase in activity and in pattern were reported for ali- and arylesterases. For instance, 14 bands characterized the brain of mature rat versus 7 in the 1-day-old animal (Bernsohn, Barron, Hess, and Hedrick, 1963). In man and in the rat or guinea pig, the ontogenetic occurrence and/or rapid increase of quantity and the number of ali-esterase isozymes rather coincided with the development of white matter and the process of myelinization (Bernsohn et al., 1963; Bernsohn and Barron, 1964; Barron and Bernsohn, 1968; Frey, Riekinnen, Rinne, and Arstila, 1970; Frey, Arstila, Rinne, and Riekinnen, 1971). However, some isozymes disappeared or decreased in activity during development (Bernsohn et al., 1963; Frey et al., 1971). It is of interest that, as in the case of the muscle, these latter results, as well as some of the redistribution patterns of the ali-esterase isozymes, may be explained by the presence of repressors, their changes during the development, and their redistribution (to myelin, for instance; Frey et al., 1971).

Even more complex data pertain to the pre- and postnatal ontogenesis of the isozymes of BuChE and AChE. Maynard (1966) reported in the chick brain relatively small, quantitative ontogenetic changes involving what she considered isozymes of AChE. On the other hand, the Hines-Loyola group indicated a possible appearance of additional BuChE and/or AChE

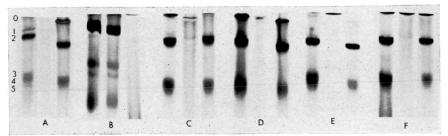

FIG. 1. Disc electrophoresis of cholinesterases during development.
A: Saline-treated adult mother; *B*: 10-day old embryo; *C*: 1-day old mouse; *D*: 3-day old mouse; *E*: 5-day old mouse; *F*: 10-day old mouse.

Numbers at left indicate enzyme band described in text. 0 is origin. For each set of three gels, the left gel is the control: the center and the right electrophoretogram developed with 5×10^{-6} M mytelase and with 10^{-6} M DFP, indicating BuChE and AChE bands, respectively. For methods, see Karczmar et al., 1972*a,b*

bands in the course of rat, mouse, and human development (Bernsohn et al., 1963; Bernsohn and Barron, 1964; Barron and Bernsohn, 1965, 1968; Karczmar et al., 1972*b,c*). Our data also indicated a major shift in the pattern and characterization of ChE isozymes.

In the study of the pre- and postnatal development of the mouse, we found strong activity and multiplicity of the isozymes of BuChE at 10 days of gestation; only one isozyme of AChE seemed present at that time. In the course of subsequent development, BuChE activity and the number of its isozymes declined, whereas the opposite occurred in the case of AChE; altogether, at 1 day of age, the AChE-BuChE pattern became reversed compared to that observed early in gestation (Karczmar et al., 1972*b,c*; Srinivasan, Karczmar, and Bernsohn, 1972; Figs. 1–4). Subsequently, however, additional BuChE bands developed (Figs. 1–4).

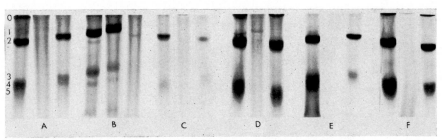

FIG. 2. The zymographs of mouse brain at various stages of development; mother treated with DFP on 10th day of pregnancy. Gel *A*: BuChE (Band 1) is absent in DFP-treated mother's brain as well as in the 1-day-old newborn. Middle gel in *C*: the development of pseudo enzyme (Band 1) is absent as compared to normal. For other explanation, see Fig. 1.

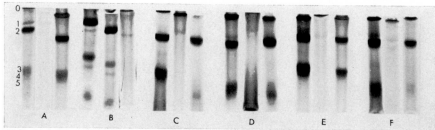

FIG. 3. Adult mother was treated with physostigmine on 10th day of pregnancy. Note the decrease in BuChE of the 10-day embryo (*B*); otherwise enzyme pattern similar to that of controls. For further explanation, see Fig. 1.

An interesting suggestion may be made with regard to BuChE isozymes on the basis of the results dealing with the development of the fetus following the treatment of mothers at various periods of pregnancy with DFP and physostigmine (Karczmar et al., 1972*b,c*). The treatment at the 10th day of gestation with DFP but not with physostigmine blocked the embryonic appearance of one of the BuChE isozymes and prevented altogether the appearance of one of the BuChE patterns at birth; subsequently, however (at the 5th day of the postnatal development), the two BuChE isozymes characteristic for the normal development became apparent. It may be hypothesized, therefore, that there is no synthetic mechanism available at birth for the formation of the two postnatal BuChE bands. Therefore, the DFP destruction via phosphorylation of one of the embryonic BuChE isozymes prevents the early appearance of the postnatal BuChE isozymes; this effect cannot occur with the competitive, short-acting BuChE blocker physostigmine. On the other hand, some mechanism for the molecular organization and for the synthesis of the adult BuChE isozymes seems to emerge postnatally.

Several additional features of our experiments deserve mention. First,

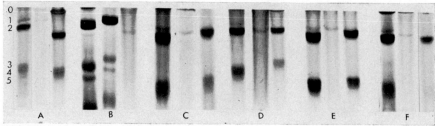

FIG. 4. Brains of scopolamine-treated mother (10th day of pregnancy) and of the newborns. Enzyme pattern similar to that of control. For further explanation, see Fig. 1.

the receptor mechanisms were not involved in the phenomena described as atropinic substances did not have any effect on the ontogenesis of BuChE and AChE isozymes (Fig. 4). Second, the high prenatal activity of BuChE shown at present by the electrophoretic technique is a novel finding not necessarily corroborated by the results obtained with manometric and other methods. The differences in the data obtained by the two types of methods were pointed out by others (see, for instance Maynard, 1966; also this section, below).

Arylesterase

Arylesterase and its molecular forms present special difficulties. While the ontogenetic presence of ali-esterases and the development of their isoforms may be hypothetically related to myelination and related processes of lipid formation, the function of arylesterases is even more enigmatic. Organophosphorus-insensitive forms may occur in the rat brain first postnatally (1-day-old rat; Bernsohn et al., 1963). The same appears true for the postnatal human brain; for instance, a marked proportion of esterases appeared to be organophosphorus-insensitive at 5 and 10 days of postnatal development, but this fraction seemed to decrease with maturation (Barron and Bernsohn, 1968), and its isozymes appeared to constitute some 11% of the total esterase (Estrugo et al., 1969).

In the case of the muscle, the very interesting finding is that of high activity of arylesterase isozymes in neonatal rat (Barron et al., 1966, 1967, 1968). The localization of these enzymic forms in the end plates seemed to overlap with that of AChE. Their activity and multiplicity decreased postnatally (Barron et al., 1966, 1967). The only suggestion as to their function was made on the basis of their cellular location in the lysozymes (Shnitka and Seligman, 1961); this localization seems to characterize actively anabolizing tissues (Adams, 1963).

Significance of the ontogenesis of various esterase forms

First, certain special difficulties inherent in the electrophoretic and related preparative methods should be stressed. The isozymes differ as to their extractability (and its pH dependence), their solubility, and as to whether their fractions are free or bound; this subject has been dealt with at length elsewhere (Bernsohn, Barron, and Hess, 1964; Barron and Bernsohn, 1966; Bernsohn, Barron, Doolin, Hess, and Hedrick, 1966; Koeppen,

Barron, and Bernsohn, 1969). In our recent work, for instance, a BuChE and/or AChE fraction incapable of going into the gel was described; this fraction seemed to increase during the development. The biological signifi- cance of these biophysical corollaries of the differences in the structure of the various enzymic forms is not clear; at any rate, these complexities render the comparison of the data from various laboratories difficult. The clarifica- tion of the functional significance of the data must await further develop- ment of our knowledge. Several investigators suggested that the appear- ance of certain isozymes of AChE is particularly important for function such as EEG maturation (see above). The marked qualitative shift in the patterns of BuChE and AChE isozymes shown in our laboratories (Karczmar et al., 1972b,c) should be mentioned in this context. Furthermore, we described above the possible role of ali-esterases in myelination and lipid metabolism (see above; Barron and Bernsohn, 1965; Frey et al., 1971). The significance of arylesterases is still more puzzling; possibilities such as that of their role in transacetylations (Franz and Krish, 1968) are among many that should be explored.

GENERAL DISCUSSION

Relationship between neurogenesis, the ACh system, and the effects of cholinergic and anti-cholinergic drugs

The above description illustrates that while generally in ontogenesis the components of the ACh system increase rather markedly at the begin- ning of neurogenesis, and subsequently at the onset of nerve function and overt behavior, this relationship is frequently not ideal, and often simply absent. Indeed, the precocious non-neural appearance of ACh, ChAc, and AChE during the development of many forms seems well documented. Fur- thermore, subsequent to the pre-neural stages of development, neurogenesis and development of nerve function coincide only in the general sense with neurochemical development of the ACh system. For instance, it is obvious that the appearance of the EEG and particularly of its mature pattern in the chick or rat occurs very late compared to the appearance of ACh or AChE in the CNS rudiment, and the first response of the latter to cholinergic drugs as well as the first appearance of its mature pattern again do not relate to any particular moment in ontogenesis of ACh or AChE, or even to the steep rate of their synthesis. Similarly, the maturation of the rhythmicity of the heart does not readily coincide with the ontogenesis of the ACh system, and the responses of the heart to cholinergic agents antedate the development of the cardiac innervation. Similar inconsistencies seem to characterize the ontogenesis of the ACh system in relation to neural function and to the cholinergic drug response in many invertebrate forms, particularly in insects. Finally, not only may components of the ACh system not appear synchronously with the neural function in the areas where cholinergic synapses occur finally in the adult, but, conversely, AChE and even ChAc may appear ontogenetically in certain neural structures which ultimately are not cholinergic; the spinal ganglion is a prime example of this phenomenon.

Perhaps these cautionary statements are superfluous. Indeed, while no one doubts that ACh, AChE, and ChAc are necessary for function at the cholinergic synapses, no one will claim that these substances are able to effect transmission without appropriate anatomical structurization. Additionally, the maintenance of neuronal transmission may require, besides appropriate morphogenesis, the presence of non-cholinergic substances and mechanisms (Karczmar and Nishi, 1971; Karczmar, Nishi, and Blaber, 1970). This general conceptualization must be applied, in a different way to the brain and the CNS on the one hand, and to certain peripheral synapses and junctions on the other. Indeed, in the case of the former, the cholinergic synapses identified at present are few, and there is suspicion that even when the pertinent work is finished, they will still constitute the minority among the central synapses. Perhaps it may then be claimed that the imperfect ontogenetic parallelism between the ACh system and nerve function is exactly what we can expect. However, it should also be kept in mind that the cholinergic synapses, as few as these may be, and/or cholinoceptivity of non-cholinergic central neurons (see Introduction) are very important for the organizational and functional aspects of the CNS (Karczmar, 1970; Karczmar and Nishi, 1971; Karczmar et al., 1970; Karczmar, Nishi, and Blaber, 1972a).

What then about the peripheral sites where the "pure" cholinergic synapses exist in the adult—as in the case of the sympathetic ganglia and of the cardiovagal and skeletal neuromyal junctions? There seems to be a divergence of opinion in the case of the latter, as Filogamo and Marchisio (1971) felt that ontogenesis of the ACh system coincides with that of neuromyal function, while Koelle (1963) and Gerebtzoff (1959) opined that the ACh system—particularly AChE—is precocious compared to function (see also Karczmar, 1963a). There is no doubt that the response of the junction to ACh is precocious, while frequently postnatal maturation is needed before it acquires the adult pattern (see Kupfer and Koelle, 1951; Wise and McQuillen, 1970; Mann and Salatsky, 1970). Fewer data are available with regard to the relationship between neurogenesis, functionalization, and the development of ACh system in the sympathetic ganglia. It is, however, pertinent in this context that, as stated by Giacobini (Giacobini et al., 1970), monoamine oxidase and other components of the adrenergic system other than AChE and ChAc, are important in the ganglion not only with regard to the functionalization of the post-ganglionic sympathetic nerve endings, but also with regard to the cell bodies, and the maximal activity of these enzymes corresponds to the synaptizations and "maturational activity" within the ganglion. It may therefore be stated altogether that the ACh system is just one of the components of the multiple maturation process. One more aspect of this multiplicity should be stressed.

Isozymes and AChE fractions

Certain data were adduced above (Iqbal and Talwar, 1971; Karczmar et al., 1972*b,c*) which may suggest that the ontogenesis of the isozymes of AChE may be a better marker of the development of function than AChE taken as an entity. Particularly, a drastic shift in the total pattern of AChE and BuChE isozymes could have such a meaning (Karczmar et al., 1972*b,c*). The isozymes may exhibit differential localization in certain membrane and receptor structures, and their appearance in ontogenesis may indicate the emergence of certain functional patterns dependent upon stereochemical isozyme-subcellular couplings. Their physical characteristics may dictate the patterns of their migration in the axon, their localization with regard to cell constituents, and their incorporation in the neuronal membranes; this suggestion of Koelle, Hossaini, Akbarzadek, and Koelle (1970) may embrace both isozymes and subfractions of AChE independent of its isozymal differentiation. Moreover, the same reasoning may be applied to ChAc, which was not studied from this particular viewpoint, or for that matter to ACh and its various forms (free, releasable, or stored, vesicular or extravesicular).

Although further ontogenetic studies along these lines will offer pertinent and important data, certain aspects of the problem raised above seem beyond this approach, such as, for instance, those of the ephemeral ontogenetic appearance of ChAc and AChE in non-cholinergic neurons, of the preneural presence of these substances, or of their inductive and related functions. On at least some occasions, the components of the ACh system may have nothing to do with the cholinergic synapses; as expressed by Filogamo (Filogamo and Marchisio, 1971), this system at the earlier stages of neuroblast development "is independent of synaptic contacts . . . and . . . is a primitive and peculiar property of neuroblasts."

What may be these "independent" functions, not related to transmission? What may be, furthermore, the role of ephemeral or non-neuronal AChE and ChAc?

Morphogenetic, trophic, and transport function

In the body of this review, morphogenetic functions of AChE and/or ACh and morphogenetic effects of cholinergic agents are emphasized. It appears that the ACh system may play an inductor role in the formation of the end plate and the structuralization of its AChE, ChE, and their isozymes, in the embryogenetic cell movements of such diverse forms of echinoderms (see above) and chick (Drews and Kussätzer, 1971), or in the formation of the CNS, at least as indicated by the blocking effect of hemicholiniums on neurogenesis (Becker, Linder, and Gibson, 1967). In fact, induction of the CNS by the chorda-mesoderm implant during amphibian development leads also to the induction of ChE (Boell and Shen, 1944; Boell, 1948); it is regrettable that the inductive capacity of the components of the ACh system was apparently never tested. It is difficult to say whether or not the role of the cholinergic system in regeneration and in growth (trophic action) is related to its morphogenetic role. In any event, 25 years ago, I (Karczmar, 1946), as well as Giacobini, Filogamo, and others more recently, strongly suggested that the ontogenetic presence of the ACh system may be required not only for the future cholinergic synapses but for differentiation, maturation, and growth. It should be pointed out in this context that a factor independent of the ACh system and of the cholinergic innervation may be concerned in regeneratives and trophic phenomena (see above).

Even more generally, it must be remembered that ACh and/or AChE may be involved in and needed for secretory, transport and metabolic phenomena. Koelle (1963) describes a number of systems in which ACh or AChE may regulate membrane permeability; in fact, this may explain the presence of AChE and/or ACh in a number of adult non-neuronal systems, including certain types of skin and membranes, and the red blood cells of certain vertebrates. It is particularly interesting that ACh and anti-ChE agents affected the permeability of the latter as well as of the frog skin to cations (see Koelle, 1963). The mechanism underlying the role of ACh in permeability and in transport phenomena concerning both micro- (ions) and macromolecular transport was laid down by Hokin (Hokin and Hokin, 1960; Hokin, 1969). The process in question involves phosphate incorporation into the phosphaditic acid molecule, as well as changes in phospholipids. In fact, ACh was shown to increase the phospholipid turnover as well as the phosphate incorporation into phosphaditic acid (Schramm, 1968; Lockwood and Williams-Ashman, 1970). This mechanism may then explain the presence of the ACh system not only in various membranes subserving transport (see Koelle, 1963) but also in organs concerned with secretory activity such as seminal vesicles (Lockwood and Williams-Ashman, 1970), parotid gland, and others (Schramm, 1967, 1968). In our context, one may hypothesize that macromolecular and ionic transport may require the cellular presence of the ACh system independently of its role in transmission, synaptization, or morphogenesis.

Altogether, it seems obvious that today it would be simplistic to account for the appearance of the ACh system in ontogenesis or phylogenesis as the single concomitant of transmittive function. The cholinergic synapses require, obviously, more than just the chemical presence of this system, which in addition seems necessary for certain nonsynaptic processes. Furthermore, the system itself appears to be more complex than ever, since its pattern of function may depend not just on AChE and ChAc as single entities but on their isozymes. Nevertheless, tremendous strides have been made in the past few years in the pertinent areas, and the time seems near when all these aspects of the problem will be fully clarified, and when the earlier reference of this author (Karczmar, 1967) to the "exasperatingly . . . complex picture," most difficult to understand, of the cholinergic system will become a "grandfather-clock" statement.

ACKNOWLEDGMENT

The published and unpublished results from the laboratories of the senior author were supported in part by NIH research grant IROI NB 06455, NIH training grant GM 00077, and Illinois Mental Health Research Grant 17-176.

REFERENCES

Adams, R. L. P. (1963): Periodical activation of lysosomal enzymes during regeneration of liver. *Biochemical Journal,* 87:532-536.

Adlard, B. P. F., and Dobbing, J. (1971): Elevated acetylcholinesterase activity in adult rat brain after undernutrition in early life. *Brain Research*, 30:198-199.

Agarwal, I. P., and Monga, J. N. (1958): Morphogenetic effects of eserine sulphate. *Journal of the Anatomical Society of India*, 7:15-18.

Ancel, P. (1945): L'achondroplasie. Sa réalisation éxperimentale, sa pathogénie. *Annales d'Endocrinologie*, 6:1-24.

Axelsson, J., and Thesleff, S. (1959): A study of supersensitivity in denervated mammalian skeletal muscle. *Journal of Physiology*, 147:178-193.

Bacq, Z. M. (1935): Recherches sur la physiologie et al pharmacologie du système nerveux autonome, XVII. Les esters de la choline dans les extraits de tissus des invertébres. *Archives Internationales de Physiologie*, 42:24-42.

Barron, K. D., Ordinario, A. T., Bernsohn, J., Hess, A. R., and Heduck, M. T. (1968): Cholinesterases and non-specific esterases of developing and adult (normal and atrophic) rat gastrocnemius. I. Chemical assay and electrophoresis. *Journal of Histochemistry and Cytochemistry*, 16:346-361.

Barron, K. D., and Bernsohn, J. (1965): Brain esterases and phosphatases in multiple sclerosis. *Annals of the New York Academy of Sciences*, 122:369-399.

Barron, K. D., and Bernsohn, J. (1968): Esterase of developing human brain. *Journal of Neurochemistry*, 15:273-284.

Barron, K. D., Bernsohn, J., and Hess, A. R. (1963): Abnormalities in brain esterases in multiple sclerosis. *Proceedings of the Society for Experimental Biology and Medicine*, 113:521-524.

Barron, K. D., Bernsohn, J., and Hess, A. R. (1966): Esterases and proteins of normal and atrophic feline muscle. *Journal of Histochemistry and Cytochemistry*, 14:1-24.

Barron, K. D., Bernsohn, J., and Ordinario, A. T. (1967): Proteins, non-specific and cholinesterases of rat gastrocnemius and effects of tenotomy and denervations. *Journal of Histochemistry and Cytochemistry*, 15:782-783.

Becker, B. A., Linder, J., and Gibson, J. E. (1967): Effect of hemicholinium on the morphology of the developing chick embryo. *Toxicology and Applied Pharmacology*, 10:27-39.

Begliomini, A., and Moriconi, A. (1960): On the time of appearance and localization of cholinesterase in the striped muscle of the chick embryo. *Rivista di Biologia*, 51:517-531.

Bennett, E. L., and Rosenzweig, M. R. (1969): Central cholinergic transmission; Comments and general discussion. In: *Symposium on Central Cholinergic Transmission and Its Behavioral Aspects*, edited by A. G. Karczmar. *Federation Proceedings*, 28:158-159.

Bernsohn, J., and Barron, K. D. (1964): Multiple molecular forms of brain hydrolases. *International Review of Neurobiology*, 7:297-344.

Bernsohn, J., Barron, K. D., Doolin, R. F., Hess, A. R., and Hedrick, M. T. (1966): Subcellular localization of rat brain esterases. *The Journal of Histochemistry and Cytochemistry*, 14:455-472.

Bernsohn, J., Barron, K. D., and Hess, A. R. (1964): Esterase activity and zymogram pattern in developing rat brain. In: *Progress in Brain Research*, edited by Williamina A. Himwich and Harold E. Himwich, 9:161-164. Elsevier Publishing Company, Amsterdam.

Bernsohn, J., Barron, K. D., Hess, A. R., and Hedrick, M. T. (1963): Alterations in properties and isoenzyme patterns of esterases in developing rat brain. *Journal of Neurochemistry*, 10:783-794.

Boell, E. J. (1948): Biochemical differentiation during amphibian development. *Annals of the New York Academy of Sciences*, 49:773-800.

Boell, E. J., Greenfield, P., and Shen, S. C. (1955): Development of cholinesterase in the optic lobes of the frog (*Rana pipiens*). *The Journal of Experimental Zoology*, 129:415-452.

Boell, E. J., and Shen, S. C. (1944): Functional differentiation in embryonic development. I. Cholinesterase activity of induced neural structures in *Amblystoma punctatum*. *Journal of Experimental Zoology*, 97:21-44.

Boréus, L. O. (1967): Pharmacology of the human fetus: Dose-effect relationships for acetylcholine during ontogenesis. *Biologia Neonatorum*, 11:328-337.

Boréus, L. O. (1968): Demonstration of a receptor reserve for acetylcholine in the human fetus. *Acta Physiologica Scandinavica*, 72:194-199.

Boréus, L. O., Malmfors, T., McMurphy, D. M., and Olson, L. (1969): Demonstration of adrenergic receptor function and innervation in the ductus arteriosus of the human fetus. *Acta Physiologica Scandinavica*, 77:316-321.

Boréus, L. O., and McMurphy, D. M. (1971): Ontogenetic development of cholinergic receptor function in guinea pig ileum. *Acta Physiologica Scandinavica*, 81:143-144.

Bracha, P., and O'Brien, R. D. (1966): The relation between physical properties and uptake of insecticides by eggs of the large milkweed bug. *Journal of Economic Entomology*, 59:1255-1264.

Brzin, M., and Tennyson, V. (1967): Microgasometric and ultracytochemical study of cholinesterase development in the embryonic and adult rabbit. *Journal of Cell Biology*, 35:18A.

Bull, G., Hebb, C., and Ratkovic, D. (1956): Choline acetylase in the central nervous system of man and some other mammals. *Journal of Physiology*, 134:718-728.

Bull, G., Hebb, C., and Ratkovic, D. (1970): Choline acetyltransferase activity of human brain tissue during development and at maturity. *Journal of Neurochemistry*, 17:1505-1516.

Bunge, R. P., and Bunge, M. B. (1965): Ultrastructural characteristics of synapses forming in cultured spinal cord. *Anatomical Record*, 151A:329.

Burdick, C. J., and Strittmatter, G. F. (1965): Appearance of biochemical components related to acetylcholine metabolism during the embryonic development of chick brain. *Archives of Biochemistry and Biophysics*, 109:293-301.

Burt, A. M. (1968): Acetylcholinesterase and choline acetyltransferase activity in the developing chick spinal cord. *Journal of Experimental Zoology*, 169:107-112.

Burt, A. M., and Narayanan, C. H. (1970): Effect of extrinsic neuronal connections on development of acetylcholinesterase and choline acetyltransferase activity in the ventral half of the chick spinal cord. *Experimental Neurology*, 29:201-210.

Buznikov, G. A., Chudakova, I. V., Berchysheva, L. V., and Vyazmina, N. M. (1968): The role of neurohumors in early embryogenesis. *Journal of Embryology and Experimental Morphology*, 20:119-128.

Buznikov, G. A., Chudakova, I. V., and Zvezdina, N. D. (1964): The role of neurohumours in early embryogenesis. I. Serotonin content of developing embryos of sea urchin and loach. *Journal of Embryology and Experimental Morphology*, 12:563-573.

Buznikov, G. A., Kost, A. N., Kucherova, N. F., Mndzhoyan, A. L., Suvorov, N. N., and Berchysheva, L. V. (1970): The role of neurohumors in early embryogenesis. III. Pharmacological analysis of the role of neurohumors in cleavage divisions. *Journal of Embryology and Experimental Morphology*, 23:549-570.

Cantino, D. (1969): Proc. Ital. Eighth Congr. Electron Microscopy, p. 287.

Cantino, D. (1970): An histochemical study of the nerve supply to the developing alimentary tract. *Experientia*, 26:766-767.

Chadwick, L. E. (1963): Actions on insects and other invertebrates. In: *Handbuch der experimentellen Pharmakologie*, Vol. 15; *Cholinesterases and Anticholinesterase Agents*, edited by G. B. Koelle. Springer-Verlag, Berlin, pp. 741-798.

Chino, H., and Yushima, T. (1953): On the occurrences of an acetylcholine-like substance in some insect eggs. 2. The changes in acetylcholine-like substance during embryonic development in some insect eggs. *Annotationes Zoologicae Japonenses*, 26:233-237.

Coghill, G. E. (1933): Somatic myogenic action in embryos of *Fundulus heteroclitus*. *Proceedings of the Society for Experimental Biology and Medicine*, 31:62-64.

Cohn, P., and Richter, D. (1956): Enzymic development and maturation of the hypothalamus. *Journal of Neurochemistry*, 1:166-172.

Coraboeuf, E., LeDouarin, G., and Obrecht-Coutris, G. (1970): Release of acetylcholine by chick embryo heart before innervation. *Journal of Physiology*, 206:383-395.

Corner, M. A., and Bot, A. P. C. (1967): Developmental patterns in the central nervous system of birds. III. Somatic motility during the embryonic period and its relation to behavior after hatching. In: *Progress in Brain Research: Developmental Neurology*, edited by C. G. Bernhard and J. P. Schadé. 26:214-236. Elsevier, Amsterdam.

Corner, M. A., Schadé, J. P., Sedlacek, J., Stoeckart, R., and Bot, A. P. C. (1967): Developmental patterns in the central nervous system of birds. I. Electrical activity in the cerebral hemisphere, optic lobe, and cerebellum. In: *Progress in Brain Research: Developmental Neurology*, edited by C. T. Bernhard and J. P. Schadé. 26:145-192. Elsevier, Amsterdam.

Couteaux, R. (1955): Localizations of cholinesterase at neuromuscular junctions. *International Review of Cytology*, 4:335-375.

Dewhurst, S. A., McCaman, R. E., and Kaplan, W. D. (1970): The time course of development of acetylcholinesterase and choline acetyltransferase in *Drosophila melanogaster*. *Biochemical Genetics*, 4:499-508.

Diamond, J., and Miledi, R. (1962): A study of foetal and newborn rat muscle fibers. *Journal of Physiology*, 162:393-408.

Drachman, D. B. (1964): Atrophy of skeletal muscle in chick embryos treated with botulinum toxin. *Science*, 145:719-721.

Drachman, D. B. (1967): Is acetylcholine the trophic neuromuscular transmitter? *Archives of Neurology*, 17:206-218.

Drachman, D. B., and Coulombre, A. J. (1962): Experimental clubfoot and arthrogryposis multiplex congenita. *Lancet*, II:523-526.

Drachman, D. B., and Romand, F. C. A. (1970): Effect of neuromuscular blockade on enzymatic activities of muscles. *Archives of Neurology*, 23:85-89.

Drachman, D. B., and Singer, M. (1971): Regeneration in botulinum-poisoned forelimbs of the newt, *Triturus*. *Experimental Neurology*, 32:1-11.

Drews, U., and Kussäther, E. (1971): Cholinesterase bei der Knorpelen-entwicklung *in vitro*. *Anatomischer Anzeiger*, 128: (Suppl.) 453-454.

Dryden, W. F. (1970): Development of acetylcholine sensitivity in cultured skeletal muscle. *Experientia*, 26:984-986.

Duffy, P. E., Tennyson, V. M., and Brzin, M. (1967): Cholinesterase in adult and embryonic hypothalamus. A combined cytochemical electron microscopic study. *Archives of Neurology*, 16:385-403.

Durante, M. (1956): Cholinesterase in the development of the ascidian, *Ciona intestinalis*. *Experientia*, 12:307-308.

Durante, M. (1957): Cholinesterase in the anterior and posterior hemiembryos of *Ciona intestinalis*. *Acta Embryologiae et Morphologiae Experimentalis*, 1:131-133.

Eccles, J. C. (1972): Possible synaptic mechanisms subserving learning. In: *Symposium on the Brain and Human Behavior*, edited by A. G. Karczmar and J. C. Eccles. Springer-Verlag, Berlin, pp. 39-61.

Engel, W. K. (1961): Cytochemical localization of cholinesterase in cultured skeletal muscle. *Journal of Histochemistry and Cytochemistry*, 9:66-72.

Estrugo, S. F., Bernsohn, J., Barron, K. D., and Hess, A. (1969): Isolation and properties of some molecular species of human brain esterases. *Biochimica et Biophysica Acta*, 171:265-276.

Fahn, S., and Cote, L. J. (1968): Regional distribution of choline acetylase in the brain of the rhesus monkey. *Brain Research*, 7:323-325.

Ferrand, R., and LeDouarin, G. (1971): Cholinesterase activities demonstrated in the chick embryo in adenohypophyseal tissue differentiated in situ or as a chorioallontoic graft. *Comptes Rendus Hebdomaires des Séances de L'Academie des Sciences: Serie D,* 272:1531-1533.

Filogamo, G. (1960a): *Bulletin de l'Association des Anatomistes,* 44:251.

Filogamo, G. (1960b): Experimental research on the activity of specific and non-specific cholinesterases in the development of the optic lobe of the chicken. *Archives de Biologie,* 71:159-198.

Filogamo, G. (1963): *Bulletin de l'Association des Anatomistes,* 48:115.

Filogamo, G., Giacobini, E., Giacobini, G., and Noré, B. (1971): Developmental changes of DOPA decarboxylase in chick embryo and chick spinal and sympathetic ganglia. *Journal of Neurochemistry,* 18:1589-1591.

Filogamo, G., and Marchisio, P. C. (1971): Acetylcholine system and development. In: *Neurosciences Research,* edited by S. Ehrenpreis and O. C. Solnitsky. Academic Press, New York, pp. 29-64.

Filogamo, G., and Mussa, A. (1967): Effects of spinal cord removal on the earliest AChE activity of the myotomes in the chick embryo. *Acta Embryologiae et Morphologia Experimentalis,* 9:274-279.

Filogamo, G., and Robecchi, M. G. (1969): Neuroblasts in the olfactory pits in mammals. *Acta Anatomica,* 56 (Suppl.): 182-187.

Filogamo, G., and Strumia, E. (1958): Ricerche sperimentali sulle correlazioni interneuroniche nello sviluppo dei centri e delle vie ottiche nel pollo. *Rendiconti Accademia Nazionale dei Lincei,* 25:119-120.

Fischback, G. D., Nameroff, M., and Nelson, R. G. (1970): Electrical properties of chick skeletal muscle fibers developing in tissue culture. *Biophysical Society Abstracts,* 14th Annual Meeting, 76a.

Francis, C. M. (1953): Cholinesterase in the retina. *Journal of Physiology,* 120:435-439.

Franz, W., and Krish, K. (1968): Acylgruppenüberträgung auf aromatische Amine durch Carboxylesterasen. *Hoppe-Seylers' Zeitschrift für Physiologische Chemie,* 349: 1413-1422.

Frey, H. J., Riekinnen, P. J., Rinne, U. K., and Arstila, A. U. (1970): Peptidase activity of myelin during the myelination period in guinea pig brain. *Brain Research,* 22:243-248.

Frey, H. J., Arstila, A. U., Rinne, U. K., and Riekinnen, P. J. (1971): Esterases in developing CNS myelin. *Brain Research,* 30:159-167.

Geiger, R. S. (1960): Effects of LSD-25, serotonin and sera from schizophrenic patients on adult mammalian brain cultures. *Journal of Neuropsychiatry,* 1:185-199.

Geiger, R. S. (1962): Localization of cholinesterases in adult mammalian brain. *International Journal of Neuropharmacology,* 1:295-302.

Gennsner, G., and Nilsson, E. (1970): Response to adrenaline, acetylcholine and change of contraction frequency in early human hearts. *Experientia,* 26:1105-1107.

Gerebtzoff, M. A. (1954): Appareil cholinestérasique á l'insertion tendineuse des fibres musculaires striées. *Comptes Rendus des Séances de la Société de Biologie,* 148:632-634.

Gerebtzoff, M. A. (1959): *Cholinesterases.* Pergamon Press, New York.

Giacobini, G. (1970a): Development changes of choline acetyltransferase in chick muscles and peripheral nerves of the chick embryo. *Bollettino della Societa Italiana di Biologia Sperimentale,* 46:807-869.

Giacobini, G. (1970b): Development of choline acetyltransferase activity in wing muscles and peripheral nerves of the chick embryo. *Bollettino della Societa Italiana di Biologia Sperimentale,* 46:867-869.

Giacobini, E. (1971): Biochemistry of the developing autonomic neuron. In: *Chemistry and Brain Development,* edited by R. Paoletti and A. N. Davison. Plenum Press, New York, pp. 145-155.

Giacobini, G., Marchisio, P. C., Giacobini, E., and Koslow, S. H. (1970): Developmental changes of cholinesterase and monoamine oxidase in chick embryo spinal and sympathetic ganglia. *Journal of Neurochemistry*, 17:1177-1185.

Gibson, J. E., and Becker, B. A. (1969): Impairment of motor function of neonatal chicks by hemicholinium treatment during incubation. *Toxicology and Applied Pharmacology*, 14:380-932.

Glees, P., and Sheppard, B. L. (1964): Electron microscopical studies of the synapse in the developing chick spinal cord. *Zeitschrift für Zellforschung*, 62:356-362.

Goedde, H. W., Doenicke, A., and Altland, K. (1967): *Pseudocholinesterasen*. Springer-Verlag, Berlin.

Goodwin, B. C., and Sizer, I. W. (1965): Effects of spinal cord and substrate on acetylcholinesterase in chick embryonic skeletal muscle. *Developmental Biology*, 11:136-153.

Gustafson, T. (1963): Cellular mechanisms in the morphogenesis of the sea urchin embryo. *Experimental Cell Research*, 32:570-589.

Gustafson, T. (1969): Cell recognition and cell contacts during sea urchin development. In: *Cellular Recognition*, edited by T. Smith and R. A. Good. Appleton-Century-Crofts, New York, pp. 47-60.

Gustafson, T., and Toneby, M. I. (1970): On the role of serotonin and acetylcholine in sea urchin morphogenesis. *Experimental Cell Research*, 62:108-117.

Gustafson, T., and Toneby, M. I. (1971): How genes control morphogenesis. The role of serotonin and acetylcholine in morphogenesis. *American Scientist*, 59:452-462.

Gustafson, T., and Wolpert, L. (1967): Cellular movement and contact in sea urchin morphogenesis. *Experimental Cell Research*, 62:102-117.

Guth, L. (1969): Trophic effects of vertebrate neurons. *Neurosciences Research Program Bulletin*, 7:1-70.

Guth, L., Albers, R. W., and Brown, W. C. (1964): Quantitative changes in cholinesterase activity of denervated muscle fibers and sole plates. *Experimental Neurology*, 10:236-250.

Guttman, E. (1963): Evidence for the trophic function of the nerve cell in neuromuscular relations. In: *The Effect of Use and Disuse on Neuromuscular Functions*, edited by P. Hník. Elsevier, Amsterdam, pp. 29-34.

Hagopian, M., Tennyson, V. M., and Spiro, D. (1969): Cytochemical localization of cholinesterase in embryonic rabbit cardiac muscle. *Journal of Histochemistry and Cytochemistry*, 18:38-43.

Hebb, C. O. (1957): Biochemical evidence for the neural function of acetylcholine. *Physiological Reviews*, 37:196-220.

Hebb, C. O. (1963): Formation, storage and liberation of acetylcholine. In: *Handbuch der experimentellen Pharmakologie*, Vol. 15; *Cholinesterases and Anticholinesterase Agents*, edited by G. B. Koelle. Springer-Verlag, Berlin, pp. 55-88.

Hebb, C., and Silver, A. (1956): Choline acetylase in the central nervous system of man and some other mammals. *Journal of Physiology*, 134:718-728.

Hess, A. (1960): The effects of eye removal on the development of cholinesterase in the superior colliculus. *Journal of Experimental Zoology*, 144:11-24.

Hess, A. (1961): The effect of unilateral eye removal on the cholinesterase activity of the optic tectum of adult frogs. *Anatomical Record*, 140:295-305.

Hirano, H. (1967): Ultrastructural study on the morphogenesis of the neuromuscular junction in the skeletal muscle of the chick. *Zeitschrift für Zellforschung*, 79:198-208.

Hokin, L. E., and Hokin, M. R. (1960): Studies on the carrier function of phosphatidic acid in sodium transport. I. The turnover of phosphatidic acid and phosphoinositide in the avian salt gland on stimulation of secretion. *Journal of General Physiology*, 44:61-85.

Hokin, L. E. (1969): Functional activity in glands and synaptic tissue and the turnover of phosphatidyl inositol. *Annals of the New York Academy of Sciences,* 165:695-709.

Holmes, R. S., and White, G. S. ((1970): Developmental genetics of the esterase isozymes of *Fundulus heteroclitus. Biochemical Genetics,* 4:47-480.

Holmstedt, B., and Sjöqvist, F. (1961): Some principles about histochemistry of cholinesterase with special reference to the thiocholine method. In: *Symposium on Histochemistry of Cholinesterase,* Basel, 2:1-10. *Bibliotheca Anatomica.*

Hösli, E., and Hösli, L. (1971): Acetylcholinesterase in cultured rat spinal cord. *Brain Research,* 30:193-197.

Hui, E., and Smith, A. (1970): Regeneration of the amputated amphibian limb: Retardation by hemicholinium-3. *Science,* 170:1313-1314.

Iqbal, Z., and Talwar, G. P. (1970): Acetylcholinesterase in developing chick embryo brain. *Journal of Neurochemistry,* 18:1261-1267.

James, D. W., and Tresman, R. L. (1969): An electron-microscopic study of the de novo formation of neuromuscular junctions in tissue culture. *Zeitschrift für Zellforschung,* 100:126-140.

Juntunen, J., and Teravainen, H. (1970): Morphogenesis of myoneural junctions induced postnatally in the tibialis anterior muscle of the rat. *Acta Physiologica Scandinavica,* 79:462-468.

Kano, M., Shimada, Y., and Ishikawa, K. (1971): Acetylcholine sensitivity of skeletal muscle cells differentiated *in vitro* from chick embryo. *Brain Research,* 25:216-219.

Karczmar, A. G. (1946): The role of amputation and nerve resection in the regressing limbs of urodele larvae. *Journal of Experimental Zoology,* 103:401-427.

Karczmar, A. G. (1955): Limb regeneration and differentiation of "overt behavior" in urodeles as studied by means of their response to chemical agents. *Annals of the New York Academy of Sciences,* 60:1108-1135.

Karczmar, A. G. (1963a): Ontogenesis of cholinesterases. In: *Handbuch der experimentellen Pharmakologie,* Vol. 15; *Cholinesterases and Anticholinesterase Agents,* edited by G. B. Koelle, pp. 129-186. Springer-Verlag, Berlin.

Karczmar, A. G. (1963b): Ontogenetic effects of anti-cholinesterase agents. In: *Handbuch der experimentellen Pharmakologie,* Vol. 15; *Cholinesterases and Anticholinesterase Agents,* edited by G. B. Koelle, pp. 799-832. Springer-Verlag, Berlin.

Karczmar, A. G. (1967): Pharmacologic, toxicologic, and therapeutic properties of anti-cholinesterase agents. In: *Physiological Pharmacology,* edited by W. S. Root and F. G. Hofmann. Academic Press, New York, pp. 163-322.

Karczmar, A. G. (1969): Is the cholinergic central nervous system over-exploited? In: *Symposium on Central Cholinergic Transmission and Its Behavioral Aspects,* edited by A. G. Karczmar. *Federation Proceedings,* 28:147-157.

Karczmar, A. G. (1970): Central cholinergic pathways and their behavioral implications. In: *Principles of Psychopharmacology,* edited by W. G. Clark and J. del Giudice, Academic Press, New York, pp. 57-86.

Karczmar, A. G., and Berg, G. G. (1951): Alkaline phosphatase during limb development and regeneration of *Amblystoma opacum* and *Amblystoma punctatum. Journal of Experimental Zoology,* 117:319-364.

Karczmar, A. G., and Berg, G. G. (1952): Effects of dibenzanthracene and methylcholanthrene on forelimb regeneration of urodele larvae. *Journal of Morphology,* 91:479-514.

Karczmar, A. G., and Koppanyi, T. (1953): Central effects of diisopropylfluorophosphonate (DFP) in urodele larvae. *Archiv für Experimentelle Pathologie und Pharmakologie,* 219:263-272.

Karczmar, A. G., and Nishi, S. (1971): The types and sites of cholinergic receptors. In: *Advances in Cytopharmacology,* Vol. 1, edited by F. Clementi and B. Ceccarelli. Raven Press, New York, pp. 301-317.

Karczmar, A. G., Nishi, S., and Blaber, L. C. (1970): Investigations, particularly by means of the anti-cholinesterase agents, of the multiple peripheral and central cholinergic mechanisms. *Acta Vitaminologica et Enzymologica,* 24:131-189.

Karczmar, A. G., Nishi, S., and Blaber, L. C. (1972*a*): Synaptic modulations. In: *Brain and Human Behavior,* edited by A. G. Karczmar and J. C. Eccles. Springer-Verlag, Berlin, pp. 63-92.

Karczmar, A. G., Srinivasan, R., and Bernsohn, J. (1972*b*): Effects of drugs on ontogenesis of mouse acetyl- and butyrylcholinesterase isozymes. *Neuropharmacology* (*in press*).

Karczmar, A. G., Srinivasan, R., and Bernsohn, J. (1972*c*): Ontogenesis of isozymes of acetylcholinesterase and butyrylcholinesterase of the mouse. *Neuropharmacology* (*in press*).

Kelly, A. M., and Zacks, S. I. (1969): The fine structure of motor endplate morphogenesis. *Journal of Cell Biology,* 42:154-169.

Kerr, W. P., and Brazzel, J. R. (1960): Laboratory tests of insecticides against eggs and larvae of the cabbage looper. *Journal of Economic Entomology,* 53:991-992.

Khera, K. S., LaHam, Q. N., Ellis, C. F. G., Zawidzka, Z. Z., and Grice, H. C. (1966): Foot deformity in ducks from injections of EPN during embryogenesis. *Toxicology and Applied Pharmacology,* 8:540-549.

Kling, A., Finer, S., and Nair, V. (1965): Effects of early handling and light stimulation on the acetylcholinesterase activity of the developing rat brain. *International Journal of Neuropharmacology,* 4:353-357.

Kling, A., Finer, S., and Gilmour, J. (1969): Regional development of acetylcholinesterase activity in the maternally reared and maternally deprived cat. *International Journal of Neuropharmacology,* 8:25-31.

Koelle, G. B. (1963): Cytological distribution and physiological functions of cholinesterases. In: *Handbuch der experimentellen Pharmakologie,* Vol. 15; *Cholinesterases and Anticholinesterase Agents,* edited by G. B. Koelle, pp. 187-298. Springer-Verlag, Berlin.

Koelle, G. B. (1969): Significance of acetylcholinesterase in central synaptic transmission. In: *Symposium on Central Cholinergic Transmission and Its Behavioral Aspects,* edited by A. G. Karczmar, *Federation Proceedings,* 28:147-157.

Koelle, W. A., Hossaini, K. S., Akbarzadek, P., and Koelle, G. B. (1970): Histochemical evidence and consequences of the occurrence of isoenzymes of acetylcholinesterase. *Journal of Histochemistry and Cytochemistry,* 18:812-819.

Koelle, G. B., Wolfand, L., Friedenwald, J. S., and Allen, R. A. (1952): Localization of specific cholinesterase in ocular tissues of the cat. *American Journal of Ophthalmology,* 35:1580-1584.

Koenig, E. (1965): Synthetic mechanisms in the axon. II. RNA in myelin-free axons of the cat. *Journal of Neurochemistry,* 12:357-361.

Koenig, E. (1967): Synthetic mechanisms in the axon. III. Stimulation of acetylcholinesterase synthesis by actinomycin-D in the hypoglossal nerve. *Journal of Neurochemistry,* 14:429-435.

Koenig, E., and Koelle, G. B. (1961): Mode of regeneration of acetylcholinesterase in cholinergic neurons following irreversible inactivation. *Journal of Neurochemistry,* 8:1969-1988.

Koenig, J., and Pecot-Dechavassine, M. (1971): Relations entre l'apparition des potentials miniature spontanés et l'ultrastructure des plaques motrices en voie de reinnervation et de neoformation chez le rat. *Brain Research,* 27:43-57.

Koeppen, A. H., Barron, K. D., and Bernsohn, J. (1969): Redistribution of rat brain esterases during subcellular fractionation. *Biochimica et Biophysica Acta,* 183:253-264.

Koppanyi, T., and Karczmar, A. G. (1947): Pharmacological methods in the study of overt behavior. *Federation Proceedings,* 6:346.

Kovács, T., Kover, A., and Balogh, C. (1961): Localization of cholinesterase in various types of muscle. *Journal of Cellular and Comparative Physiology*, 57:63-71.

Krysan, J. L., and Guss, P. L. (1971): Paraoxon inhibition of an insect egg lipase. *Biochimica et Biophysica Acta*, 239:349-352.

Kupfer, C., and Koelle, G. B. (1951): A histochemical study of cholinesterase during formation of the motor end plate of the albino rat. *Journal of Experimental Zoology*, 116:397-415.

Landauer, W. (1949): Le problème de l'électivité dans les expériences de la tératogenèse biochimique. *Archives d'Anatomie Microscopique et de Morphologie Experimentale*, 38:184-189.

Landauer, W. (1954): On the chemical production of developmental abnormalities and of phenocopies in chicken embryos. *Journal of Cellular and Comparative Physiology*, 43:261-305.

Landauer, W. (1960): Nicotine-induced malformations of chicken embryos and their bearing on the phenocopy problem. *Journal of Experimental Zoology*, 143:107-122.

Larrabee, M. G., Partlow, M. L., and Brown, W. T. (1969): Abstr, 2nd Int. Meet. International Society for Neurochemistry, Milano, pp. 261.

Lebowitz, P., and Singer, M. (1970): Neurotrophic control of protein synthesis in the regenerating limb of the newt *Triturus*. *Nature*, 225:824-827.

Lehrer, G. M., Maliner, R., and Gioia, M. (1966): The electron microscope localization of acetylcholinesterase in the guinea pig organ of Corti. *Journal of Histochemistry and Cytochemistry*, 14:816A.

Lentz, T. L. (1969a): Cytological studies of muscle dedifferentiation and differentiation during limb regeneration of the newt *Triturus*. *American Journal of Anatomy*, 124:447-479.

Lentz, T. L. (1969b): Development of the neuro-muscular junction. I. Cytological and cytochemical studies on the neuromuscular junction of differentiating muscle in the regenerating limb of the newt *Triturus*. *Journal of Cell Biology*, 42:431-443.

Lentz, T. L. (1970): Development of the neuromuscular junction. II. Cytological and cytochemical studies on the neuromuscular junction of dedifferentiating muscle in the regenerating limb of the newt *Triturus*. *Journal of Cell Biology*, 47:423-436.

Lentz, T. L. (1971): Nerve trophic function: *In vitro* assay of effects of nerve tissue on muscle cholinesterase activity. *Science*, 171:187-189.

Lentz, T., and Barrnett, R. (1963): The role of the nervous system in regenerating hydra: The effect of neuropharmacological agents. *Journal of Experimental Zoology*, 154:305-328.

Leplat, G., and Gerebtzoff, M. A. (1956): Localization de l'acétylcholinesterase et des médiateurs diphénoliques dans la retine. *Annales d'Oculistique*, (Paris), 189: 121-128.

Levi-Montalcini, R., and Hamburger, V. (1953): A diffusible agent of mouse sarcoma producing hyperplasia of sympathetic ganglia and hyperneurotization of viscera in chick embryo. *Journal of Experimental Zoology*, 165:233-278.

Liddell, J., Newman, G. E., and Brown, D. F. (1963): A pseudocholinesterase variant in human tissue. *Nature*, 198:1090-1091.

Lindeman, V. F. (1947): The cholinesterase and acetylcholine content of the chick retina with special reference to functional activity as indicated by the pupillary constrictor reflex. *American Journal of Physiology*, 148:40-44.

Lissak, M., Toro, I., and Pasztor, J. (1942): Untersuchungen über den Zusamenhang des Acetylcholingehaltes und der Innervation des Herzmuskels in Gewebe-Kulturen. *Pflügers Archiv für die gesamte Physiologie des Menschen und der Tiere*, 245:794-801.

Lockwood, D. H., and Williams-Ashmann, H. G. (1970): Cholinergic-stimulated alkaline phosphatase secretion and phospholipid synthesis in guinea pig seminal vesicles. *Journal of Cellular Physiology*, 77:7-16.

Lustig, E. S. De (1942): Estudio del automatismo muscular en cultivos in vitro con eserina, acetilcolina, adrenalina y atropina. *Revista de la Sociedad Argentina de Biologia,* 18:524-531.

Lustig, E. S. De (1943): Accion de substacias curarizantes sobre cultivos de musculo de embrion de pollo. *Revista de la Sociedad Argentina de Biologia,* 19:159-169.

Maletta, G. J., Vernadakis, A., and Timiras, P. S. (1966): Pre- and post-natal development of the spinal cord: Increased acetylcholinesterase activity. *Proceedings of the Society for Experimental Biology and Medicine,* 121:1210-1211.

Maletta, G. J., and Timiras, P. S. (1966): Acetyl- and butyrylcholinesterase activity of selected brain areas in developing rats after neonatal X-irradiation. *Journal of Neurochemistry,* 13:75-84.

Mann, E., Pleul, O., and Kewitz, H. (1971): Free and structurally bound acetylcholine in the developing rat brain. *Naunyn-Schmiedebergs Archiv für Pharmakologie,* 269A: 473.

Mann, W. S., and Salafsky, B. (1970): Development of the differential response to succinylcholine in the fast and slow twitch skeletal muscle of the kitten. *Journal of Physiology,* 210:581-592.

Marchisio, P. C. (1969): Choline acetyltransferase (ChAc) activity in developing chick optic centres and the effects of monolateral removal of retina at an early embryonic stage and at hatching. *Journal of Neurochemistry,* 16:665-671.

Marchisio, P. C., and Consolo, S. (1968): Developmental changes of choline acetyltransferase (ChAc) activity in chick embryo spinal and sympathetic ganglia. *Journal of Neurochemistry,* 15:759-764.

Marchisio, P. C., and Giacobini, G. (1969): Choline acetyltransferase activity in the central nervous system of the developing chick. *Brain Research,* 15:301-304.

Massoulie, J., Rieger, R. F., and Bon, S. (1971): Espèces acetylcholinésterasiques globulaires et allongées des organes électriques des poissons. *European Journal of Biochemistry,* 21:542-551.

Mathews, A. P. (1902): The action of pilocarpine and atropine on the embryos of the starfish and of the sea urchin. *American Journal of Physiology,* 6:207-215.

Maynard, E. A. (1966): Electrophoretic studies of cholinesterases in brain and muscle of the developing chicken. *Journal of Experimental Zoology,* 161:319-336.

McCaman, M. W. (1966): Biochemical effects of denervation on normal and dystrophic muscle: acetylcholinesterase and choline acetyltransferase. *Life Sciences,* 5:1459-1465.

McGeer, R. L., and McGeer, E. G. (1971): Cholinergic enzyme systems in Parkinson's disease. *Archives of Neurology,* 25:265-268.

Miledi, R. (1960a): The acetylcholine sensitivity of frog muscle fibers after complete or partial denervation. *Journal of Physiology,* 151:1-23.

Miledi, R. (1960b): Junctional and extra-junctional acetylcholine receptors in skeletal muscle fibers. *Journal of Physiology,* 151:24-30.

Mumenthaler, M., and Engel, W. K. (1961): Cytochemical localization of cholinesterases in developing chick embryo skeletal muscle. *Acta Anatomica,* 47:174-299.

Muslin, B. S. (1968): Blood pseudo and true cholinesterase activity during the ontogenesis of rats. *Biulleten Eksperimental Noi Biologii I Meditsiny,* 65:19-22.

Myslivecek, J., Hassmannova, J., Rokyta, R., Sobotka, P., and Zahlava, J. (1965): Peculiarities of influencing cortical synapses at early periods of postnatal life. *Plzensky Lekarsky Sbornik,* 25:9-34.

Nachmansohn, D. (1938a): Cholinestérase dans le tissus embryonnaires. *Comptes Rendus des Séances de la Société de Biologie,* 127:670-673.

Nachmansohn, D. (1938b): Changement de la cholinestérase dans le muscle strié. *Comptes Rendus des Séances de la Société de Biologie,* 128:599.

Nachmansohn, D. (1940): On the physiological significance of cholinesterase. *Yale Journal of Biology and Medicine,* 12:565-589.

Nachmansohn, D. (1963): Actions on axons, and evidence for the role of acetylcholine in axonal conduction. In: *Handbuch der experimentellen Pharmakologie*, Vol. 15; *Cholinesterases and Anticholinesterase Agents*, edited by G. B. Koelle. 15:701-740. Springer-Verlag, Berlin.

Nachmansohn, D. (1970): Proteins in excitable membranes. *Science*, 168:1059-1066.

Nair, V. (1966): Effect of in utero x-irradiation on the ontogenesis of brain enzymes (carbonic anhydrase and acetylcholinesterase). In: *Proc. Third International Congress of Radiation Research*, p. 164.

Nelson, P. G., Peacock, J. H., Amano, T., and Minna, J. (1971a): Electrogenesis in mouse neuroblastoma cells *in vitro*. *Journal of Cell Physiology*, 77:337-352.

Nelson, P. G., Peacock, J. H., and Amano, T. (1971b): Responses of neuroblastoma cells to iontophoretically applied acetylcholine. *Journal of Cell Physiology*, 77:353-362.

Nichols, C. W., and Koelle, G. B. (1968): Comparison of the localization of acetylcholinesterase and non-specific cholinesterase activities in mammalian and avian retinas. *Journal of Comparative Neurology*, 133:1-16.

Nickel, E., and Waser, P. G. (1968): Elektronenmikroskopische Untersuchungen am Diaphragma der Maus nach einseitiger Phrenikotomie. I. Die degenerierende motorische Endplatte. *Zeitschrift für Zellforschung*, 88:278.

Numanoi, H. (1953): Studies on the fertilization substance. IV. Presence of acetylcholine-like substance and cholinesterase in echinoderm germ cells during fertilization. *Tokyo University of Education: Science Reports*, 3:193-200.

Obrecht-Coutris, G., and Coraboeuf, E. (1967): Sensibilité á la noradrénaline et á l'acétylcholine du myocarde de Poulet. *Journal of Physiology*, 59:275-276.

O'Brien, R. R. (1960): *Toxic Phosphorus Esters*. Academic Press, New York.

Ozand, P., Artvinis, S., and Yarimagan, S. (1970): Investigation of the kinetic characteristics of red blood cell acetylcholinesterase in ABO, Rh hemolytic disease of the newborn and thalassemia major cases. *Turkish Journal of Pediatrics*, 12:1-7.

Page, E. (1967): The occurrence of inclusions within membrane-limited structures that run longitudinally in the cells of mammalian heart muscle. *Journal of Ultrastructure Research*, 17:63-71.

Pakhomov, A. N., Aronshtam, A. A., and Margulis, B. A. (1970): Electrophoretic investigation of esterases during the development of chick skeletal muscles. *Journal of Evolutionary Biochemistry and Physiology*, 6:502-506.

Pantelouris, E. M., and Arnason, A. (1966): Ontogenesis of serum esterases in *Mus musculus*. *Journal of Embryology and Experimental Morphology*, 16:55-64.

Poulson, D. E., and Boell, E. J. (1946): The development of cholinesterase activity in embryos of normal genetically deficient strains of *Drosophila melanogaster*. *Anatomical Record*, 96:508.

Redfern, P. A. (1970): Neuromuscular transmission in newborn rats. *Journal of Physiology*, 209:701-709.

Reger, J. F. (1959): Studies on the fine structure of normal and denervated neuromuscular junctions from mouse gastrocnemius. *Journal of Ultrastructure Research*, 2:269-282.

Resketnikova, N. A. (1970): Acetylcholine content in developing eggs of the frog *Rana temporaria*. *Journal of Evolutionary Biochemistry and Physiology*, 6:14-18.

Richardson, D. L., Karczmar, A. G., and Scudder, C. L. (1972): Effects of pre-natal cholinergic drug treatment on post-natal behavior and brain chemistry in mice. *Federation Proceedings*, 31:596.

Rizzoli (1964): L'attivitá acetilcolinesterasica negli emisferi cerebrali del pollo: I. Nell'animale normale durante l'embriogenesi ed i primi venti giorni di vita postnatale. *Atti della Societa Medico-Chirurgica di Padova*, 40:5-19.

Robbins, N., and Yonezawa, T. (1971): Developing neuromuscular junctions: First signs of chemical transmission during formation in tissue culture. *Science*, 172:395-397.

Robert, E. D., and Oester, Y. T. (1970a): Absence of supersensitivity to acetylcholine in innervated muscle subjected to a prolonged pharmacologic nerve block. *Journal of Pharmacology and Experimental Therapeutics*, 174:133-140.

Robert, E. D., and Oester, Y. T. (1970b): Electrodiagnosis of nerve-impulse deprived skeletal muscle. *Journal of Applied Physiology*, 28:439-443.

Roberts, G. M., Gimeno, M. S., and Webb, J. R. (1965): On the role of acetylcholine in regulating the rate of the early chick embryo heart. *Journal of Cellular and Comparative Physiology*, 66:267-272.

Rogers, K. T., De Vries, L., Kepler, J. A., Kepler, C. R., and Speidel, E. R. (1960): Studies on chick brain of biochemical differentiation related to morphological differentiation and onset of function. II. Alkaline phosphatase and cholinesterase levels and onset of function. *Journal of Experimental Zoology*, 144:89-103.

Rose, S., and Glow, P. H. (1967): Denervation effects on the presumed de novo synthesis of muscle cholinesterase and the effects of acetylcholine availability on retinal cholinesterase. *Experimental Neurology*, 18:267-275.

Rosenzweig, M. R., Bennett, E. L., and Diamond, M. C. (1967): Experimental complexity, cerebral change, and behavior. *Brain Chemistry and Behavior Research Project Newsletter*, 14:1-14.

Rozanova, V. D. (1967): On the role of cholinergic mechanisms of activation and inhibition of the electrical activity of the cortex in ontogenesis of dogs. *Zhurnal Evolyutsionnoi Biokhimii i Fiziologii*, 3:47-54.

Rubin, R. (1903): Versuche über die Beziehung des Nervensystems zur Regeneration bei Amphibien. *Wilhelm Roux Archiv für Entwicklungs-mechanik der Organismen*, 16:21-75.

Salkeld, E. H. (1965): Electrophoretic separation and identification of esterases in eggs and young nymphs of the large milkwood bug, *Oncopeltus fasciatus* (Dallas). *Canadian Journal of Zoology*, 43:593-602.

Sawyer, C. H. (1943a): Cholinesterase and behavior problem in *Amblystoma*. I. The relationship between the development of the enzyme and early motility. II. The effects of inhibiting cholinesterase. *Journal of Experimental Zoology*, 92:1-27.

Sawyer, C. H. (1943b): Cholinesterase and behavior problem in *Amblystoma*. III. The distribution of cholinesterase in nerve and muscle throughout development. IV. Cholinesterase in nerveless muscle. *Journal of Experimental Zoology*, 94:1-31.

Sawyer, C. H. (1944): Nature of the early somatic movements in *Fundulus heteroclitus*. *Journal of Cellular and Comparative Physiology*, 24:71-84.

Sawyer, C. H. (1947): Cholinergic stimulation of the release of melanophore hormone by the hypophysis in salamander larvae. *Journal of Experimental Zoology*, 106:145-180.

Schotté, O. E. (1922): Influence des nerfs sur la regénération des pattes antérieures de Tritons adultes. *Compte Rendu des Séances: Société de Physique et d'Histoire Naturelle de Genève*, 39:67-70.

Schotté, O. E., and Butler, E. G. (1941): Morphological effects of denervation and amputation of limbs in urodele larvae. *Journal of Experimental Zoology*, 87:279-322.

Schotté, O. E., and Karczmar, A. G. (1944): Limb parameters and regression rates in denervated and amputated limbs of urodele larvae. *Journal of Experimental Zoology*, 97:43-70.

Schotté, O. E., and Karczmar, A. G. (1945): Temperature and regression rates in denervated amputated limbs of urodele larvae. *Journal of Experimental Zoology*, 99:235-261.

Schramm, M. (1967): Secretion of enzymes and other macromolecules. *Annual Review of Biochemistry*, 36:307-320.

Schramm, M. (1968): Amylase secretion in rat parotid slices by apparent activation of endogenous catecholamines. *Biochimica et Biophysica Acta*, 165:546-549.

Scudder, C. L., Akers, T. K., and Karczmar, A. G. (1963): Effects of drugs on the tunicate electrocardiogram. *Comparative Biochemistry and Physiology,* 9:307-312.

Scudder, C. L., Akers, T. K., and Karczmar, A. G. (1966): Effects of cholinergic drugs on tunicate smooth muscle. *Comparative Biochemistry and Physiology,* 17:559-567.

Scudder, C. L., and Karczmar, A. G. (1966): Histochemical studies of cholinesterases in *Ciona intestinalis. Comparative Biochemistry and Physiology,* 17:553-558.

Sedlacek, J. (1967): Development of optic evoked potentials in chick embryos. *Physiologia Bohemoslovaca,* 16:531-537.

Sharma, K. N., Dua, S., Singh, B. K., and Anand, B. K. (1964): Electro-ontogenesis of cerebral and cardiac activities in the chick embryo. *Electroencephalography and Clinical Neurophysiology,* 16:503-509.

Shen, S. C., Greenfield, P., and Boell, E. J. (1956): Localization of acetylcholinesterase in chick retina during histogenesis. *Journal of Comparative Neurology,* 106:433-461.

Shnitka, T. K., and Seligman, A. M. (1961): Role of esteratic inhibition on localization of esterase and the simultaneous cytochemical demonstration of inhibitor-sensitive and resistant enzyme species. *Journal of Histochemistry and Cytochemistry,* 9:504-527.

Silva, D. G., and Ikeda, M. (1971): Ultrastructural and acetylcholinesterase studies on the innervation of the ductus arteriosus, pulmonary trunk, and aorta of the fetal lamb. *Journal of Ultrastructure Research,* 34:358-374.

Singer, M. (1960): Nervous mechanisms in the regeneration of body parts in vertebrates. In: *Developing Cell Systems and their Control.* The Ronald Press Company, New York, pp. 115-133.

Singer, M., Davis, M. H., and Arkovitz, E. S. (1960a): Acetylcholinesterase activity in the regenerating forelimb of the adult newt *Triturus. Journal of Embryology and Experimental Morphology,* 8:98-111.

Singer, M., Davis, M. H., and Scheuing, M. R. (1960b): The influence of atropine and other neuropharmacological substances on regeneration of the forelimb in the adult Urodele *Triturus. Journal of Experimental Zoology,* 143:33-46.

Siou, G. (1958): Distribution normale et variation expérimentale de l'activité cholinestérasique au niveau des tubercules quadrijumeaux antérieures chez la Souris. *Comptes Rendus Hebdomaires des Séances de l'Académie des Sciences,* 246:315-317.

Siou, G. (1962): L'activité cholinestérasique dans les tubercules quadrijumeaux antérieurs au cours du développement postnatal chez le lapin. *Archives d'Anatomie Microscopique et de Morphologie Expérimentale,* 51:287-324.

Sippel, T. O. (1955): Properties and development of cholinesterase in the hearts of certain vertebrates. *Journal of Experimental Zoology,* 128:165-184.

Smith, E. H., and Salkeld, E. H. (1966): The use and action of ovicides. *Annual Review of Entomology,* 11:331-368.

Smith, R. W., Morris, J. A., and Assali, N. S. (1964): Effects of chemical mediators on the pulmonary and ductus arteriosus circulation in the fetal lamb. *American Journal of Obstetrics and Gynecology,* 89:252-260.

Sobotka, P., Myslivecek, J., and Springer, V. (1964): The effect of acetylcholine on the steady potential of the brain during the ontogenetic development. *Activitas Nervosa Superior,* 6:49-50.

Sollmann, T. L. (1904): The simultaneous action of pilocarpine and atropine on the developing embryos of the sea urchin and starfish. A contribution to the study of the antagonistic action of poisons. *American Journal of Physiology,* 10:352-361.

Srinivasan, R., Karczmar, A. G., and Bernsohn, J. (1972): Developmental cholinesterase levels and isozyme patterns in offspring after injection of some CNS-active drugs into pregnant mice. *Transactions of the American Society for Neurochemistry,* 3:124.

Staley, A. N., and Benson, E. S. (1968): The ultrastructure of frog ventricular cardiac muscle and its relationship to mechanisms of excitation-contraction coupling. *Journal of Cell Biology,* 38:99-114.

Stephenson, M., and Rowatt, E. (1947): The production of acetylcholine by a strain of *Lactobacillus planatarum*. *Journal of General Microbiology*, 1:279-298.

Stromblad, B. C. R. (1960): Cholinesterase activity in skeletal muscle after botulinum toxin. *Experientia*, 16:458-460.

Strumia, E., and Baima-Bollone, P. L. (1964): AChE activity in the spinal ganglia of the chick embryo during development. *Acta Anatomica*, 57:281-293.

Szafran, Z., and McCarty, K. S. (1968): Esterase activity in embryonic development. *Proceedings of the Society for Experimental Biology and Medicine*, 128:116-120.

Szepsenwohl, J. (1947): Electrical excitability and spontaneous activity in explants of skeletal and heart muscle of chick embryo. *Anatomical Record*, 98:67-85.

Tauc, L., and Gerschenfeld, H. M. (1961): Cholinergic transmission mechanisms for both excitation and inhibition in molluscan central synapses. *Nature*, 192:366-367.

Tennyson, V. M. (1970): The fine structure of the developing nervous system. In: *Developmental Neurobiology*, edited by W. A. Himwich. C. C. Thomas, Springfield, Ill., pp. 47-116.

Tennyson, V. M. (1971): Cytochemical localization of cholinesterase activity in adult rabbit heart. *Journal of Histochemistry and Cytochemistry*, 19:376-381.

Tennyson, V. M., and Brzin, M. (1970): The appearance of acetylcholinesterase in the dorsal root neuroblast of the rabbit embryo. *Journal of Cell Biology*, 46:64-80.

Tennyson, V. M., Brzin, M., and Duffy, P. (1966): Cholinesterase localization in the developing nervous system of the rabbit embryo and human fetus by electron microscopic histochemistry. *Anatomical Record*, 154:432A.

Tennyson, V. M., Brzin, M., and Duffy, P. (1968): Electron microscopic cytochemistry and microgasometric analysis of cholinesterase in the nervous system. In: *Progress in Brain Research, Brain Barrier System*, edited by A. Lajtha and D. H. Ford. Elsevier, Amsterdam, pp. 15-35.

Teräväinen, H. (1968): Development of the myoneural junction in the rat. *Zeitschrift für Zellforschung*, 87:249-265.

Thesleff, S. (1960): Supersensitivity of skeletal muscle produced by botulinum toxin. *Journal of Physiology*, 151:598-607.

Tibbs, J. (1960): Acetylcholinesterase in flagellated systems. *Biochimica et Biophysica Acta*, 41:115-122.

Torre, C. (1970): Azione del DFP sull 'embrione di pollo. Prime osservazione. *Bollettino della Societa Italiana di Biologia Sperimentale*, 46:523-526.

Tweedle, C. (1971): Transneuronal effects on amphibian limb regeneration. *Journal of Experimental Zoology*, 177:13-30.

Usdin, E. (1970): Reactions of cholinesterases with substrates, inhibitors and reactivators. In: *Anti-cholinesterase Agents*, edited by A. G. Karczmar, Int. Encyclop. Pharmacol. Therap., Section 13, 1:45-354. Pergamon Press, Oxford.

Youngstrom, K. A. (1941): Acetylcholinesterase concentration during the development of the human fetus. *Journal of Neurophysiology*, 4:473-477.

Van Der Kloot, W. G. (1955): The control of neurosecretion and diapause by physiological changes in the brain of the *Cecropia* silkworm. *Biological Bulletin*, 109:276-294.

Van Der Kloot, W. G. (1960): Neurosecretion in insects. *Annual Review of Entomology*, 5:35-52.

Weis, J. S., and Weiss, P. (1970): The effect of nerve growth factor on limb regeneration in *Amblystoma*. *Journal of Experimental Zoology*, 174:73-78.

Weiss, P., and Hiscoe, H. B. (1948): Experiments on the mechanism of nerve growth. *Journal of Experimental Zoology*, 107:315-395.

Werner, I., Peterson, G. R., and Shuster, L. (1971): Choline acetyltransferase and acetylcholinesterase in cultured brain cells from chick embryos. *Journal of Neurochemistry*, 18:141-151.

Whiting, H. P. (1955): Functional development in the nervous system. In: *Biochemistry of the Developing Nervous System*, edited by H. Waelsh. Academic Press, New York, pp. 85-103.

Willmer, E. N. (1970): Cytology and Evolution. Academic Press, New York.

Wilson, B. W., Montgomery, M. A., and Asmundson, R. V. (1968): Cholinesterase activity and inherited muscular dystrophy of the chicken. *Proceedings of the Society for Experimental Biology and Medicine,* 129:199-206.

Wilson, B. W., Mettler, M. A., and Asmundson, R. V. (1969): Acetylcholinesterase and non-specific esterases in developing avian tissues: Distribution and molecular weights of esterases in normal and dystrophic embryos and chicks. *Journal of Experimental Zoology,* 172:49-58.

Wise, G. A., and McQuillen, M. P. (1970): Transient myasthenia. Clinical and electromyographic studies. *Archives of Neurology,* 22:556-565.

Yntema, C. (1959): Regeneration in sparsely innervated and aneurogenic forelimb of Amblystoma larvae. *Journal of Experimental Zoology,* 140:101-129.

Zahlava, J. (1965): Functional development of the cortical areas of the auditory analyzer. Doctoral dissertation, Plzen.

Zelena, J. (1962): The effect of denervation on muscle development. In: *The Denervated Muscle,* edited by E. Gutman. Publishing House of the Czechoslovak Academy of Science, Prague, p. 103.

Zschintzsch, J., O'Brien, R. D., and Smith, E. H. (1965): The relation between uptake and toxicity of organophosphates for eggs of the large milkweed bug. *Journal of Economic Entomology,* 58:614-621.

Zsigmond, E. K., and Downs, J. R. (1971): Plasma cholinesterase activity in newborns and infants. *Canadian Anaesthetists Society Journal,* 18:278-285.

DISCUSSION

PAOLETTI: Have your drugs any effect on the function of the placenta? The high level of cholinergic activity in the placenta may be affected by DFP or physostigmine with subsequent effects on behavior of the offspring.

KARCZMAR: This is an interesting possibility. Indeed, the placenta is an ephemeral organ with high acetylcholine and cholinesterase levels. It resembles some other tissues which are "ephemerally" cholinergic, such as spinal ganglia, as shown by Giacobini. Such organs may be expected to respond to cholinergic drugs during the time of persistence of their cholinergicity. We have at present no pertinent experiments as to this point.

CALDEYRO-BARCIA: What is your explanation for the fact that both anticholinergic and anticholinesterase drugs given to the mother on the 10th day have similar effects on the development of the cholinergic system?

KARCZMAR: I can speculate only. We and others showed that atropinics decrease brain acetylcholine levels. This, in turn, seems related to the presence of free acetylcholine when anticholinergics are administered—presumably because receptors are occupied by the atropinics. There may be additionally increased release (and turnover) of acetylcholine. These factors may tend to induce an increase in cholinesterase activity, and this may be the reason for the similar effect, an augmentation, on cholinesterase of both anticholinergics and anticholinesterases. I would like to add also that the behavioral effect on the offspring of mothers treated with anticholinergics and anticholinesterases is also paradoxical; first, because both types of drugs induce a similar effect on aggression, and second, as anticholinergics, which are antiaggressive in the adult animal, are "proaggressive" in the offspring when given to pregnant mice.

DRABKOVA: An anesthesiological observation on neonates to myasthenic mothers, treated with acetylcholinesterase inhibitors, is that the airways of these neonates contain a considerable amount of viscous secretion which is difficult to suck out during resuscitation.

KARCZMAR: Thank you for this information. There are several cases of a temporary neonatal myasthenia-like syndrome. We can obtain a similar effect in animals if we treat pregnant mothers with neuromyal blockers or with hemicholinium: the offspring shows then a short-lived myasthenia-like muscle weakness, antagonizable with anticholinesterases. The methods which we employed to test behavioral effects in the offspring after pharmacological treatment of mothers are rather subtle, and they deal with specific behaviors—aggression, learning, exploration. Without appropriate psychologic tests, and without controls, which will be difficult to obtain in the case of human material, these effects would not be apparent in man. Of course, I do not know at present if these effects are reversible in later life.

Fetal Pharmacology, edited by L. Boréus
Raven Press, New York © 1973

Histochemical and Pharmacological Evidence of Amine Mechanisms in Human Fetal Vascular Shunts

C. Owman, S. Aronson, G. Gennser, and N.-O. Sjöberg

Departments of Histology, Pediatrics, and Obstetrics and Gynecology at Malmö, University of Lund, Lund, Sweden

The ductus venosus and the ductus arteriosus are unique vascular areas in the fetus showing special hemodynamic features in shunting part of the oxygenized blood past the hepatic and pulmonary vascular beds. It has for a long time been assumed that the flow through these bypasses is monitored by specific vasomotor mechanisms. Thus, based on the findings of smooth-muscle fibers around the beginning of the ductus venosus, Amoroso and Barron suggested in 1942 that a sphincter was located at the junction between the umbilical vein and the ductus venosus (see Barclay, Franklin, and Prichard, 1944). The hypothesis was later supported by angiographic studies on fetuses and newborns, where Lind, Stern, and Wegelius (1964) demonstrated a temporary filling defect in this region. With regard to the ductus arteriosus, the direct fetal communication between the pulmonary trunk and aorta, its closure after birth is regarded to take place in two steps: first, a contraction of the vessel with narrowing of its lumen, and then intimal proliferation causing final obliteration. Much evidence has been suggested that the oxygen tension of the blood passing this muscular artery plays an important role during its closure. The observations that noradrenaline and acetylcholine restored the patency of the ductus venosus in newborn lambs in which it is normally closed (Peltonen and Hirvonen, 1965), and that such amines were found to contract the ductus arteriosus of lamb fetuses (Born, Dawes, Mott, and Rennick, 1956; Kovalcik, 1963), indicated that amine mechanisms might also normally be involved in the hemodynamics of the ductus venosus and ductus arteriosus. Investigations were therefore performed on the histochemical localization of autonomic nerves and on the *in vitro* contractile response to vasoactive amines in these and adjacent vascular areas of human fetuses.

Catecholamine-containing nerves in *the umbilical vein system and ductus venosus* (Ehinger, Gennser, Owman, Persson, and Sjöberg, 1968) were visualized in 20- to 24-week-old previable fetuses obtained at legal abortions, using the fluorescence histochemical method of Falck and Hillarp (for methodological details, see Falck and Owman, 1965). This kind of histochemical approach is based on the fact that adrenergic nerves begin to synthesize and store high levels of catecholamines already at a very early stage of their development (Enemar, Falck, and Hakanson, 1965; De Champlain, Malmfors, Olson, and Sachs, 1970; Owman, Sjöberg, and Swedin, 1971). The cholinesterase method of Koelle (1963) in combination with appropriate inhibitors (Holmstedt, 1957) was employed in the histochemical demonstration of cholinergic nerves in mid-term fetuses.

The umbilical cord (tissue preparations also taken at full term) revealed the presence of fluorescent nerves only within a short segment close to the umbilical ring, thus probably constituting aberrant fibers from the abdominal wall. No cholinesterase-containing nerves were found (only fetal half of the cord studied). This would indicate that the nerve elements previously claimed to occur in the umbilical cord and placenta on the basis of methylene blue and other stainings (see ten Berge, 1962; Fox and Jacobson, 1969) are at least not adrenergic. Immediately inside the abdominal wall, the umbilical vein was devoid of histochemically visible nerve fibers. Adrenergic nerves were found in varying numbers in the rest of the umbilical vein. In the free-running intra-abdominal portion, they ran at some distance from the umbilical vein, being rather more related to the small arteries and veins present in the surrounding mesenchyme. This intra-abdominal part of the umbilical vein showed no cholinesterase-containing fibers. Near the intrahepatic portion of the umbilical vein, an increasing number of fluorescent nerve fascicles were found, some splitting up into smaller branches which extended toward the wall of the vein. In the intrahepatic part, these branches formed a characteristic plexus superimposed on the vein. At the origin of

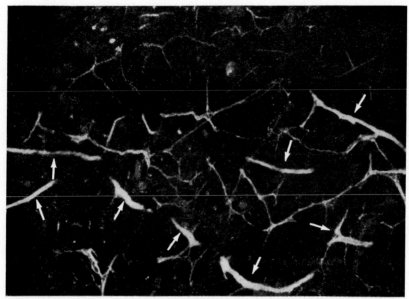

FIG. 1. Human fetus, 23-cm length. Demonstration of adrenergic nerves in the first part of ductus venosus, at the junction with the umbilical vein. The vessel has been cut open, flattened, and sectioned from the outside. Rich plexus formation in the vessel wall of green-fluorescent adrenergic fibers, running in small bundles (arrows) or isolated. When isolated, the fibers are seen to have a varicosed appearance. Fluorescence micrograph. ×100

the ductus venosus, the amount of fluorescent nerves in the plexus suddenly increased concomitant with a reduction of the lumen diameter and thickening of the vessel wall which, after staining with hematoxylin—van Gieson, revealed a clear accumulation of smooth-muscle fibers. The nerve fibers had a beaded appearance in this region, suggesting that they participated in a terminal innervation apparatus in the sphincter-like structure at the junction between the umbilical vein and ductus venosus (Fig. 1). Within a short distance toward the caval vein, the amount of nerves in the ductus wall gradually decreased so that only few fluorescent nerves remained more distally where the lumen became wider. The same scarcity of fluorescent nerves was found at the junction with the caval vein. The only cholinesterase fibers present in the ductus preparations ran in the mesenchyme at some distance from the vessel proper (Fig. 2).

Pharmacological tests on the isolated umbilical vein were performed on its final free-running abdominal part (fetuses 20- to 23-weeks-old). Nor-

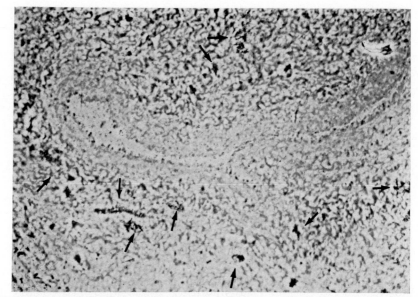

FIG. 2. Human fetus, 21 weeks old. Demonstration of cholinergic nerves in first part of ductus venosus. Longitudinally and transeversely sectioned nerve trunks (arrows) lie in the connective tissue around the vessel, but not in direct contact with it. Incubation time 21 hr. Mipafox. Phase-contrast micrograph. ×200

adrenaline and serotonin (5-HT) elicited a marked circular contraction in this preparation. The contraction was reproduced with tyramine, whose effect was blocked by cocaine, indicating that the transmitter in the adrenergic nerves was present in sufficient amount to produce a local contraction of the vascular smooth musculature. Also, acetylcholine contracted the vessel, and the effect was abolished by atropine.

The part of the ductus venosus studied (fetuses 20- to 23-weeks-old) included the supposed sphincter. The noradrenaline contraction (Fig. 3)

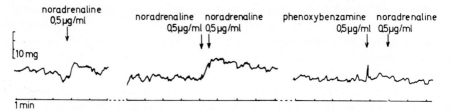

FIG. 3. Human fetus, 22 weeks old, ductus venosus. Contractile response to noradrenaline abolished by phenoxybenzamine.

was not constant and could be demonstrated only in preparations from two out of eight fetuses. However, both acetylcholine and 5-HT contracted the ductus venosus. Against the background of the findings that the ductus venosus was well supplied by adrenergic nerve terminals, the failing nor-adrenaline response was somewhat unexpected. There are several possible explanations to the result: it could be due to the simultaneous action of some antagonizing mechanism, or to an uneven distribution of adrenergic receptors in the vascular system (Lemtis, 1955), and/or to an insufficient degree of maturity of, for example, the enzyme mechanisms constituting the receptor (Ariëns, 1966). A related discrepancy has been reported for the mouse vas deferens in which functional transmission (indicated by the registration of excitatory junction potentials) did not occur until 18 days postpartum, although structurally the adrenergic nerves are already fully developed before that stage (Furness, McLean, and Burnstock, 1970).

A somewhat unexpected observation was that neither catechol-O-methyl-transferase (COMT) nor monoamine oxidase (MAO) activities in the human umbilical vein system were correlated with the amount of adrenergic nerve terminals present in the corresponding vascular regions at the corresponding fetal ages (Gennser and von Studnitz, 1969). If, in the fetus, the amount of these enzymes does not reflect the amount of catecholamine-containing nerve terminals, they may then rather be involved in the control of the quantities of catecholamines reaching a given receptor area at a given stage of development. According to such an assumption, high MAO (and/or COMT) activities would mean a more pronounced catecholamine degrada-tion and, physiologically, a less pronounced catecholamine-induced con-traction of the vessel. Similar considerations have been made from studies on MAO and COMT activities in the fetal heart as related to the heart rate (Ignarro and Shideman, 1968).

Histochemical evidence for the presence of adrenergic nerves in the *ductus arteriosus* of the human fetus (10 to 24 weeks gestational age) has been reported by Aronson, Gennser, Owman, and Sjöberg (1968, 1970) and by Boréus, Malmfors, McMurphy, and Olson (1969). In preparations from fetuses older than 15 weeks, a large number of varicosed fluorescent nerve fibers (probably terminals) were found throughout the entire thick-ness of the wall (Fig. 4, left) with a particular concentration in the middle of the media. The nerves closely followed the direction of the muscle cells. There was a tendency to an increase of the nerve supply in the middle third of the ductus length (Fig. 4, right). The terminal nerve plexus appeared to arise from several large bundles of moderately fluorescent, smooth nerves coursing along the outside of the ductus arteriosus and adjacent parts of the

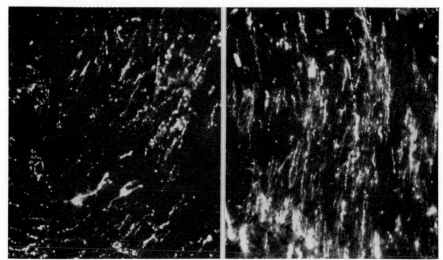

FIG. 4. *Left:* Fetus, 18 weeks old, transverse section of ductus arteriosus. Large number of varicose adrenergic nerve terminals following the direction of the muscle cells which run essentially in circular direction. Fluorescence micrograph. ×125

Right: Fetus, 17 weeks old, transverse section from the middle portion of ductus arteriosus. Accumulation of green-fluorescent adrenergic nerve terminals running in the essentially circular direction of the muscle fibers and distributed throughout the entire thickness of the vascular media. Fluorescence micrograph. ×125

pulmonary trunk and aorta. These bundles were also observed in ductus preparations from 14- to 15-week-old fetuses, but, in contrast, these fetuses had only few, scattered nerve fibers within the ductus wall. Fluorometrically, the ductus arteriosus contained 0.18 to 0.57 µg/g noradrenaline (method of Bertler, Carlsson, Rosengren, and Waldeck, 1958, as modified by Häggendal, 1963); neither adrenaline nor dopamine was found. Similar findings have since been made in fluorescence histochemical studies on the ductus arteriosus of the fetal lamb (Ikeda, 1970), and they are in accordance with earlier evidence that the region receives sympathetic nerves from the superficial cardiac sympathetic plexus (Nonidez, 1937; Boyd, 1941; Allan, 1955). Cholinesterase staining revealed the presence of the enzyme only in scattered thick bundles running in the periphery of ductus arteriosus of 18- to 20-week-old fetuses (Aronson et al., 1970). Electron-microscopic studies on lamb fetuses near term have confirmed the presence of both adrenergic and cholinergic nerve terminals in the media of the ductus arteriosus; furthermore, the distance to the smooth-muscle cells indicates the existence of a functionally important autonomic neuro-effector apparatus (Silva and Ikeda, 1971).

The effect of certain vasoactive compounds has been tested on isolated ductus arteriosus from 10- to 21-week-old human fetuses (Aronson et al., 1970). Graded, dose-dependent contractile responses were obtained with acetylcholine, histamine, 5-HT, and bradykinin (Fig. 5), as well as with noradrenaline and adrenaline; isoprenaline was without effect. The responses were antagonized by the respective specific inhibitors (Fig. 5). Some of the amines were tested separately on the aortic and pulmonary half of the ductus, and were found to produce a similar contraction (Fig. 6). It was notable that acetylcholine was about 15 times more potent in its contractile effect than were the catecholamines. The action of tyramine resembled that of noradrenaline. The intensity of the amine-induced contraction was proportional to the size of the vessel, being less in the younger fetuses. Using a

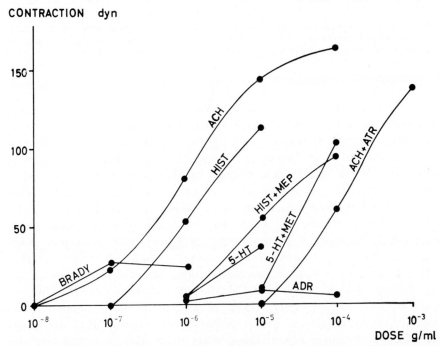

FIG. 5. Fetus, 20 weeks old. Contractile response to acetylcholine (ACH), histamine (HIST), bradykinin (BRADY), 5-hydroxytryptamine (5-HT), adrenaline (ADR). The specific antagonists atropine (ATR), mepyramine (MEP), and methysergide (MET) were all added in the same concentration (10^{-6} g/ml) together with the agonist.

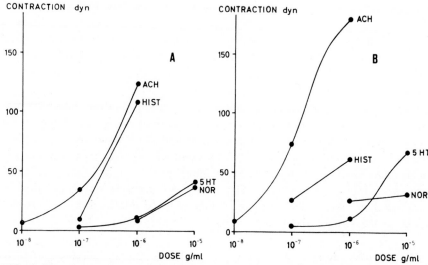

FIG. 6. Fetus, 18 weeks old. The contractile responses to acetylcholine (ACH), histamine (HIST), 5-hydroxytryptamine (5-HT), and noradrenaline (NOR) were similar in the aortic half (A) and the pulmonary half (B) of the ductus arteriosus.

perfusion technique and spiral strips, Boréus et al. (1969) observed that the isolated human ductus arteriosus (from fetuses aged 10 to 24 weeks) responded more intensely to acetylcholine than to noradrenaline, and that the latter contraction was blocked by an α-adrenergic receptor blocking agent. A marked tachyphylaxis to noradrenaline was noted by both groups of workers. It was recently demonstrated by McMurphy and Boréus (1971) that the contractile response of perfused human ductus arteriosus to acetylcholine could be obtained already at 12 weeks. The configuration of the dose-response curve did not change with advancing fetal age, indicating an early full development of the cholinergic (atropine-sensitive) receptor mechanism in this vessel. Alterations in the oxygen tension (40 to 760 mm Hg) did not elicit *per se* any contractile response, nor did they influence the acetylcholine-induced contraction (McMurphy and Boréus, 1971). In contrast to this, Aronson (1971), using isolated preparations, obtained small contractions by oxygen in several preparations of human fetal ductus arteriosus. Furthermore, a potentiating effect by oxygen on contractures induced by acetylcholine was noted. Tension always increased by a mean of 1½ times when aeration of the bath was changed from 95% N_2 to 95% O_2 in the presence of 5% CO_2 (Fig. 7). The response to noradrenaline was

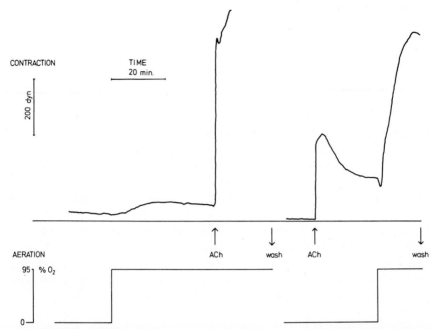

FIG. 7. Isolated ductus arteriosus from fetus aged 19.5 weeks. Notice the small contractile response to oxygen alone. The contraction by 10^{-6} g/ml of acetylcholine (ACh) is potentiated by oxygen.

potentiated in a similar way. On the other hand, a branch of the pulmonary artery—contracted with acetylcholine—always relaxed when the aeration was changed to 95% O_2 + 5% CO_2.

The presently reported as well as earlier results (Boréus, 1967; Mc-Murphy and Boréus, 1968) show that both adrenergic and cholinergic receptor functions in smooth musculature are well developed early in human fetal life. There is strong histochemical and pharmacological evidence that the hemodynamic mechanisms involved in the two fetal bypasses—ductus venosus and ductus arteriosus—may operate through a neural adrenergic mechanism. It is unlikely that the few cholinergic nerves visualized play an important vasomotor role in these areas (provided that the cholinesterase technique discloses the presence of cholinergic nerves which, of course, is not necessarily true for the fetus since the enzyme activity may develop comparatively late). Judging from the pharmacological experiments, it is possible that also in the fetal organism circulating, non-neural acetylcholine may have a physiologically significant action in the regulation of flow through ductus venosus and ductus arteriosus.

SUMMARY

Amine mechanisms in the two vascular shunts—ductus venosus and ductus arteriosus—and adjacent vascular areas were investigated by a combination of histochemical and pharmacological methods.

Fluorescence histochemistry (formaldehyde method) revealed no adrenergic nerves in the umbilical cord (except aberrant fibers in its abdominal insertion). A small number of fluorescent nerves occurred in the free-running, intra-abdominal part of the umbilical vein. The sphincter-like area in the ductus venosus had a rich supply of adrenergic nerves in a terminal plexus formation. A prominent adrenergic innervation was also found in the ductus arteriosus where these nerves occurred throughout the vascular media, particularly in the mid-portion of the vessel. Only scattered cholinergic fibers (cholinesterase technique) were found in preparations from ductus venosus and ductus arteriosus.

Both vascular shunts were studied *in vitro* and found to contract with acetylcholine, noradrenaline, and 5-HT. The noradrenaline response was blocked by phenoxybenzamine and the acetylcholine response by atropine. The effect of noradrenaline was reproduced with tyramine. Adrenaline, histamine, and bradykinin also contracted the ductus arteriosus. In this vessel, the acetylcholine and noradrenaline contractile responses could also be obtained in anoxia, and they were markedly potentiated by increased oxygen tension. There is thus strong histochemical and pharmacological evidence that the hemodynamic mechanisms involved in the two investigated fetal bypasses may operate through a neural adrenergic mechanism. It is unlikely that the few cholinergic nerves visualized play an important vasomotor role in these areas (provided that the cholinesterase technique discloses the presence of cholinergic nerves, which is not necessarily true for the fetus since the enzyme activity may develop comparatively late). Judging from the pharmacological experiments, it is possible that in the fetal organism also non-neural acetylcholine may have a physiologically significant action in the regulation of flow through ductus venosus and ductus arteriosus.

ACKNOWLEDGMENT

This investigation was supported by the Association for the Aid of Crippled Children, New York.

REFERENCES

Allan, F. D. (1955): The innervation of the human ductus arteriosus. *Anatomical Record,* 122:611.

Aronson, S. (1971): Different effects of oxygen on the human foetal ductus arteriosus. Proceedings of the 3rd Meeting of German Society of Perinatal Medicine, Berlin.

Aronson, S., Gennser, G., Owman, C., and Sjöberg, N.-O. (1968): Amine mechanisms in the contractility of the human ductus arteriosus. First Scandinavian Meeting of Perinatal Medicine, Lund, Sweden.

Aronson, S., Gennser, G., Owman, C., and Sjöberg, N.-O. (1970): Innervation and contractile response of the human ductus arteriosus. *European Journal of Pharmacology,* 11:178-186.

Barclay, A. E., Franklin, K. J., and Prichard, M. M. L. (1944): *The Foetal Circulation.* Blackwell, Oxford.

ten Berge, B. S. (1962): Nervenelemente in der Plazenta und Nabelschnur. *Geburtshilfe und Frauenheilkunde,* 22:1228-1233.

Bertler, A., Carlsson, A., Rosengren, E., and Waldeck, B. (1958): A method for the fluorimetric determination of adrenaline, noradrenaline, and dopamine in tissues. *Kungliga Fysiografiska Sällskapets i Lund Förhandlingar,* 28:121.

Boréus, L. O. (1967): Pharmacology of the human fetus: Dose-effect relationships for acetylcholine. *Biologia Neonatorum,* 11:328-337.

Boréus, L. O., Malmfors, T., McMurphy, D. M., and Olson, L. (1969): Demonstration of adrenergic receptor function and innervation in the ductus arteriosus of the human fetus. *Acta Physiologica Scandinavica,* 77:316-321.

Born, G. V. R., Dawes, G. S., Mott, J. C., and Rennick, B. R. (1956): The constriction of the ductus arteriosus caused by oxygen and by asphyxia in newborn lambs. *Journal of Physiology,* 132:304.

Boyd, J. D. (1941): The nerve supply of the mammalian ductus arteriosus. *Journal of Anatomy,* 75:457.

De Champlain, J., Malmfors, T., Olson, L., and Sachs, C. (1970): Ontogenesis of peripheral adrenergic neurons in the rat: pre- and postnatal observations. *Acta Physiologica Scandinavica,* 80:276-288.

Ehinger, B., Gennser, G., Owman, C., Persson, H., and Sjöberg, N.-O. (1968): Histochemical and pharmacological studies on amine mechanisms in the umbilical cord, umbilical vein and ductus venosus of the human fetus. *Acta Physiologica Scandinavica,* 72:15-24.

Enemar, A., Falck, B., and Hakanson, R. (1965): Observations on the appearance of norepinephrine in the sympathetic nervous system of the chick embryo. *Developmental Biology,* 11:268-283.

Falck, B., and Owman, C. (1965): A detailed methodological description of the fluorescence method for the cellular demonstration of biogenic monoamines. *Acta Universitatis Lundensis II,* 7:1-23.

Fox, H., and Jacobson, H. N. (1969): Nerve fibers in the umbilical cord and placenta of two species of sub-human primates (*Macaca phillipensis* and *Galago crassicaudatus*). *Acta Anatomica,* 73:48-55.

Furness, J. B., McLean, J. R., and Burnstock, G. (1970): Distribution of adrenergic nerves and changes in neuromuscular transmission in the mouse vas deferens during postnatal development. *Developmental Biology,* 21:491-505.

Gennser, G., and von Studnitz, W. (1969): Monoamine oxidase and catechol-O-methyltransferase activity in umbilical vessels of the human fetus. *Experientia,* 25:980-981.

Häggendal, J. (1963): An improved method for fluorimetric determination of small amounts of adrenaline and noradrenaline in plasma and tissues. *Acta Physiologica Scandinavica,* 59:242.

Holmstedt, B. (1957): A modification of the thiocholine method for the determination of cholinesterase. II: Histochemical application. *Acta Physiologica Scandinavica,* 40:331.

Ignarro, L. J., and Shideman, F. E. (1968): Catechol-O-methyl-transferase and monoamine oxidase activities in the heart and liver of the embryonic and developing chick. *Journal of Pharmacology and Experimental Therapeutics,* 159:29-37.

Ikeda, M. (1970): Adrenergic innervation of the ductus arteriosus of the fetal lamb. *Experientia,* 26:525-526.

Koelle, G. B. (1963): Cytological distributions and physiological functions of cholinesterases. In: *Handbuch der Experimentellen Pharmacologie,* vol. 15. Springer-Verlag, Berlin, p. 187.

Kovalcik, V. (1963): The response of the isolated ductus arteriosus to oxygen and anoxia. *Journal of Physiology,* 169:185.

Lemtis, H. (1955): Über die Architektonik. des Zottengefässapparates der menschlichen Placenta. *Anatomischer Anzeiger,* 102:106-133.

Lind, J., Stern, L., and Wegelius, C. (1964): *Human Foetal and Neonatal Circulation.* Charles C Thomas, Springfield, Ill., pp. 1-54.

McMurphy, D. M., and Boréus, L. O. (1968): Pharmacology of the human fetus: Adrenergic receptor function in the small intestine. *Biologia Neonatorum,* 13:325-339.

McMurphy, D. M., and Boréus, L. O. (1971): Studies on the pharmacology of the perfused human fetal ductus arteriosus. *American Journal of Obstetrics and Gynecology,* 109:937-942.

Nonidez, R. (1937): Distribution of the aortic nerve fibers and epitheloid bodies (Supracardial ganglia) in the dog. *Anatomical Record,* 69:299.

Owman, C., Sjöberg, N.-O., and Swedin, G. (1971): Histochemical and chemical studies on pre- and postnatal development of the different systems of "short" and "long" adrenergic neurons in peripheral organs of the rat. *Zeitschrift für Zellforschung,* 116:319-341.

Peltonen, T., and Hirvonen, L. (1965): Experimental studies on fetal and neonatal circulation. *Acta Paediatrica* (Uppsala), Stockholm Suppl. 161:1-55.

Silva, D. G., and Ikeda, M. (1971): Ultrastructural and acetylcholinesterase studies on the innervation of the ductus arteriosus, pulmonary trunk and aorta of the fetal lamb. *Journal of Ultrastructural Research,* 34:358-374.

DISCUSSION

LIND: We have studied the closure of the ductus venosus at birth. In the full-term stillborn infant, the opening of the ductus venosus into the portal sinus is wide open, but if the infant has lived 2 to 3 days it is already halfway closed and the so-called sphincter is clearly seen. In cross-section, no or few muscle fibers were seen in the sphincter, however. But the wall of the portal sinus is rich in musculature and might well contribute to the closure of the distal end of the ductus.

OWMAN: I agree that it might contribute to the closure. I want to point out that in our *in vitro* studies it is difficult to interpret exactly the components involved in the *in situ* closure mechanism since the reactions we test are defined by the part of the vessel we remove for analysis.

MIRKIN: What evidence exists to support the statement that the adrenergic neurons are functional early in pregnancy?

OWMAN: The following data have led us to suggest that neural adrenergic mechanisms are involved in the two bypasses studied: (1) adrenergic nerves are present prenatally in structures which are functioning only early in life; (2) the nerves are constituting a plexus formation of the kind we generally associate with a functioning neuro-effector apparatus; (3) the neuro-effector apparatus fulfills ultrastructural criteria for a functioning unit (Silva and Ikeda, 1971); (4) tryptamine (like noradrenaline) exerts a contraction in the vessel; and (5) stimulation of the nerves to the ductus arteriosus in the guinea pig produces a contraction (Barcroft, J., Kennedy, J. A., and Mason, M. F. (1938): The relation of the vagus nerve to the ductus arteriosus in the guinea-pig. *Journal of Physiology,* 92:p. 1).

Fetal Pharmacology, edited by L. Boréus
Raven Press, New York © 1973

Differentiation of the Catecholamine-Storing Cells

Antti Hervonen and Lasse Kanerva

Department of Anatomy, University of Helsinki, Helsinki, Finland

The embryological experiments of Yntema and Hammond (1947) led to the concept that the paraganglia and adrenal medulla, the main catecholamine stores of the fetal period, were derived from a common origin called the neural crest. The differentiation of the catecholamine-storing cells of the human fetus has been described by several investigators (see Coupland, 1965; Hervonen, 1971). The primitive sympathetic cell (PSC) (or sympathetic neuroblast) which originates from the neural crest gives rise to four types of catecholamine-containing cells (Owman, Sjöberg, and Swedin, 1971: intra-adrenal catecholamine-storing cells, extra-adrenal catecholamine-storing cells (the paraganglia, intraganglionic catecholamine-storing cells), classical "long" adrenergic neurons, and finally the "short" adrenergic neurons.

The differentiational inductions directioning the development toward each of these lines are not known. Recently, however, more light has been shed on this problem. Lempinen (1964) first described the effect of hydrocortisone on the differentiation of chromaffin cells. The total amount of newborn-rat catecholamine-storing cells increased tremendously after treatment with hydrocortisone. New chromaffin cells appeared also within the sympathetic ganglia. These findings were recently confirmed by Eränkö and Eränkö (1971, 1972) who used fluorescence microscopy for documentation of the changes in the catecholamine stores in newborn rats. They found about a 10-fold increase in the number of small, intensively fluorescent cells in the superior cervical ganglion of the rat. Further, the total amount of the paraganglionic tissue increased greatly. As suggested by Lempinen (1964), hydrocortisone probably exerts its effect on some still primitive cell types inducing the differentiation toward the catecholamine storage line.

Parallel indirect evidence was found during the studies on the differentiation of human fetal catecholamine-storing cells (Hervonen, 1971). The differentiation of PSC directed toward the catecholamine-storing cell type only if the microcirculatory patterns of the region were sufficient. The absence of capillaries evidently directed the development toward the neuronal line of differentiation. This choice of differentiational line was very clearly demonstrated in the human fetal adrenal medulla. Results supporting this concept were presented although not discussed from the differentiational point of view by Diner (1965) in her comprehensive study on the development of rat adrenal medulla. Recently, Kanerva (*unpublished data*) showed clearly that the treatment with glucocorticoids induced the appearance of catecholamines in the satellite cells of the paracervical ganglion of the newborn-rat uterus. The satellites of the sympathetic ganglia are known to originate also from the PSC (Smitten, 1962). The glucocorticoid effect in other ganglia seems to be identical; new fluorescent cells appear randomly scattered over the entire area of the sympathetic trunk. Their localization corresponds to that of the satellite cells in the control material. Thus the effect of glucocorticoids seems to be powerful enough even to change the direction of differentiation of the PSC-derived cells.

Although the changes induced by glucocorticoids in the catecholamine-storage patterns of the rat might be due to the unspecific and general stimulation of cellular metabolism leading to activation of the catecholamine synthesis, the possibility of a specific humoral induction mechanism should be emphasized. The steroid pattern of human fetal adrenal cortex also includes glucocorticoids during the stage of differentiation when the first signs of catecholamines were detectable by means of fluorescence microscopy (Hervonen, 1971). In human fetal paraganglia, the involution of rat catecholamine stores other than adrenal medulla after birth might be due to the decrease of the glucocorticoid level if compared with the level during pregnancy (Lempinen, 1964). Recent evidence from tissue cultures of human fetal primitive sympathetic cells supports the concept that glucocorticoids are of decisive importance when the direction of differentiation of PSC is determined (Hervonen, Hervonen, and Rechardt, 1971).

The final conclusions from the data presented must await further experimental work. However, regulatory events in many respects similar to the suggested inductive action of glucocorticoids on the developing primitive sympathetic cells, are functioning otherwhere in the fetal organism (sex differentiation, as the best example). The adrenocortical regulation of the adrenaline synthesis (see Pohorecky and Wurtman, 1971) may be the final form of these inductive effects on the mature catecholamine-storing cells.

The variety of catecholamine-storing cells listed at the beginning of this chapter may be results of different degrees of humoral induction at different localizations within the sympathetic nervous tissue.

REFERENCES

Coupland, R. E. (1965): *The Natural History of the Chromaffin Cells.* Longmans, London.

Diner, O. (1965): Observations sur le developpement de le médullosurrenale du rat: L'evolution de la partie non chromaffine. *Archives d'Anatomie Microscopique,* 54:671-718.

Eränkö, O., and Eränkö, L. (1971): Small, intensely fluorescent granule containing cells in the superior cervical ganglion of the rat. *Progress in Brain Research,* 34:39-51.

Eränkö, L., and Eränkö, O. (1972): Effect of hydrocortisone on histochemically demonstrable catecholamines in the sympathetic ganglia and extra-adrenal chromaffin tissue of the rat. *Acta Physiologica Scandinavica,* 84:125-133.

Hervonen, A. (1971): Development of catecholamine storing cells in human fetal paraganglia and adrenal medulla. *Acta Physiologica Scandinavica,* suppl. 368:1-94.

Hervonen, A., Hervonen, H., and Rechardt, L. (1971): Axonal growth from the primitive sympathetic elements of human fetal adrenal medulla. *Experientia,* 28:178-180.

Lempinen, M. (1964): Extra-adrenal chromaffin tissue of the rat and the effect of cortical hormones on it. *Acta Physiologica Scandinavica,* 62, suppl. 231.

Owman, C., Sjöberg, N.-O., and Swedin, G. (1971): Histochemical and chemical studies on pre- and postnatal development of the different systems of "short" and "long" adrenergic neurons in peripheral organs of the rat. *Zeitschrift für Zellforschung und Mikroskopischen Anatomie,* 116:319-341.

Pohorecky, L., and Wurtman, R. (1971): Adrenocortical control of epinephrine synthesis. *Pharmacological Reviews,* 23:1-35.

Smitten, N. A. (1962): A cytological analysis of the origin of chromaffino-blasts in some mammals. *Journal of Embryology and Experimental Morphology,* 10:152-166.

Yntema, C., and Hammond, W. S. (1947): The development of autonomic nervous system. *Biological Reviews,* 22:344-359.

DISCUSSION

RÄIHÄ: Would you care to speculate on whether the effects you see by corticosteroid hormones are due to an increase in the amount of catecholamine-storing cells or whether they are due to an "induction" of the enzymes in the noradrenaline-biosynthesizing pathway, for example, tyrosine hydroxylase, or both. We have observed a marked increase in phenylalanine-hydroxylating activity in the liver of newborn rats after administration of the synthetic glucocorticoid triamcinolone.

HERVONEN: We believe that the effect of glucocorticoids on the developing primitive sympathetic cells is a direct effect on the enzyme level. The best candidate in this respect would be tyrosine hydroxylase which is known to be the rate-limiting enzyme of the catecholamine synthesis. Work to confirm this is proceeding. The other possible explanation would be the acceleration of the cellular metabolism leading to detectable catecholamine synthesis in the previously only latently differentiated cells.

Raven Press, New York © 1973
Fetal Pharmacology, edited by L. Boréus

Some Effects of Adrenaline on the Vessels of the 17-Day-Old Rat Fetus

Alfred Jost, Jean-Paul Maltier, and Claude Petter

*Laboratory of Comparative Physiology, University of Paris VI,
9 quai Saint-Bernard, Paris (5e), France.*

A large dose of adrenaline injected into the rat or the rabbit fetus at certain stages produces in 6 hr edema and hemorrhages at the level of the extremities (Jost, 1953*a,b*; Jost, Roffi, and Courtat, 1969). The affected parts become necrotic and fall off. This results in congenital amputations or limb deformities. In the rat fetus, this effect is observed if adrenaline is given between days 15 and 17 inclusive, but not on day 18 or thereafter. Efforts were made to explore the vascular changes occurring after the injection of adrenaline in the 17.5-day-old rat fetus. One approach was histological, and some observations will be summarized here; further details are reported elsewhere by J. P. Maltier who is responsible for the histological part of this study.

MATERIALS AND METHODS

Under ether anesthesia of the mother, a volume of 5 μl containing 1 μg of l-adrenaline at pH 2 to 3 was injected intravenously into a vitelline vein through the uterine wall without damaging the fetal membranes (technique of Jost, Petter, Duval, Maltier, and Roffi, 1964). The uterus was rapidly replaced into the maternal abdominal cavity until sacrifice of the fetus. Under continued (or renewed) maternal ether anesthesia, the uterus was gently opened, without damaging the fetal membranes. In case of accidental rupture of the membranes, the fetus was discarded. A ligature was rapidly placed between the placenta and the entire fetal membranes in order to interrupt the feto-placental exchange of blood. After the membranes were opened, the cord was again ligated and sectioned between the two ligatures. Ligating the umbilical cord is essential to the procedure in order to prevent leakage of blood and reduction of the fetal blood volume.

The 17.5-day-old rat fetus weighs approximately 800 mg, and it is very soft and watery. The penetration of the fixative fluid is probably rapid but it is not immediate, and alterations in the tone of the blood vessels due to the fixative fluid itself cannot be excluded. The freezing method of Hörnblad and Larsson (1967) seems more reliable, although Hörnblad, Larsson, and Marsk (1969) do not exclude that freezing of larger fetuses might elicit vasomotor effects. Moreover, fixation in Bouin's fluid and embedding the fetus in paraffin produces a loss of weight and shrinkage of the whole body, and certainly of the vessels as well. Nevertheless, in fetuses fixed 1, 3, or 10 min or 3 hr after the injection of adrenaline, independent modifications in the diameter of various vessels were observed; this seems to validate the method. It was also verified that an injection of 12 μl of saline at pH 2 to 3 does not significantly alter the blood vessels after 3 min.

In other experiments, the blood volume contained in the normal 17.5-day-old rat fetus and its adnexa was determined with ^{131}I-labeled albumin injected intravenously; it was approximately 130 μl.

RESULTS

In fetuses fixed 1 min after the injection of adrenaline, the diameter of most of the explored vessels was reduced in the histological sections (Table 1). The most striking reduction was seen in the umbilical vein at the level where it runs through the belly wall (Fig. 1). Very few blood cells were present in the hepatic area and the inferior vena cava (Fig. 2). The diameters of the veins were very reduced; it is difficult to assess whether this results from a vasomotor effect of adrenaline or from the diminished amount of blood. The constriction of the umbilical vein might also be a factor in causing the pale color of the whole fetus immediately after the injection of adrenaline.

As soon as 3 min after the injection, the diameter of the umbilical vein

TABLE 1. *Influence of 1 μg of l-adrenaline on diameter (or surface of section of some vessels in histological sections (external diameter or area unless otherwise stated).*

Vessel		Controls	1 min	3 hr
Umbilical vein (ring)	(μm)	230 ± 95 (4)	26 ± 15 (8)	159 ± 74 (9)
Sphincter ductus venosus	(μm)	198 ± 57 (4)	96 ± 37 (7)	110 ± 21 (12)
Inferior vena cava (diaphragm)	($10^3 \mu m^2$)	169 ± 82 (4)	47 ± 22 (8)	160 ± 25 (12)
Ascending aorta (lumen)	(μm)	228 ± 60 (4)	169 ± 24 (8)	197 ± 18 (11)
Pulmonary artery (lumen)	(μm)	194 ± 53 (4)	110 ± 20 (8)	160 ± 24 (11)
Ductus arteriosus (lumen)	(μm)	222 ± 50 (4)	91 ± 36 (8)	107 ± 45 (9)
Descending aorta (lumen)	(μm)	295 ± 84 (4)	231 ± 36 (8)	229 ± 48 (11)
External carotid	(μm)	160 ± 10 (8)	140 ± 14 (16)	131 ± 8 (24)
External jugular vein	($10^3 \mu m^2$)	255 ± 50 (8)	65 ± 12 (6)	164 ± 27 (23)
Central limb artery (fibula)	(μm)	42 ± 7 (9)	20 ± 14 (4)	47 ± 5 (9)
Central limb vein (fibula)	(μm)	56 ± 6 (12)	49 ± 9 (6)	133 ± 36 (4)

Number of fetuses studied in parentheses.
± confidence interval for $p = 0.05$.

had somewhat increased although it remained narrowed (Table 2). Blood cells were again seen in the inferior vena cava and in other hepatic veins, and the diameters of these veins had returned to nearly normal values. Probably as results of the diminished diameter of the sphincter of the ductus venosus (Fig. 2), more blood entered the liver, and the sinus intermedius was patent (Table 2). This was especially conspicuous in the fetuses fixed after 10 min.

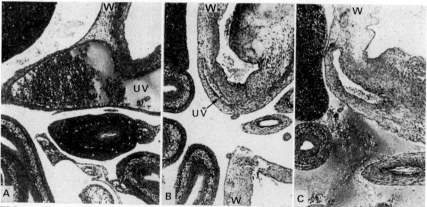

FIG. 1. Histological sections through the abdominal wall (W) at the level of the umbilical ring, showing the umbilical vein (UV) in a control fetus (*A*) and in fetuses injected with adrenaline 1 min (*B*) and 3 hr (*C*) before fixation. The umbilical vein had returned to an almost normal condition in other fetuses in the 3-hr group. ×47

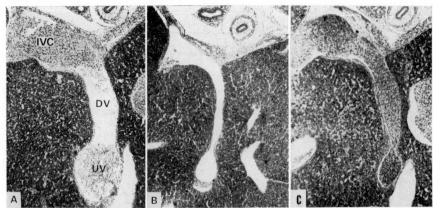

FIG. 2. Sections at the level of the ductus venosus (DV) between the umbilical vein (UV) and the inferior vena cava (IVC) in a control fetus (*A*) and in fetuses injected with adrenaline 1 min (*B*) or 3 hr (*C*) before fixation. The sphincter of the ductus venosus was nearly normal in other fetuses in the 3-hr group. ×30

Immediately after the injection of adrenaline, the ductus arteriosus and the sphincter of the ductus venosus contracted (diameter reduced by approximately one-half; Table 1). Three hr later, the diameter of the ductus arteriosus was still reduced in the nine fetuses examined (Fig. 3). The sphincter of the ductus venosus was still contracted (Fig. 1) in nine out of

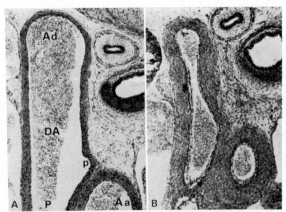

FIG. 3. Sections at the level of the ductus arteriosus (DA) in a control fetus (*A*) and in a fetus given adrenaline 3 hr before fixation (*B*). The origin of the pulmonary arteries (p) is seen in the control fetus. Aa and Ad, aorta ascendens and descendens; P, main pulmonary artery. ×54

TABLE 2. *Effects of adrenaline on some veins at various times after an injection of adrenaline*

Vein		Control	1 min	3 min	10 min	3 hr
Umbilical vein	(μm)	230 ± 95 (4)	26 ± 15 (8)	32–126[a]	86 ± 21 (4)	159 ± 74 (9)
Sphincter ductus venosus	(μm)	198 ± 37 (4)	96 ± 37 (7)	78–138[a]	142 ± 46 (4)	110 ± 21 (12)
Inferior vena cava	(10^3 μm^2)	169 ± 82 (4)	47 ± 22 (8)	185–239[a]	205 ± 30 (5)	160 ± 25 (12)
Sinus intermedius	(μm)	242–432[a]	268 ± 60 (7)	464–638[a]	425 ±161 (4)	411 ±106 (12)

Number of fetuses studied in parentheses.
± confidence interval for $p = 0.05$.
[a] Extreme values of only three determinations.

12 fetuses, and the umbilical vein in five (Fig. 1) out of nine.

Meanwhile, for one reason or another, blood cells seemed to accumulate in the venous system and heart atria, whereas edema developed in several areas. This was especially clear in the limbs where the main vein was distended after 3 hr (Table 1) and filled with blood cells; the connective tissue was edematous and sometimes blebs would appear. It could be verified that blood did not circulate, or only very little, in the limbs; when india ink was given intravenously to fetuses treated with adrenaline 1 or 2 hr before, the limbs remained whitish whereas the body blackened; in controls, the india ink was rapidly seen in the limbs as well as throughout the body.

CONCLUSION

The techniques used in these experiments on very small fetuses can probably be assumed to give some information on the repartition of blood in the fetus and on the condition of the vessels since differences were observed between control and adrenaline-injected fetuses and since these differences changed with the period of time elapsed after the injection. However, the possibility that artifacts intervene cannot be excluded.

Adrenaline given *in vivo* seems to have long-lasting effects on the ductus arteriosus and probably also on the umbilical vein and on the sphincter of the ductus venosus. This might be due to the important adrenergic innervation of these vessels reported in other animal species (Ehinger, Gennser, Owman, Persson, and Sjöberg, 1968; Boréus, Malmfors, McMurphy, and Olson, 1969; Aronson, Gennser, Owman, and Sjöberg, 1970; Lachenmayer, 1971). The various parts of the vascular bed on which adrenaline might have similar effects have to be explored further.

The hemodynamic consequences of these (and possibly other) effects of adrenaline on fetal hemodynamics in the 17-day-old rat fetus and their bearing on the problem of teratogenic hemorrhages remain to be assessed.

REFERENCES

Aronson, S., Gennser, G., Owman, C., and Sjöberg, N. O. (1970): Innervation and contractile response of the human ductus arteriosus. *European Journal of Pharmacology*, 11:178-186.

Boréus, L. O., Malmfors, T., McMurphy, D. M., and Olson, L. (1969): Demonstration of adrenergic receptor function and innervation in the ductus arteriosus of the human fetus. *Acta Physiologica Scandinavica*, 77:316-321.

Ehinger, B., Gennser, G., Owman, C., Persson, H., and Sjöberg, N. O. (1968): Histochemical and pharmacological studies on amine mechanisms in the umbilical cord, umbilical vein and ductus venosus of the human fetus. *Acta Physiologica Scandinavica,* 72:15.

Hörnblad, P. Y. (1969): Effect of oxygen and umbilical cord clamping on closure of the ductus arteriosus in the guinea pig and the rat. Studies on the closure of the ductus arteriosus. VI. *Acta Physiologica Scandinavica,* 76:58.

Hörnblad, P. Y., and Larsson, K. S. (1967): Studies on closure of the ductus arteriosus. I. Whole-body freezing as improvement of fixation procedures. *Cardiologia,* 51:231-241.

Hörnblad, P. Y., Larsson, K. S., and Marsk, L. (1969): Studies on closure of the ductus arteriosus. VII. Closure rate and morphology of the ductus arteriosus in the lamb. *Cardiologia,* 54:336-342.

Jost, A. (1953a): Dégénérescence des extrémités du foetus de rat provoquée par l'adrénaline. *Comptes Rendus Hebdomadaires des Séances de l'Académie des Sciences* (Paris), 236:1510-1512.

Jost, A. (1953b): La dégénérescence des extremites du foetus de rat sous des actions hormonales (acroblapsie expérimentale) et la théorie des bulles myélencéphaliques de Bonnevie. *Archives Françaises de Pédiatrie,* 10:855-860.

Jost, A., Petter, C., Duval, G., Maltier, J. P., and Roffi, J. (1964): Action de l'adrénaline sur le partage du sang entre le foetus et le placenta. Facteurs hémodynamiques de certaines lésions congénitales des extrémités. *Comptes Rendus Hebdomadaires des Séances de Académie des Sciences* (Paris), 259:3086-3088.

Jost, A., Roffi, J., and Courtat, M. (1969): Congenital amputations determined by the br gene and those induced by adrenaline injection in the rabbit foetus. In: *Limb Development and Deformity: Problems of Evaluation and Rehabilitation,* edited by C. A. Swinyard. C. C. Thomas Publ., Springfield, Ill., pp. 187-189.

Lachenmayer, L. (1971): Adrenergic innervation of the umbilical vessels. Light and fluorescence microscopic studies. *Zeitschrift für Zellforschung,* 120:120-136.

NOTE ADDED IN PROOF

Recent observations *in vivo* confirm the previous histological studies. With 12 μl of diluted india ink added (or not), 2 μg of adrenaline was injected intravenously as described in the text. The alive fetuses were placed under a magnifier, regularly moistened with tepid saline, and observed for 15 to 20 min. The heart continued beating: constriction could be observed in the adrenaline-treated fetuses at the level of the ductus arteriosus after opening the chest, and at the level of the umbilical vein after reclining the abdominal wall.

DISCUSSION

TERAMO: I should like to make a comment on the flow through the ductus venosus. Recently, Rudolph et al. (*Pediat. Res.,* 5:452, 1971) observed a very large range (18 to 19%) in the proportion of umbilical venous return through the ductus venosus in human fetuses in early gestation. The measurements were done using the isotope-labeled microsphere method during hysterotomies for legal abortions. The flow through the ductus venosus was unrelated to weight. In the same fetus, the flow through the ductus remained almost unchanged, although during the same observation period the actual umbilical blood flow decreased and the distribution of the cardiac output changed markedly.

JOST: I have no experience in that field. Could variations in the fetal p_{O_2} be a factor?

DAWES: Aren't the injected doses of adrenaline very large?

JOST: Of course they are. We used such large doses because they produce limb abnormalities in practically 100% of the treated young; the purpose of the observations was to explore the mode of development of the limb abnormalities.

McBRIDE: You mentioned the very limited period (15th to 17th day of rat gestation) that the injection of noradrenaline could produce deformities. Did earlier injections produce any effects or is it merely technically too difficult?

JOST: Earlier injections are difficult to perform in a satisfactory way. In some fetuses given adrenaline intraperitoneally earlier, I observed blebs on various parts of the body, for example, the back (Jost, 1953b).

Fetal Pharmacology, edited by L. Boréus
Raven Press, New York © 1973

Adenosine 3',5'-Monophosphate During Fetal and Postnatal Development

Benjamin Weiss* and Samuel J. Strada**

Laboratory of Preclinical Pharmacology, National Institute of Mental Health, Saint Elizabeths Hospital, Washington, D.C. 20032

Any discussion of the role adenosine 3',5'-monophosphate (cyclic AMP) plays in the ontogeny of the fetus should be prefaced by a statement indicating the sparcity of data showing a causal relationship between cyclic AMP and developmental processes. On the other hand, cyclic AMP has been shown to elicit such a wide variety of biochemical effects and enjoys such a central position in many regulatory mechanisms that it may not be too great an extrapolation to predict that it is also an important component of the mechanisms governing fetal growth. (For recent reviews and monographs, see Robison, Butcher, and Sutherland, 1968; Sutherland, Robison, and Butcher, 1968; Weiss and Kidman, 1969; Breckenridge, 1970; Greengard and Costa, 1970; Weiss and Crayton, 1970a; Weiss, 1970; Hardman, Robison, and Sutherland, 1971; Robison, Butcher, and Sutherland, 1971; Weiss, 1971a; Jost and Rickenberg, 1971; Weiss and Strada, 1972.) It is within this context that we outline some of the biochemical actions of cyclic AMP, particularly as they may relate to the growth and differentiation of cells, and discuss the factors influencing the concentration of cyclic

* Present address: Department of Pharmacology, Medical College of Pennsylvania, Philadelphia, Pa.
** Present address: Department of Pharmacology, Houston Medical School, Houston, Texas.

AMP during postnatal development. We also pose what we feel are the unanswered questions and what we think may be the fruitful avenues for future research.

EFFECTS OF CYCLIC AMP ON THE GROWTH, PROLIFERATION, AND DIFFERENTIATION OF CELLS

There are many possible mechanisms available for regulating cellular growth and differentiation, the most obvious being genetic control of protein synthesis. Hormonal and environmental (particularly nutritional) factors may also play a role, although the mechanisms by which these effects occur are poorly understood. One intriguing possibility is that the cyclic AMP system, and, more specifically, the development of the sensitivity of the cyclic AMP system to hormone action may be causally related to those cellular events associated with cell proliferation and differentiation.

Only recently has evidence become available to support the notion that cyclic AMP is involved in the processes of cellular growth and proliferation. Not only has it been shown that pure cultures of mammalian cells contained the enzymatic machinery required to synthesize and degrade cyclic AMP (Makman, 1970; Weiss, Shein, and Snyder, 1971; Perkins, MacIntyre, Riley, and Clark, 1971; Peery, Johnson, and Pastan, 1971), but also that these cells possessed an adenylate cyclase system that was sensitive to hormonal stimulation (Makman, 1970, 1971) and contained a cyclic AMP-dependent protein kinase activity (Klein and Makman, 1971). However, the amount of adenylate cyclase activity and its sensitivity to hormones depended on the type of cell, the conditions in which the cells were grown, and the rates of growth of the cells. For example, rat hepatoma cells grown in suspension culture contained less adenylate cyclase activity than cells grown in stationary culture (Makman, 1970). These results were recently confirmed with other cell lines (Makman, 1971a), suggesting that one means of regulating adenylate cyclase activity could be through either a cell-to-surface or a cell-to-cell interaction.

Malignant cells grown in culture characteristically have unregulated growth and loss of contact inhibition. Cyclic AMP and its dibutyryl derivative have been shown to promote contact inhibition of cell growth (Ryan and Heidrick, 1968; Heidrick and Ryan, 1970, 1971), to reestablish this property of contact-inhibited growth to cultures of transformed cells (Sheppard, 1971), and to restore the abnormal morphology and replication pattern

TABLE 1. *Adenylate cyclase activity of astrocytes and virally transformed astrocytoma cells of the hamster.*

Tissue	Adenylate Cyclase (pmoles cyclic AMP formed/mg protein/min $\pm$ SE)
Normal astrocytes	75 ± 9
Astrocytoma cells	29 ± 1 [a]

Cultures of normal newborn hamster astrocytes and SV_{40} virus-transformed astrocytoma cells were prepared and assayed for adenylate cyclase activity.
[a] $p < 0.001$ compared with normal astrocytes (from Weiss et al., 1971).

of transformed cells to that more characteristic of normal growth (Johnson, Friedman, and Pastan, 1971; Hsie, Jones, and Puck, 1971; Yang and Vas, 1971; Hsie and Puck, 1971).

Another interesting finding is that, generally, malignant cells have less hormone-sensitive adenylate cyclase activity than nonmalignant cells (Burk, 1968; Weiss et al., 1971; Makman, 1971a; Perkins et al., 1971; Peery et al., 1971). As an example, it is shown in Table 1 that normal, newborn hamster astrocytes had almost three times the adenylate cyclase activity compared with that of SV_{40} virus-transformed astrocytoma cells.

The obvious inference to be drawn from these studies is that changes in the intracellular concentration of cyclic AMP can alter the growth and transformational properties of these cells. In support of this notion, Otten, Johnson, and Pastan (1971) measured the concentration of cyclic AMP in several different strains of transformed and nontransformed fibroblasts, and found an inverse relationship between the growth rate of these cells and the concentration of cyclic AMP. Moreover, they showed that the cyclic AMP levels were increased at confluency in a cell line having the property of contact-inhibited growth, and were decreased in a cell line devoid of contact-inhibited growth. These experiments suggest that cyclic AMP may regulate the rate of proliferation of cells, perhaps by mediating the contact inhibition of growth, and that the increased rate of growth and loss of contact inhibition characteristic of transformed, malignant cells may result from a reduced concentration of cyclic AMP. Measurement of the concentration of cyclic AMP in other normal and transformed cell types should help clarify these points.

Definitive evidence that cyclic AMP is the causative agent in cellular differentiation is not yet available. However, there are several indications that cyclic AMP influences the differentiation of cells. For example, Castaneda and Tyler (1968) showed that adenylate cyclase activity of sea urchin eggs is increased after fertilization. Moreover, dibutyryl cyclic AMP has been reported to induce the differential mitosis of melanoblasts into melanocytes in cultured explants of the caudal fin of the goldfish (Chen and Tchen, 1970), and to induce the formation of axons in mouse neuroblastoma cells (Prasad and Hsie, 1971). The experiments of Bonner, Konijn, and their colleagues (Konijn, Van de Meene, Bonner, and Barkley, 1967; Konijn, Barkley, Chang, and Bonner, 1968; Konijn, Van de Meene, Chang, Barkley, and Bonner, 1969; Bonner, 1970) who showed that cyclic AMP induces the morphogenesis of the cellular slime mold *Dictyostelium discoideum* perhaps by a chemotactic action, and the work of Yokota and Gots (1970), who found that cyclic AMP is essential for the formation of flagella in coliform bacteria provide further fuel for the concept of a role for cyclic AMP in cellular differentiation.

Epinephrine, certain prostaglandins, and several polypeptide hormones including parathyroid hormone, growth hormone, and vasopressin stimulate the proliferation of rat thymic lymphocytes. These compounds also increase DNA synthesis and enhance the flow of cells into the mitotic stage (MacManus and Whitfield, 1969, 1970; Rixon, Whitfield, and MacManus, 1970; Whitfield, MacManus, and Gillan, 1970a; Whitfield, MacManus, and Rixon, 1970b; MacManus, Whitfield, and Youdale, 1971; Franks, MacManus, and Whitfield, 1971). These effects are thought to be mediated through a change in the concentration of cyclic AMP. Thus, the action of these hormones can be mimicked both *in vivo* and *in vitro* by the exogenous administration of either cyclic AMP or dibutyryl cyclic AMP; their effects are enhanced by phosphodiesterase inhibitors such as caffeine and are diminished by imidazole which stimulates phosphodiesterase activity; and the actions of epinephrine and prostaglandins on DNA synthesis, thymocyte proliferation, and mitosis are preceded by an increase in the intracellular concentration of cyclic AMP. In addition, there is evidence that cyclic AMP mediates the isoproterenol-induced cellular proliferation of mouse parotid gland. The *in vivo* administration of isoproterenol raised the concentration of cyclic AMP several-fold in mouse parotid gland, and the increase preceded the enhanced incorporation of thymidine into DNA induced by isoproterenol (Guidotti, Weiss, and Costa, 1971).

EFFECTS OF CYCLIC AMP ON ENZYME INDUCTION

In 1965, Makman and Sutherland reported that *Escherichia coli* could synthesize cyclic AMP from ATP through the action of adenylate cyclase and that the intracellular concentration of cyclic AMP depended upon the nutrients in the culture medium. In the presence of glucose, cyclic AMP rapidly disappeared from the cells and appeared in the medium. However, an abrupt rise in the concentration of cyclic AMP occurred in the organisms coincident with the complete utilization of glucose. On the basis of these findings, they speculated that the cyclic nucleotide was involved in controlling the availability of endogenous reserves, in synthesizing inducible enzymes, and for other specialized functions such as motility. This general role for cyclic AMP in bacterial physiology has been supported by the more recent evidence showing that this nucleotide counteracts catabolite repression in *Escherichia coli* and is required for synthesizing and inducing a number of enzymes in these organisms. Thus, cyclic AMP increases the synthesis of β-galactosidase and other inducible enzymes such as tryptophanase, galactonase, glycerokinase, D-serine deaminase, and thymidine phosphorylase, (Pastan and Perlman, 1968, 1969, 1970; Perlman and Pastan, 1968a,b; deCrombrugghe, Varmus, Perlman, and Pastan, 1969, 1970; Varmus, Perlman, and Pastan, 1970a,b; Miller, Varmus, Parks, Perlman, and Pastan, 1971). The effects of cyclic AMP on enzyme induction are not limited to bacteria but occur in mammalian systems as well (Yeung and Oliver, 1968; Jost, Hsie, and Rickenberg, 1969; Jost, Hsie, Hughes, and Ryan, 1970; Jost and Sahib, 1971; Wicks, 1968, 1969, 1971; Linarelli, Weller, and Glinsman, 1970; Chuah and Oliver, 1971).

EFFECTS OF CYCLIC AMP ON PROTEIN KINASES

Cyclic AMP-dependent protein kinases have been isolated from many mammalian and non-mammalian systems (Walsh, Perkins, and Krebs, 1968; Kuo and Greengard, 1969a,b; Miyamoto, Kuo, and Greengard, 1969a,b; Kuo, Krueger, Sanes, and Greengard, 1970; Gill and Garren, 1970; Tao, Salas, and Lipmann, 1970; Reimann, Walsh, and Krebs, 1971), and it has been proposed that the biological effects of cyclic AMP are mediated through the activation of protein kinases. One of the prominent actions of the cyclic AMP dependent kinases is the phosphorylation of histones (Langan, 1969a,b; Kuo and Greengard, 1970; Greengard and Kuo, 1970). Basic cellular proteins such as histones are characteristic components of the DNA genome and serve to regulate gene transcription. It is generally held that the phosphorylation of histones uncovers gene sequences allowing the DNA molecule to be transcribed (Georgiev, 1969). A general scheme has evolved that the cyclic AMP-dependent protein kinases consist of two subunits—a catalytic subunit and a regulatory (inhibitory) subunit that binds cyclic AMP. Cyclic AMP activates the protein kinase by removing the inhibitory subunit, thereby freeing the active (cyclic AMP-independent) form of the enzyme (Greengard and Kuo, 1970; Tao et al., 1970; Miyamoto, Petzold, Harris, and Greengard, 1971; Reimann et al., 1971; Tao, 1971; Walton, Gill, Abrass, and Garren, 1971; Anderson, Schneider, Emmer, Perlman, and Pastan, 1971). Thus, by activating protein kinases, cyclic AMP induces the phosphorylation of histones. These phosphorylated histones in turn act as derepressors, allowing transcription (and therefore protein synthesis) to take place.

Having emphasized the importance of cyclic AMP as a regulator of the growth, proliferation, and differentiation of cells, we can now turn our attention to the postnatal changes which take place in the enzymes which actually control the intracellular concentration of cyclic AMP in the organism during these critical periods of growth and development.

DEVELOPMENT OF ADENYLATE CYCLASE ACTIVITY AND THE ACQUISITION OF HORMONAL SENSITIVITY

The ontogenetic development of adenylate cyclase activity in various parts of the rat brain is illustrated in Fig. 1. In each brain area studied, enzyme activity increased from birth; however, the pattern of development varied with the structure. For example, adenylate cyclase activity of brainstem and cerebrum increased rapidly from birth to 15 days of age, then declined substantially between 15 and 60 days. Enzyme activity of cerebellum increased more slowly and reached a maximum at about 30 days.

In these studies, enzyme activity was assayed in the presence of sodium fluoride which stimulates adenylate cyclase activity maximally. However, there is now ample evidence showing that adenylate cyclase is not a simple discrete molecule but rather that it possesses different sites at which stimulators can act. This conclusion, suggested originally by the early work of Sutherland and Rall (1960), is supported largely by studies showing that the adenylate cyclase of different tissues can be activated by specific hormones. For example, hormonal specificity for activating adenylate cyclase has now been shown for leutinizing hormone in the corpus luteum (Marsh, Butcher, Savard, and Sutherland, 1966), for ACTH in the adrenal cortex (Grahame-Smith, Butcher, Ney, and Sutherland, 1967), for thyroid-stimulating hormone in thyroid homogenates (Pastan and Katzen, 1967), for catecholamines in pineal gland (Weiss and Costa, 1968a), and for hypothalamic extracts in

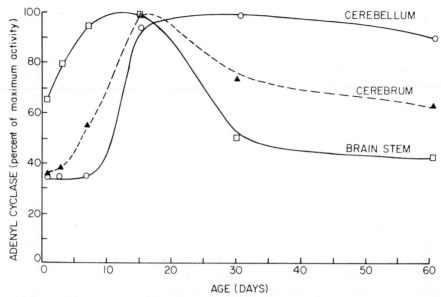

FIG. 1. Ontogenetic development of adenylate cyclase activity of rat brain. Adenylate cyclase activity of rat brain homogenates was determined by the method of Krishna, Weiss, and Brodie (1968). Maximum activity for cerebellum was 480 pmoles of cyclic AMP formed per mg protein per min, for cerebrum 420, and for brainstem 350. (Data taken from Weiss, 1971b.)

the anterior pituitary (Zor, Kaneko, Schneider, McCann, Lowe, Bloom, Borland, and Field, 1969).

The question of whether this specificity is due to different enzymes or to different receptors on the same enzyme is still open. There is, however, general agreement that there are different sites on the adenylate cyclase system that can respond to different activators. This has been shown in pineal gland (Weiss, 1969a), fat cells (Rodbell, Birnbaumer, and Pohl, 1970), thyroid (Burke, 1970), and heart (Drummond, Severson, and Duncan, 1971). Evidence has also been presented (Bitensky, Russell, and Robertson, 1968; Ray, Tomasi, and Marinetti, 1970; Reik, Petzhold, Higgins, Greengard, and Barrnett, 1970) for the existence of two discrete adenylate cyclases of rat liver. Moreover, recent studies with *Streptococcus salivarius* have shown that there are different adenylate cyclases separable by Sephadex column chromatography (Khandelwal and Hamilton, 1971). On the other hand, in fat cells there is evidence for a single adenylate cyclase with different receptor proteins associated with it (Birnbaumer, Pohl, and Rodbell, 1969; Birnbaumer and Rodbell, 1969).

Experiments with pineal gland have shown that there are at least two types of adenylate cyclase activities: a basal adenylate cyclase activity (i.e., enzyme activity measured in the absence of activator) and a catecholamine-sensitive adenylate cyclase activity. This hormone-sensitive enzyme can be altered without affecting the basal activity. Thus, sympathetically denervating the pineal gland (Weiss and Costa, 1967; Weiss, 1969b), exposing rats to continuous illumination (Weiss, 1969b), or ovariectomizing rats (Weiss and Crayton, 1970b) all increased the norepinephrine-sensitive adenylate cyclase without affecting the basal activity.

By studying the ontogenetic development of pineal adenylate cyclase activity, we showed that a norepinephrine-sensitive adenylate cyclase can develop without a concomitant change in the basal enzyme activity. Adenylate cyclase of pineal gland of newborn rats was not activated by norepinephrine; the responsiveness to the catecholamine developed a few days after birth, reached a maximum by about 20 days, and then declined slightly thereafter (Weiss, 1971b). This is similar to the results of Rosen and Erlichman (1969), who reported that the catecholamine-induced stimulation of tad-pole erythrocyte adenylate cyclase increased with age.

Schmidt, Palmer, Dettbarn, and Robison (1970) studied the effect of age on the increased concentration of cyclic AMP in rat brain slices in response to norepinephrine. Norepinephrine failed to increase the concen-tration of cyclic AMP in brain slices of newborn rats but raised the level of the cyclic nucleotide several-fold in rats 6 days of age and older. In more recent work, Schmidt and Robison (1971) found that the extent to which norepinephrine increased the concentration of cyclic AMP varied both with age and with the brain area studied. In general, the sensitivity to norepineph-rine increased for the first 2 weeks after birth and then declined.

Several other investigators have also shown differences in adenylate cyclase activity as a function of age. Forn, Schonhofer, Skidmore, and Krishna (1970) reported a lower norepinephrine-stimulated adenylate cy-clase activity in fat cell homogenates of old rats than in those of younger animals. Bitensky, Russell, and Blanco (1970) showed that the glucagon and epinephrine-responsive adenylate cyclase of rat liver declined with in-creasing age. Similarly, Makman (1971b) reported that the catecholamine-stimulated adenylate cyclase activity of mouse thymocytes decreased with age.

An important question still to be answered is what factors are respon-sible for changes in the development of hormone-sensitive adenylate cyclase activities. Along these lines, we have shown that a norepinephrine-sensitive adenylate cyclase can develop in the pineal gland even in the absence of its primary innervation, i.e., the sympathetic nervous system (Weiss, 1970, 1971a; Strada and Weiss, 1972). Thus, removing the sympathetic input to the pineal gland in newborn animals by ganglionectomy, immuno-sympathectomy, or chemical sympathectomy with 6-hydroxydopamine failed to prevent the development of a hormone-sensitive adenylate cyclase in pineal gland; the sensitivity of the cyclic AMP system to norepinephrine in these animals was, in fact, greater than in that of control animals.

Makman (1971a) recently reported that several hormones stimulated adenylate cyclase activity to a greater extent in stationary cell cultures than in suspension cultures. Moreover, Seeds and Gilman (1971) showed that the norepinephrine-sensitive adenylate cyclase appeared in cultured fetal mouse brain cells only after several days of culture, at which time the cell density was greatly increased. These interesting observations suggest that cell-to-cell interactions may be important for the acquisition of hormonal sensitivity.

DEVELOPMENT OF PHOSPHODIESTERASE ACTIVITY

The postnatal development of phosphodiesterase activity has been the subject of several investigations. Schmidt et al. (1970) reported a several-fold increase in phosphodiesterase activity of rat brain between birth and 23 days of age; the ratio of the enzyme activity in the soluble and particulate fractions did not change significantly with age. Gaballah and Popoff (1971) also studied the development of the total phosphodiesterase activity in different subcellular fractions of rat brain. They found that enzyme activity increased two- to threefold between 10 and 20 days of age. All subcellular fractions examined (i.e., mitochondria, nerve endings, and nerve ending membrane) increased by about the same extent.

Figure 2 illustrates that the postnatal development of phosphodiesterase activity varies with the brain area. In the rat, enzyme activity of brain-stem and cerebrum increased several-fold between 2 and 16 days of age. However, phosphodiesterase of cerebellum did not increase during this period and actually showed a slight decline with age.

MULTIPLE PHOSPHODIESTERASE ACTIVITIES

As in the case with adenylate cyclase, we no longer consider phosphodiesterase as a single enzyme, but rather as a group of enzymes with an

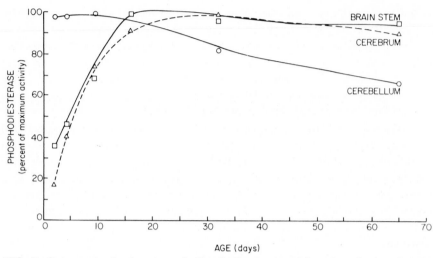

FIG. 2. Ontogenetic development of phosphodiesterase activity of rat brain. Phosphodiesterase activity of rat brain homogenates was determined by the method of Butcher and Sutherland (1962). Maximum activity for cerebellum was 15 nmoles cyclic AMP hydrolyzed per mg protein per min, for cerebrum 28, and for brainstem 27. (Data taken from Weiss, 1971*b*.)

extremely complex array of molecular forms, each having different physical, chemical, and kinetic properties. For example, by using agarose gel filtration, Thompson and Appleman (1971*a,b*) found one phosphodiesterase with a relatively high molecular weight (approximately 400,000) and an apparent K_m of about 1×10^{-4} M and one phosphodiesterase with a lower molecular weight (about 200,000) and a K_m of about 5×10^{-6} M. The higher molecular weight fraction hydrolyzed cyclic 3′,5′-guanosine monophosphate (cyclic GMP) as well as cyclic AMP. Other investigators have also shown— using kinetic analyses and electrophoretic separation procedures—that several tissues, including brain, have multiple forms of phosphodiesterase activity (Rosen, 1970; Huang and Kemp, 1971; Monn and Christiansen, 1971; Kakiuchi, Yamazaki, and Teshima, 1971; Uzunov and Weiss, 1972).

Phosphodiesterase activities with relatively high specificities for cyclic 3′,5′-uridine monophosphate (Hardman and Sutherland, 1965; Klotz and Stock, 1971) and for cyclic GMP have also been demonstrated (Beavo, Hardman, and Sutherland, 1970), and there are apparently phosphodiesterases that can be activated by different, endogenously occurring substances (Kakiuchi and Yamazaki, 1970; Cheung, 1971).

Our own studies of the different phosphodiesterase activities have been carried out using a simple micromethod recently developed in our laboratory (Weiss, Lehne, and Strada, 1972). In this procedure, the 5′-AMP formed from the hydrolysis of cyclic AMP is converted stoichiometrically to ATP with the addition of myokinase and pyruvate kinase. The ATP is determined by the luminescence generated by the addition of a firefly luciferin-luciferase preparation. This assay is sensitive enough to measure the phosphodiesterase activity in a homogenate of brain containing as little as 0.1 μg of tissue. Using this procedure we have studied the distribution of the multiple forms of phosphodiesterase in the various parts of the rat brain and the rate at which these enzyme activities develop postnatally.

The kinetic analyses of the data were evaluated as decribed earlier (Weiss and Strada, 1972). Briefly, phosphodiesterase activity is determined in the presence of varying concentrations of cyclic AMP. The data are plotted according to Lineweaver and Burk (1934). If the data allow two straight lines to be drawn through the experimental points, this can be

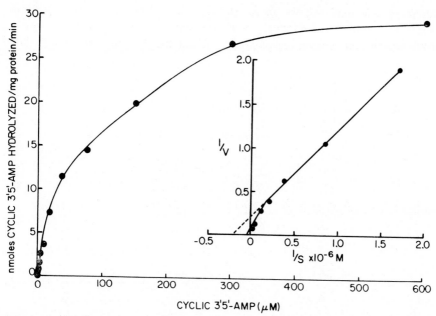

FIG. 3. Phosphodiesterase activities of pig cerebrum as a function of the substrate concentration. Varying concentrations of cyclic AMP were incubated with an enzyme partially purified from pig cerebrum (equivalent to 1 μg of protein). (From Weiss et al., 1971.)

TABLE 2. *Regional distribution of the phosphodiesterase activities of rat brain.*

Tissue	Phosphodiesterase activity (nmoles/mg protein/min)		
	V total	V high K_m	V low K_m
Caudate nucleus	150	146	4
Hippocampus	130	123	7
Olfactory tubercle	130	126	4
Parietal cortex	100	96	4
Thalamus	55	52	3
Olfactory bulb	50	47	3
Hypothalamus	50	48	2
Septum and fornix	50	47	3
Inferior colliculus	16	13	3
Superior colliculus	10	8	2
Medulla	10	8	2
Cerebellum	8.5	6.4	2.1
Pineal	8.3	5.0	3.3
Pons	8.0	6.7	1.3
Spinal cord	5.0	4.0	1.3

interpreted as evidence for the existence of two different phosphodiesterase activities—one with a relatively high apparent K_m and one with a lower K_m (Thompson and Appleman, 1971a,b). When the two lines are extrapolated

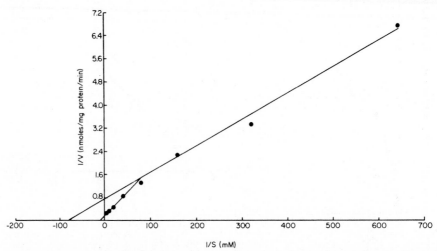

FIG. 4. Multiple phosphodiesterase activities of rat spinal cord. Spinal cord of a 60-day-old rat was homogenized and assayed for phosphodiesterase activity in the presence of varying concentrations of substrate. V total $= 5.0$ nmoles cyclic AMP hydrolyzed/mg protein/min; V high $K_m = 4.0$ nmoles cyclic AMP hydrolyzed/mg protein/min; V low $K_m = 1.3$ nmoles cyclic AMP hydrolyzed/mg protein/min.

to the ordinate, the point of intersection of the line representing the lower K_m enzyme with the ordinate represents the maximum velocity of the lower K_m enzyme (V low K_m). The point of intersection of the other line with the ordinate represents the maximum velocity of the total phosphodiesterase activity (V total). The difference between these two values indicates the maximum velocity of the higher K_m enzyme (V high K_m (see Fig. 3).

The data in Table 2 show that the different areas of the rat brain possess widely varying activities of phosphodiesterase, and that the ratio of the activities of the high and low K_m enzymes range from about 3:1 for the spinal cord (Fig. 4) to about 35:1 for the caudate nucleus (Fig. 5). The major reason for differences in the ratio of the high to low K_m enzymes is the differences in the activity of the high K_m enzyme; when compared with the high K_m enzyme, the activity of the low K_m phosphodiesterase was fairly constant throughout the various areas of the brain (Table 2).

DIFFERENTIAL DEVELOPMENT OF THE MULTIPLE PHOSPHODIESTERASE ACTIVITIES

We have chosen the cerebrum and cerebellum for investigating the ontogenetic development of the different phosphodiesterases because earlier

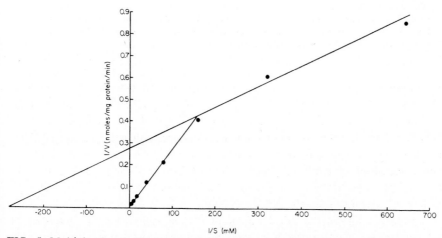

FIG. 5. Multiple phosphodiesterase activities of rat caudate nucleus. Caudate nucleus of a 60-day-old rat was homogenized and assayed for phosphodiesterase activity in the presence of varying concentrations of substrate. V total = 150 nmoles cyclic AMP hydrolyzed/mg protein/min; V high K_m = 146 nmoles cyclic AMP hydrolyzed/mg protein/min; V low K_m = 4 nmoles cyclic AMP hydrolyzed/mg protein/min.

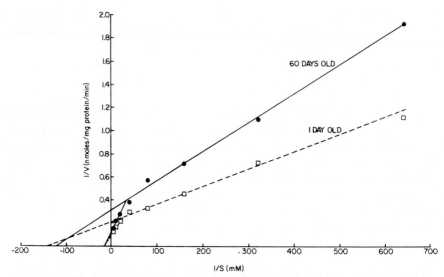

FIG. 6. Ontogenetic development of the multiple phosphodiesterase activities of rat cerebellum. The cerebellum of 1- or 60-day-old rats was homogenized and assayed for phosphodiesterase activity in the presence of varying concentrations of substrate. The relative activities of the high and low K_m phosphodiesterase activities were calculated as described in the text.

One-day-old rats: V total $= 10.5$ nmoles cyclic AMP hydrolyzed/mg protein/min; V high $K_m = 6.0$ nmoles cyclic AMP hydrolyzed/mg protein/min; V low $K_m = 4.5$ nmoles cyclic AMP hydrolyzed/mg protein/min.

Sixty-day-old rats: V total $= 10.5$ nmoles cyclic AMP hydrolyzed/mg protein/min; V high $K_m = 7.3$ nmoles cyclic AMP hydrolyzed/mg protein/min; V low $K_m = 3.2$ nmoles cyclic AMP hydrolyzed/mg protein/min.

experiments showed a distinctly different pattern of development of the total phosphodiesterase activity in these tissues. In rat cerebrum, enzyme activity increased several-fold between birth and 60 days of age, whereas in cerebellum phosphodiesterase activity failed to change with age (Weiss, 1971*b*). In addition, the present work (Table 2) showed that the cerebral cortex and cerebellum of adult rats had markedly different ratios of the high to low K_m phosphodiesterase; the cortex had a much larger ratio of the high to low K_m enzyme than did the cerebellum.

Figure 6 shows the development of the phosphodiesterase activities of rat cerebellum. Neither the total enzyme activity nor the ratio of the high to low K_m phosphodiesterase changed significantly with age. In the cerebrum, on the other hand (Fig. 7), the total phosphodiesterase activity increased more than fivefold between 1 and 60 days of age. This increase was due al-

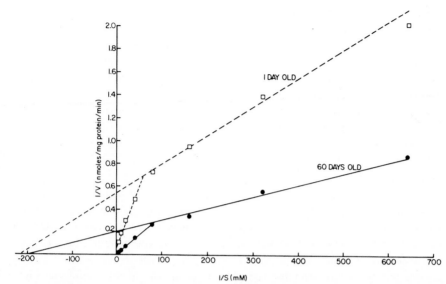

FIG. 7. Ontogenetic development of the multiple phosphodiesterase activities of rat cerebrum. The cerebrum of 1- or 60-day-old rats was homogenized and assayed for phosphodiesterase activity in the presence of varying concentrations of substrate. The relative activities of the high and low K_m phosphodiesterase activities were calculated as described in the text.

One-day-old rats: V total $= 17$ nmoles cyclic AMP hydrolyzed/mg protein/min; V high $K_m = 15$ nmoles cyclic AMP hydrolyzed/mg protein/min; V low $K_m = 2$ nmoles cyclic AMP hydrolyzed/mg protein/min.

Sixty-day-old rats: V total $= 100$ nmoles cyclic AMP hydrolyzed/mg protein/min; V high $K_m = 95$ nmoles cyclic AMP hydrolyzed/mg protein/min; V low $K_m = 5$ nmoles cyclic AMP hydrolyzed/mg protein/min.

most exclusively to a greater activity of the high K_m phosphodiesterase. Thus, whereas the low K_m phosphodiesterase activity increased from 2 to 5 nmoles/mg protein/min, the high K_m enzyme activity increased from 15 to 95 nmoles/mg protein/min.

Studies of the rat pineal gland also showed a difference in the rates at which these two enzyme activities increase with age; the high K_m phospho-diesterase increased about fivefold from 1 to 70 days of age, whereas the low K_m enzyme increased 20-fold during this same period (Weiss and Strada, 1972).

It is very tempting to speculate on the physiological significance of the different phosphodiesterase activities. Since the concentration of cyclic AMP in most tissues is on the order of 10^{-6} moles/kg of tissue (Ebadi,

Weiss, and Costa, 1971; Robison et al., 1971), perhaps the low K_m phosphodiesterase (which has a K_m of about 10^{-6} M and which probably has a higher affinity for cyclic AMP) is the enzyme that physiologically controls the basal concentrations of the cyclic nucleotide. The high K_m enzyme would become operative only when the intracellular concentrations of cyclic AMP approach 10^{-4} M, as in the case following the activation of adenylate cyclase by hormones or other stimuli (Gilman and Nirenberg, 1971; Strada, Klein, Weller, and Weiss, 1972). Tissues with low activity of the high K_m enzyme would permit a large elevation of cyclic AMP. Conversely, a high activity of the high K_m enzyme would tend to prevent any large increases in the concentration of cyclic AMP. This would explain the finding that following decapitation the concentrations of cyclic AMP increase dramatically in rat cerebellum but fail to increase significantly in the cerebrum, and would also explain why norepinephrine can increase the concentration of cyclic AMP to a greater extent in slices of rat cerebellum than in slices of cerebrum (Uzunov and Weiss, 1971). The direction for future research clearly points toward studying the physiological role of these multiple phosphodiesterases and for determining the endogenous and exogenous factors controlling their development.

CONCENTRATION OF CYCLIC AMP IN TISSUES AS A FUNCTION OF AGE

With the exception of brain, relatively little information is available relating the concentration of cyclic AMP in tissues with the age of the animals. Figure 8 shows the concentration of cyclic AMP in rat cerebrum, brainstem, and cerebellum as a function of age. The concentration of cyclic AMP increased significantly only in the cerebellum, where the levels were about three times higher in 32-day-old rats than in 1-day-old animals. Schmidt et al. (1970), studying the whole brain of the rat, showed that cyclic AMP increased more than threefold between birth and 30 days of age. However, these results are complicated by the facts that the concentration of cyclic AMP increases following decapitation (Breckenridge, 1964) and that the rate at which cyclic AMP rises differs among the brain areas. For example, between 15 sec and 2 min after decapitation, the concentration of cyclic AMP in rat cerebellum rose about fivefold, whereas the concentration in brainstem and cerebrum increased only slightly (Uzunov and Weiss, 1971). Therefore, the data represented in Fig. 8 do not accurately reflect the endogenous concentration of cyclic AMP. Indeed, Schmidt, Schmidt,

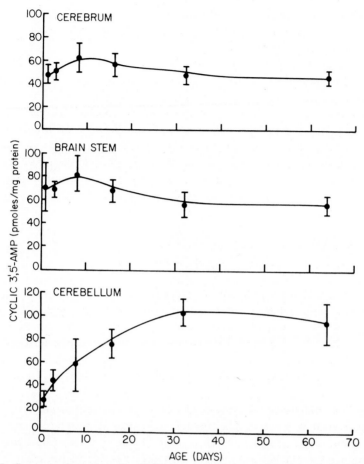

FIG. 8. Concentration of cyclic AMP in rat brain as a function of age. Rats were decapitated, and the brain was dissected and frozen in 1 min. The concentration of cyclic AMP was determined in whole homogenates of cerebrum, cerebellum, and brainstem of rats 1 to 64 days of age by the method described by Ebadi et al., (1971). Each point represents the mean value of eight experiments. Vertical brackets indicate the standard error.

and Robison (1971), using a microwave irradiation technique which prevents the postdecapitation rise in the concentration of cyclic AMP, recently reported that rat cerebellum and brainstem had similar concentrations of cyclic AMP (about 20 pmoles/mg protein). Since decapitation might cause an activation of the adenylate cyclase systems of brain, the degree to which cyclic AMP rises following decapitation may depend on the ratio of the activities of the enzymes responsible for its biosynthesis (adenylate cyclase) and hydrolysis (phosphodiesterase).

The differences that occur postnatally in the concentration of cyclic AMP in the brain areas of rats may be due to the unequal development of adenylate cyclase and phosphodiesterase. For example, we found that in the cerebrum and brainstem of rat there was a marked increase of both adenylate cyclase and phosphodiesterase activities between birth and 20 days of age. However, in cerebellum there was more than a twofold elevation of adenylate cyclase activity, but no increase in phosphodiesterase activity (Weiss, 1971*b*), and, perhaps more importantly, there was no substantial increase in the activity of the high K_m phosphodiesterase (see Fig. 6).

ADENYLATE CYCLASE, PHOSPHODIESTERASE, AND CYCLIC AMP IN HUMAN FETAL TISSUE

There are obvious problems that exist in studying human tissue, and, in particular, human fetal tissue with regard to the postmortem changes that take place in the activity of enzymes and in the concentration of endogenous materials. However, since no data on the activities of adenylate cyclase or of phosphodiesterase or on the concentration of cyclic AMP are available for human fetal tissues, we undertook such a study, fully cognizant of its limitations.

Human fetal tissues were obtained at legal abortion from Washington Hospital Research Center. The tissues were frozen within 15 min after abortion and were analyzed within 24 hr. Table 3 shows the activity of adenylate cyclase in several organs of these 10- to 14-week-old human fetuses. Of the tissues studied, the liver contained the lowest activity. This may be compared to the results of Sutherland, Rall, and Menon (1962)

TABLE 3. *Adenylate cyclase activity of human fetal tissue.*

Tissue	Cyclic AMP Formed (pmoles/mg protein/min $\pm$ SE)
Adrenal	4.1 $\pm$ 0.5 (20)
Kidney	3.6 $\pm$ 1.1 (3)
Brain	3.3 $\pm$ 0.5 (15)
Heart	3.3 $\pm$ 0.5 (23)
Liver	1.4 $\pm$ 0.2 (6)

Adenylate cyclase activity of human fetal tissue homogenates (10 to 14 weeks) was assayed in the presence of NaF (10^{-2} M). Figures in parentheses represent the number of experiments.

TABLE 4. *Cyclic AMP phosphodiesterase activity of human fetal tissue.*

Tissue	Phosphodiesterase Activity (nmoles cAMP hydrolyzed/mg protein/min $\pm$ SE)
Brain	2.8 ± 0.2 (25)
Heart	2.1 ± 0.2 (4)
Adrenal	1.9 ± 0.2 (3)
Liver	1.2 ± 1.0 (2)

Homogenates of human fetal tissue were incubated for 20 min at 37°C with 0.3 mM cyclic AMP. Figures in parentheses represent the number of experiments.

who studied the distribution of adenylate cyclase activity in dog and found that liver contained among the lowest enzyme activities. Adenylate cyclase activity of human fetal brain was only about one-tenth that reported for human adult brain (Williams, Little, and Ensinck, 1969). Unfortunately no such comparisons can be made for other tissues, as no data has been published on the distribution of adenylate cyclase in adult human tissue.

In Table 4 we present the activity of phosphodiesterase in several organs of the 10- to 14-week-old human fetus. Once more, liver contained the lowest activity, results similar to those found in the dog (Butcher and

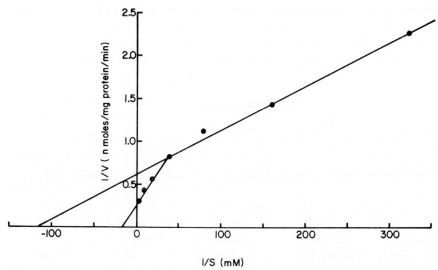

FIG. 9. Multiple phosphodiesterase activities of human fetal brain. Brains from 12-week-old human fetuses were obtained at legal abortion. The tissue was homogenized and assayed for phosphodiesterase activity in the presence of varying concentrations of substrate. V total $=$ 4.0 nmoles cyclic AMP hydrolyzed/mg protein/min; V high $K_m = 2.5$ nmoles cyclic AMP hydrolyzed/mg protein/min; V low $K_m = 1.5$ nmoles cyclic AMP hydrolyzed/mg protein/min.

TABLE 5. *Concentration of cyclic AMP in human fetal tissues.*

Tissue	Cyclic AMP (pmoles/mg protein $\pm$ SE)
Kidney	5.2 $\pm$ 1.0 (8)
Intestine	7.1 $\pm$ 1.7 (3)
Brain	8.9 $\pm$ 1.1 (8)
Heart	10.5 $\pm$ 1.0 (8)
Adrenal	12.0 $\pm$ 2.6 (5)

Tissue of 10- to 14-week-old fetuses were analyzed for cyclic AMP concentration. Figures in parentheses indicate the number of experiments.

Sutherland, 1962). A comparison with adult human brain (Williams et al., 1969; Williams, Little, Beug, and Ensinck, 1971) shows again that the fetal tissue has lower phosphodiesterase activity when calculated on the basis of protein.

Figure 9 shows that human fetal brain possesses multiple phosphodiesterase activities. The ratio of the high to low K_m phosphodiesterase was approximately 2:1, a ratio similar to that seen in brain of newborn rats.

In Table 5 we list the concentration of cyclic AMP in brain, heart, kidney, adrenal, and intestine of 10- to 14-week-old fetuses. Adrenal gland contained the highest concentration of cyclic AMP. This may reflect the relatively higher activity of adenylate cyclase compared with the activity of phosphodiesterase in this tissue (see Tables 3 and 4), and further support the concept that the relative activities of these two enzymes are a strong determinant of the intracellular concentration of cyclic AMP.

SUMMARY

Cyclic AMP is an important regulator of the growth and development of cells. It stimulates the synthesis of proteins, RNA, and DNA, perhaps by activating protein kinases. Recently, it was shown that cyclic AMP can influence the proliferation and differentiation of cells in tissue culture and can even restore the abnormal characteristics seen in virally transformed cells to those of normal cells. Our own studies have shown that virally transformed astrocytomas have less adenylate cyclase activity than do normal astrocytes, suggesting that rapidly growing cells are deficient in adenylate cyclase and cyclic AMP.

Because cyclic AMP plays such a central role in cell growth, it is important to study the ontogenetic development of the enzymes responsible for the biosynthesis (adenylate cyclase) and hydrolysis (phosphodiesterase) of cyclic AMP. Apparently, both of these enzymes exist in several forms and each can develop independently of the other. Adenylate cyclase activity of brain is very low in newborn rats. Enzyme activity increases rapidly to day 20 then declines slightly. In the pineal gland, the basal adenylate cyclase activity remains fairly constant with age but the sensitivity of the enzyme to catecholamines increases rapidly after birth.

In most brain areas studied, the total phosphodiesterase activity increases markedly after birth. However, enzyme activity in the cerebellum remains fairly constant. Like adenylate cyclase, phosphodiesterase also exists in more than one form; at least one form has a high apparent K_m for cyclic AMP and another a relatively low K_m. Different areas of the brain contain different ratios of the high to low K_m phosphodiesterase, and the rate at which these different phosphodiesterases develop varies with the tissue. For example, the high K_m phosphodiesterase increases several-fold in cerebrum, but does not increase in cerebellum.

In general, the concentration of cyclic AMP reflects the relative activities of adenylate cyclase and phosphodiesterase. Thus, the cerebellum with high adenylate cyclase and low phosphodiesterase activity has the highest concentration of cyclic AMP.

Compared with adult human or adults of other species, human fetal tissue has low activities of adenylate cyclase and phosphodiesterase and low concentrations of cyclic AMP. This is in accord with the concept that rapidly growing and undifferentiated cells have a low concentration of cyclic AMP.

REFERENCES

Anderson, W. B., Schneider, A. B., Emmer, M., Perlman, R. L., and Pastan, I. (1971): Purification of and properties of the cyclic adenosine 3',5'-monophosphate receptor protein which mediates cyclic adenosine 3',5'-monophosphate-dependent gene transcription in *Escherichia coli. Journal of Biological Chemistry,* 246:5929-5937.

Beavo, J. A., Hardman, J. G., and Sutherland, E. W. (1970): Hydrolysis of cyclic guanosine and adenosine 3',5'-monophosphates by rat and bovine tissues. *Journal of Biological Chemistry,* 245:5649-5655.

Birnbaumer, L., Pohl, S. L., and Rodbell, M. (1969): Adenyl cyclase in fat cells. I. Properties and the effects of adrenocorticotropin and fluoride. *Journal of Biological Chemistry,* 244:3468-3476

Birnbaumer, L., and Rodbell, M. (1969): Adenyl cyclase in fat cells. II. Hormone receptors. *Journal of Biological Chemistry,* 244:3477-3482.

Bitensky, M. W., Russell, V., and Blanco, M. (1970): Independent variation of glucagon and epinephrine responsive components of hepatic adenyl cyclase as a function of age, sex and steroid hormones, *Endocrinology,* 86:154-159

Bitensky, M. W., Russell, V., and Robertson, W. (1968): Evidence for separate epinephrine and glucagon responsive adenyl cyclase systems in rat liver. *Biochemical and Biophysical Research Communications,* 31:706-712.

Bonner, J. T. (1970): Induction of stalk cell differentiation by cyclic AMP in the cellular slime mold *Dictyostelium discoideum. Proceedings of the National Academy of Sciences,* 65:110-113.

Breckenridge, B. McL. (1964): The measurement of cyclic adenylate in tissues. *Proceedings of the National Academy of Sciences,* 52:1580-1586.

Breckenridge B. McL. (1970): Cyclic AMP and drug action. *Annual Review of Pharmacology,* 10:19-34.

Burk, R. R. (1968): Reduced adenyl cyclase activity in a polyoma virus transformed cell line. *Nature,* 219:1272-1275.

Butcher, R. W., and Sutherland, E. W., (1962): Adenosine 3',5'-phosphate in biological materials. I. Purification and properties of cyclic 3',5'-nucleotide phosphodiesterase and use of this enzyme to characterize adenosine 3',5'-phosphate in human urine. *Journal of Biological Chemistry,* 237:1244-1250.

Castaneda, M, and Tyler, A. (1968): Adenyl cyclase in plasma membrane preparations of sea urchin eggs and its increase in activity after fertilization. *Biochemical and Biophysical Research Communications,* 33:782-787.

Chen, S., and Tchen, T. T. (1970): Induction of melanocytogenesis in explants of *Curassius auratus* L the xanthic goldfish by dibutyryl-cAMP. *Biochemical and Biophysical Research Communications,* 41:964-966.

Cheung, W. Y. (1971): Cyclic 3',5'-nucleotide phosphodiesterase. Evidence for and properties of a protein activator. *Journal of Biological Chemistry,* 246:2859-2869.

Chuah, C-C., and Oliver, I. T. (1971): Role of adenosine cyclic monophosphate in the synthesis of tyrosine aminotransferase in neonatal rat liver. Release of enzyme from membrane-bound polysomes *in vitro. Biochemistry,* 10:2990-3001.

deCrombrugghe, B., Perlman, R. L., Varmus, H. E., and Pastan, I. (1969): Regulation of inducible enzyme synthesis in *Escherichia coli* by cyclic adenosine 3'5'-monophosphate. *Journal of Biological Chemistry,* 244:5828-5835.

deCrombrugghe, B., Varmus, H. E., Perlman, R. L., and Pastan, I. H. (1970): Stimulation of *lac* mRNA synthesis by cyclic AMP in cell free extracts of *Escherichia coli. Biochemical and Biophysical Research Communications,* 38:894-901.

Drummond, G. I., Severson, D. L., and Duncan, L. (1971): Adenyl cyclase. Kinetic properties and nature of fluoride and hormone stimulation. *Journal of Biological Chemistry,* 246:4166-4173.

Ebadi, M. S., Weiss, B., and Costa, E. (1971): Microassay of adenosine 3', 5'-monophosphate (cyclic AMP) in brain and other tissues by the luciferin-luciferase system. *Journal of Neurochemistry,* 18:183-192.

Forn, J., Schonhofer, P. S., Skidmore, I. F., and Krishna, G. (1970): Effect of aging on the adenyl cyclase and phosphodiesterase activity of isolated fat cells of rat. *Biochimica et Biophysica Acta,* 208:304-309.

Franks, D. J., MacManus, J. P., and Whitfield, J. F. (1971): The effect of prostaglandins on cyclic AMP production and cell proliferation in thymic lymphocytes. *Biochemical and Biophysical Research Communications,* 44:1177-1183.

Gaballah, S., and Popoff, C. (1971): Cyclic 3',5'-nucleotide phosphodiesterase in nerve endings of developing rat brain. *Brain Research,* 25:220-222.

Georgiev, G. P. (1968): Histones and the control of gene action. In: *Annual Review of Genetics,* Vol. 3, edited by L. R. Herschel. Annual Reviews, Inc., Palo Alto, Calif., pp. 155-180.

Gill, G. N., and Garren, L. D. (1970): A cyclic 3',5'-adenosine monophosphate dependent protein kinase from the adrenal cortex: comparison with a cyclic AMP binding protein. *Biochemical and Biophysical Research Communications,* 39:335-343.

Gilman, A. G., and Nirenberg, M. (1971): Effect of catecholamines on the adenosine 3',5'-cyclic monophosphate concentrations of clonal satellite cells of neurons. *Proceedings of the National Academy of Sciences,* 68:2165-2168.

Grahame-Smith, D. G., Butcher, R. W., Ney, R. L., and Sutherland, E. W. (1967): Adenosine 3',5'-monophosphate as the intracellular mediator of the action of adrenocorticotropic hormone on the adrenal cortex. *Journal of Biological Chemistry,* 242:5535-5541.

Greengard, P., and Costa, E., editors (1970): *Role of Cyclic AMP in Cell Function. Advances in Biochemical Psychopharmacology,* Vol. 3. Raven Press, New York.

Greengard, P., and Kuo, J. F. (1970): On the mechanism of action of cyclic AMP. In: *Advances in Biochemical Psychopharmacology,* Vol. 3, edited by P. Greengard and E. Costa. Raven Press, New York, pp. 287-306.

Guidotti, A., Weiss, B., and Costa, E. (1971): Effect of isoproterenol (ISP) on the concentration of cyclic 3',5'-AMP (cAMP) in mouse parotid gland. *Pharmacologist,* 13:256.

Hardman, J. G., Robison, G. A., and Sutherland, E. W. (1971): Cyclic nucleotides. *Annual Review of Physiology,* 33:311-336.

Hardman, J. G., and Sutherland, E. W. (1965): A cyclic 3',5'-nucleotide phosphodiesterase from heart with specificity for uridine 3',5'-phosphate. *Journal of Biological Chemistry,* 240:PC 3704-PC 3705.

Heidrick, M. L., and Ryan, W. L. (1970): Cyclic nucleotides on cell growth *in vitro. Cancer Research,* 30:376-378.

Heidrick, M. L., and Ryan, W. L. (1971): Adenosine 3',5'-cyclic monophosphate and contact inhibition. *Cancer Research,* 31:1313-1315.

Hsie, A. W., Jones, C., and Puck, T. T. (1971): Further changes in differentiation state accompanying the conversion of Chinese hamster cells to fibroblastic form by dibutyryl adenosine cyclic 3',5'-monophosphate and hormones. *Proceedings of the National Academy of Sciences,* 68:1648-1652.

Hsie, A. W., and Puck, T. T. (1971): Morphological transformation of Chinese hamster cells by dibutyryl adenosine cyclic 3',5'-monophosphate and testosterone. *Proceedings of the National Academy of Sciences,* 68:358-361.

Huang, Y.-C., and Kemp, R. G. (1971): Properties of a phosphodiesterase with high affinity for adenosine 3',5'-cyclic phosphate. *Biochemistry,* 10:2278-2283.

Johnson, G. S., Friedman, R. M., and Pastan, I. (1971): Restoration of several morphological characteristics of normal fibroblasts in sarcoma cells treated with adenosine 3',5'-cyclic monophosphate and its derivatives. *Proceedings of the National Academy of Sciences,* 68:425-429.

Jost, J.-P., Hsie, A., Hughes, S. D., and Ryan, L. (1970): Role of cyclic adenosine 3',5'-monophosphate in the induction of hepatic enzymes. I. Kinetics of the induction of rat liver serine dehydratase by cyclic adenosine 3',5'-monophosphate. *Journal of Biological Chemistry,* 245:351-357.

Jost, J.-P., Hsie, A. W., and Rickenberg, H. V. (1969): Regulation of the synthesis of rat liver serine dehydratase by adenosine 3',5'-cyclic monophosphate. *Biochemical and Biophysical Research Communications,* 34:748-754.

Jost, J.-P., and Rickenberg, H. V. (1971): Cyclic AMP. *Annual Review of Biochemistry,* 40:741-774.

Jost, J.-P., and Sahib, M. K. (1971): Role of cyclic adenosine 3',5'-monophosphate in the induction of hepatic enzymes. II. Effect of N^6, O^2 dibutyryl cyclic adenosine 3',5'-monophosphate on the kinetics of ribonucleic acid synthesis in purified rat liver nuclei. *Journal of Biological Chemistry,* 246:1623-1629.

Kakiuchi, S., and Yamazaki, R. (1970): Calcium dependent phosphodiesterase activity and its activating factor (PAF) from brain. Studies on cyclic 3',5'-nucleotide phosphodiesterase (III). *Biochemical and Biophysical Research Communications*, 41:1104-1111.

Kakiuchi, S., Yamazaki, R., and Teshima, Y. (1971): Cyclic 3',5'-nucleotide phosphodiesterase. IV. Two enzymes with different properties from brain. *Biochemical and Biophysical Research Communications*, 42:968-974.

Khandelwal, R. L., and Hamilton, I. R., (1971): Purification and properties of adenyl cyclase from *Streptococcus salivarius*. *Journal of Biological Chemistry*, 246:3297-3304.

Klein, M. I., and Makman, M. H. (1971): Adenosine 3',5'-monophosphate-dependent protein kinase of cultured mammalian cells. *Science*, 172:863-864.

Klotz, U., and Stock, K (1971): Evidence for a cyclic nucleotide-phosphodiesterase with high specificity for cyclic uridine-3',5'-monophosphate in rat adipose tissue. *Naunyn-Schmiedebergs Archiv für Pharmakologie und Experimentelle Pathologie*, 269:117-120.

Konijn, T. M., Barkley, D. S., Chang, Y. Y., and Bonner, J. T. (1968): Cyclic AMP: A naturally occurring acrasin in the cellular slime molds. *American Naturalist*, 102:225-233.

Konijn, T. M., Van de Meene, J. G. C., Bonner, J. T., and Barkley, D. S., (1967): The acrasin activity of adenosine 3',5'-cyclic phosphates. *Proceedings of the National Academy of Sciences*, 58:1152-1154.

Konijn, T. M., Van de Meene, J. G. C., Chang, Y. Y., Barkley, D. S., and Bonner, J. T. (1969): Identification of adenosine 3',5'-monophosphate as the bacterial attractant for myxamboebae of *Dictyostelium discoideum*. *Journal of Bacteriology*, 99:510-512.

Kuo, J. F., and Greengard, P. (1969a): Cyclic nucleotide dependent-protein kinases. IV. Widespread occurrence of adenosine 3',5'-monophosphate-dependent protein kinases in various tissues and phyla of the animal kingdom. *Proceedings of the National Academy of Sciences*, 64:1349-1355.

Kuo, J. F., and Greengard, P. (1969b): An adenosine 3',5'-monophosphate-dependent protein kinase from *Escherichia coli*. *Journal of Biological Chemistry*, 244:3417-3419.

Kuo, J. F., and Greengard, P. (1970): Cyclic nucleotide dependent-protein kinases. VII. Comparison of various histones as substrates for adenosine 3',5'-monophosphate and guanosine 3',5'-monophosphate-dependent protein kinases. *Biochimica et Biophysica Acta*, 212:434-440.

Kuo, J. F., Krueger, B. K., Sanes, J. R., and Greengard, P. (1970): Cyclic nucleotide-dependent protein kinases. V. Preparation and properties of adenosine 3',5'-monophosphate-dependent protein kinase from various bovine tissues. *Biochimica et Biophysica Acta*, 212:79-91.

Langan, T. A. (1969a): Histone phosphorylation: Stimulation by adenosine 3',5'-monophosphate. *Science*, 162:579-580.

Langan, T. A. (1969b): Action of adenosine 3',5'-monophosphate-dependent histone kinase *in vivo*. *Journal of Biological Chemistry*, 244:5763-5765.

Linarelli, L. G., Weller, J. L., and Glinsmann, W. H. (1970): Stimulation of fetal rat liver tyrosine amino transferase activity *in utero* by 3',5'-cyclic nucleotides. *Life Sciences*, 9:535-539.

Lineweaver, H., and Burk, D. (1934): Determination of enzyme dissociation constants. *Journal of the American Chemical Society*, 56:658-666.

MacManus, J. P., and Whitfield, J. F. (1969: Mediation of mitogenic action of growth hormone by adenosine 3',5'-monophosphate (cyclic-AMP). *Proceedings of the Society of Experimental Biology and Medicine*, 132:409-412.

MacManus, J. P., and Whitfield, J. F. (1971): Inhibition by thyrocalcitonin of the mitogenic actions of parathyroid hormone and cyclic adenosine 3',5'-monophosphate on rat thymocytes. *Endocrinology*, 86:934-939.

MacManus, J. P., Whitfield, J. F., and Youdale, T. (1971): Stimulation by epinephrine of adenyl cyclase activity, cyclic AMP formation, DNA synthesis and cell proliferation in populations of rat thymic lymphocytes. *Journal of Cell Physiology,* 77:103-116.

Makman, M. H., (1970): Adenyl cyclase of cultured mammalian cells: Activation by catecholamines. *Science,* 170:1421-1423.

Makman, M. H. (1971a): Conditions leading to enhanced response to glucagon, epinephrine, or prostaglandins by adenylate cyclase of normal and malignant cultured cells. *Proceedings of the National Academy of Sciences,* 68:2127-2130.

Makman, M. H. (1971b): Properties of adenylate cyclase of lymphoid cells. *Proceedings of the National Academy of Sciences,* 68:885-889.

Makman, R. S., and Sutherland, E. W. (1965): Adenosine 3′,5′-phosphate in *Escherichia coli. Journal of Biological Chemistry,* 240:1309-1314.

Marsh, J. M., Butcher, R. W., Savard, K., and Sutherland, E. W. (1966): The stimulatory effect of luteinizing hormone on adenosine 3′,5′-monophosphate accumulation in corpus luteum slices. *Journal of Biological Chemistry,* 241:5436-5440.

Miller, Z., Varmus, H. E., Parks, J. S., Perlman, R. L., and Pastan, I. (1971): Regulation of *Gal* messenger ribonucleic acid synthesis in *Escherichia coli* by 3′,5′-cyclic adenosine monophosphate. *Journal of Biological Chemistry,* 246:2898-2903.

Miyamoto, E., Kuo, J. F., and Greengard, P. (1969a): Adenosine 3′,5′-monophosphate-dependent protein kinase from brain. *Science,* 165:63-65.

Miyamoto, E., Kuo, J. F., and Greengard, P. (1969b): Cyclic nucleotide-dependent protein kinases. III. Purification and properties of adenosine 3′,5′-monophosphate-dependent protein kinase from bovine brain. *Journal of Biological Chemistry,* 244:6395-6402.

Miyamoto, E., Petzold, G. L., Harris, J. S., and Greengard, P. (1971): Dissociation and concomitant activation of adenosine 3′,5′-monophosphate-dependent protein kinase by histone. *Biochemical and Biophysical Research Communications,* 44:305-312.

Monn, E., and Christiansen, R. O. (1971): Adenosine 3′,5′-monophosphate phosphodiesterase: Multiple molecular forms. *Science,* 173: 540-542.

Otten, J., Johnson, G. S., and Pastan, I. (1971): Cyclic AMP levels in fibroblasts: Relationships to growth rate and contact inhibition of growth. *Biochemical and Biophysical Research Communications,* 44:1192-1198.

Pastan, I., and Katzen, R. (1967): Activation of adenyl cyclase in thyroid homogenates by thyroid-stimulating hormone. *Biochemical and Biophysical Research Communications,* 29:792-798.

Pastan, I., and Perlman, R. L. (1968): The role of the Lac promotor locus in the regulation of β-galactosidase synthesis by cyclic 3′,5′-adenosine monophosphate. *Proceedings of the National Academy of Sciences,* 61:1336-1342.

Pastan, I., and Perlman, R. L. (1969): Stimulation of tryptophanase synthesis in *Escherichia coli* by cyclic 3′,5′-adenosine monophosphate. *Journal of Biological Chemistry,* 244:2226-2232.

Pastan, I., and Perlman, R. (1970): Cyclic adenosine monophosphate in bacteria. *Science,* 169:339-344.

Peery, C. V., Johnson, G. S., and Pastan, I. (1971): Adenyl cyclase in normal and transformed fibroblasts in tissue culture: Activation by prostaglandins. *Journal of Biological Chemistry,* 246:5785-5790.

Perkins, J. P., MacIntyre, E. H., Riley, W. D., and Clark, R. B. (1971): Adenyl cyclase, phosphodiesterase and cyclic AMP dependent protein kinase of malignant glial cells in culture. *Life Sciences,* 10:1069-1080.

Perlman, R., and Pastan, I. (1968a): Cyclic 3′,5′-AMP: Stimulation of β-galactosidase and tryptophanase induction in *Escherichia coli. Biochemical and Biophysical Research Communications,* 30:656-664.

Perlman, R. L., and Pastan, I. (1968b): Regulation of β-galactosidase synthesis in *Escherichia coli* by cyclic adenosine 3′,5′-monophosphate. *Journal of Biological Chemistry,* 243:5420-5427.

Prasad, K. N., and Hsie, A. W. (1971): Morphologic differentiation of mouse neuroblastoma cells induced *in vitro* by dibutyryl adenosine 3′,5′-cyclic monophosphate. *Nature, New Biology,* 233:141-142.

Ray, T. K., Tomasi, V., and Marinetti, G. V. (1970): Hormone action at the membrane level. I. Properties of adenyl cyclase in isolated plasma membranes of rat liver. *Biochimica et Biophysica Acta,* 211:20-30.

Reik, L., Petzold, G. L., Higgins, J. Ä., Greengard, P., and Barrnett, R. J. (1970): Hormone-sensitive adenyl cyclase: Cytochemical localization in rat liver. *Science,* 168:382-384.

Reimann, E. M., Brostrom, C. O., Corbin, J. D., King, C. A., and Krebs, E. G. (1971): Separation of regulatory and catalytic subunits of the cyclic 3′,5′-adenosine monophosphate-dependent protein kinase(s) of rabbit skeletal muscle. *Biochemical and Biophysical Research Communications,* 42:187-194.

Reimann, E. M., Walsh, D. A., and Krebs, E. G. (1971): Purification and properties of rabbit skeletal muscle adenosine 3′,5′-monophosphate-dependent protein kinase. *Journal of Biological Chemistry,* 246:1986-1995.

Rixon, R. H., Whitfield, J. F., and MacManus, J. P. (1970): Stimulation of mitotic activity in rat bone marrow and thymus by exogenous adenosine 3′,5′-monophosphate (cyclic AMP). *Experimental Cell Research,* 63:110-116.

Robison, G. A., Butcher, R. W., and Sutherland, E. W. (1968): Cyclic AMP. *Annual Review of Biochemistry,* 37:149-174.

Robison, G. A., Butcher, R. W., and Sutherland, E. W. (1971): *Cyclic AMP.* Academic Press, New York.

Rodbell, M., Birnbaumer, L., and Pohl, S. L. (1970): Adenyl cyclase in fat cells. III. Stimulation by secretin and the effects of trypsin on the receptors for lipolytic hormones. *Journal of Biological Chemistry,* 245:718-722.

Rosen, O. M. (1970): Preparation and properties of a cyclic 3′,5′-nucleotide phosphodiesterase isolated from frog erythrocytes. *Archives of Biochemistry and Biophysics,* 137:435-441.

Rosen, O. M., and Erlichman, J. (1969): The development of hormone sensitivity by the adenyl cyclase of the tadpole erythrocyte. *Archives of Biochemistry and Biophysics,* 133:171-177.

Ryan, W. L., and Heidrick, M. L. (1968): Inhibition of cell growth *in vitro* by adenosine 3′,5′-monophosphate. *Science,* 162:1484-1485.

Schmidt, M. J., Palmer, E. C., Dettbarn, W.-D., and Robison, G. A. (1970): Cyclic AMP and adenyl cyclase in the developing rat brain. *Developmental Psychobiology,* 3:53-67.

Schmidt, M. J., and Robison, G. A. (1971): The effect of norepinephrine on cyclic AMP levels in discrete regions of the developing rabbit brain. *Life Sciences,* 10:459-464.

Schmidt, M. J., Schmidt, D. E., and Robison, G. A. (1971): Cyclic adenosine monophosphate in brain areas: Microwave irradiation as a means of tissue fixation. *Science,* 173:1142-1143.

Seeds, N. W., and Gilman, A. G. (1971): Norepinephrine-stimulated increase of cyclic AMP levels in developing mouse brain cell cultures. *Science,* 174:292.

Sheppard, J. R. (1971): Restoration of contact-inhibited growth of transformed cells by dibutyryl adenosine 3′,5′-cyclic monophosphate. *Proceedings of the National Academy of Sciences,* 68:1316-1320.

Strada, S. J., Klein, D. C., Weller, J., and Weiss, B. (1972): Effect of norepinephrine on the concentration of adenosine 3′,5′-monophosphate of rat pineal gland in organ culture. *Endocrinology,* 90:1470-1475.

Strada, S. J., and Weiss, B. (1971): Sympathetic nerve activity and the cyclic 3′,5′-AMP system of the rat pineal gland. In: *Biochemistry and Physiology of the Pineal Gland*, edited by D. C. Klein. Raven Press, New York.

Sutherland, E. W., and Rall, T. W. (1960): The relation of adenosine 3′,5′-phosphate and phosphorylase to the actions of catecholamines and other hormones. *Pharmacological Reviews*, 12: 265-299.

Sutherland, E. W., Rall, T. W., and Menon, T. (1962): Adenyl cyclase. I. Distribution, preparation, and properties. *Journal of Biological Chemistry*, 237:1220-1227.

Sutherland, E. W., Robison, G. A., and Butcher, R. W. (1968): Some aspects of the biological role of adenosine 3′,5′-monophosphate (cyclic AMP). *Circulation*, 37:279-306.

Tao, M. (1971): Further studies on the properties of the rabbit reticulocyte adenosine 3′,5′-cyclic-monophosphate-dependent protein kinase I. *Archives of Biochemistry and Biophysics*, 143:151-157.

Tao, M., Salas, M. L., and Lipmann, F. (1970): Mechanisms of activation by adenosine 3′,5′-cyclic monophosphate of a protein phosphokinase from rabbit reticulocytes. *Proceedings of the National Academy of Sciences*, 67:408-414.

Thompson, W. J., and Appleman, M. M. (1971a): Multiple cyclic nucleotide phosphodiesterase activities from rat brain. *Biochemistry*, 10:311-316.

Thompson, W. J., and Appleman, M. M. (1971b): Characterization of cyclic nucleotide phosphodiesterases of rat tissue. *Journal of Biological Chemistry*, 246:3145-3150.

Uzunov, P., and Weiss, B. (1971): Effects of phenothiazine tranquilizers on the cyclic 3′,5′-adenosine monophosphate system of rat brain. *Neuropharmacology*, 10:697-708.

Uzunov, P., and Weiss, B. (1972): Separation of multiple forms of cyclic adenosine 3′,5′-monophosphate phosphodiesterase in rat cerebellum by polyacrylamide gel electrophoresis. *Biochimica et Biophysica Acta (in press)*.

Varmus, H. E., Perlman, R. L., and Pastan, I. (1970a): Regulation of *Lac* messenger ribonucleic acid synthesis by cyclic adenosine 3′,5′-monophosphate and glucose. *Journal of Biological Chemistry*, 245:2259-2267.

Varmus, H. E., Perlman, R. L., and Pastan, I. (1970b): Regulation of *Lac* transcription in *Escherichia coli* by cyclic adenosine 3′,5′-monophosphate. Studies with deoxyribonucleic acid-ribonucleic acid hybridization and hybridization competition. *Journal of Biological Chemistry*, 245:6366-6372.

Walsh, D. A., Perkins, J. P., and Krebs, E. G. (1968): An adenosine 3′,5′-monophosphate-dependent protein kinase from rabbit skeletal muscle. *Journal of Biological Chemistry*, 243:3763-3765.

Walton, G. M., Gill, G. N., Abrass, I. B., and Garren, L. D. (1971): Phosphorylation of ribosome-associated protein by an adenosine 3′,5′-cyclic monophosphate-dependent protein kinase: Location of the microsomal receptor and protein kinase. *Proceedings of the National Academy of Sciences*, 68:880-884.

Weiss, B. (1969a): Similarities and differences in the norepinephrine and sodium fluoride-sensitive adenyl cyclase system. *Journal of Pharmacology and Experimental Therapeutics*, 166:330-338.

Weiss, B. (1969b): Effects of environmental lighting and chronic denervation on the response of adenyl cyclase of rat pineal gland to norepinephrine and sodium fluoride. *Journal of Pharmacology and Experimental Therapeutics*, 168:146-152.

Weiss, B. (1970): Factors affecting adenyl cyclase activity and its sensitivity to biogenic amines. In: *Biogenic Amines as Physiological Regulators*, edited by J. J. Blum. Prentice Hall Inc., Englewood Cliffs, N.J. pp. 35-73.

Weiss, B. (1971a): On the regulation of adenyl cyclase activity in the rat pineal gland. *Annals of the New York Academy of Sciences*, 185:507-519.

Weiss, B. (1971b): Ontogenetic development of adenyl cyclase and phosphodiesterase in rat brain. *Journal of Neurochemistry*, 18:469-478.

Weiss, B., and Costa, E. (1967): Adenyl cyclase activity in rat pineal gland: Effects of chronic denervation and norepinephrine. *Science*, 156:1750-1752.

Weiss, B., and Costa, E. (1968): Selective stimulation of adenyl cyclase of rat pineal gland by pharmacologically active catecholamines. *Journal of Pharmacology and Experimental Therapeutics*, 161:310-319.

Weiss, B., and Crayton, J. W. (1970a): Neural and hormonal regulation of pineal adenyl cyclase activity. In: *Advances in Biochemical Psychopharmacology*, Vol. 3, edited by P. Greengard and E. Costa. Raven Press, New York, pp. 217-239.

Weiss, B., and Crayton, J. (1970b): Gonadal hormones as regulators of pineal adenyl cyclase activity. *Endocrinology*, 87:527-533.

Weiss, B., and Kidman, A. D. (1969): Neurobiological significance of cyclic $3',5'$-adenosine monophosphate. In: *Advances in Biochemical Psychopharmacology*, Vol. 1, edited by E. Costa and P. Greengard. Raven Press, New York, pp. 131-164.

Weiss, B., Lehne, R., and Strada, S. (1972): Rapid microassay of adenosine $3',5'$-monophosphate phosphodiesterase activity. *Analytical Biochemistry*, 45:222-235.

Weiss, B., Shein, H. M., and Snyder, R. (1971): Adenylate cyclase and phosphodiesterase activity of normal and SV_{40} virus-transformed hamster astrocytes in cell culture. *Life Sciences*, 10:1253-1260.

Weiss, B., and Strada, S. J. (1972): Neuroendocrine control of the adenosine $3',5'$-monophosphate system of brain and pineal gland. In: *Advances in Cyclic Nucleotide Research*, Vol. 1, edited by P. Greengard, G. A. Robison, and R. Paoletti. Raven Press, New York, pp. 125-142.

Whitfield, J. F., MacManus, J. P., and Gillan, D. J. (1970a): The possible mediation by cyclic AMP of the stimulation of thymocyte proliferation by vasopressin and the inhibition of this mitogenic action by thyrocalcitonin. *Journal of Cell Physiology*, 76:65-76.

Whitfield, J. F., MacManus, J. P., and Rixon, R. H. (1970b): The possible mediation by cyclic AMP of parathyroid hormone-induced stimulation of mitotic activity and deoxyribonucleic acid synthesis in rat thymic lymphocytes. *Journal of Cell Physiology*, 75:213-224.

Wicks, W. D. (1968): Tyrosine-α-ketoglutarate transaminase: Induction by epinephrine and adenosine $3',5'$-cyclic phosphate. *Science*, 160:997-998.

Wicks, W. D. (1969): Induction of hepatic enzymes by adenosine $3',5'$-monophosphate in organ culture. *Journal of Biological Chemistry*, 244:3941-3950.

Wicks, W. D. (1971): Differential effects of glucocorticoids and adenosine $3',5'$-monophosphate on hepatic enzyme systems. *Journal of Biological Chemistry*, 246:217-223.

Williams, R. H., Little, S. A., Beug, A. G., and Ensinck, J. W. (1971): Cyclic nucleotide phosphodiesterase activity in man, monkey and rat. *Metabolism*, 20:743-748.

Williams, R. H., Little, S. A., and Ensinck, J. W. (1969): Adenyl cyclase and phosphodiesterase activities in brain areas of man, monkey and rat. *American Journal of Medical Sciences*, 259:190-202.

Yang, T. J., and Vas, S. I. (1971): Growth inhibitor effects of adenosine $3',5'$-monophosphate on mouse leukemia L-5178-Y-R cells in culture. *Experientia*, 27:442-444.

Yeung, D., and Oliver, I. T. (1968): Induction of phosphopyruvate carboxylase in neonatal rat liver by adenosine $3',5'$-cyclic monophosphate. *Biochemistry*, 7:3231-3239.

Yokota, T., and Gots, J. S. (1970): Requirement of adenosine $3',5'$-cyclic phosphate for flagella formation in *Escherichia coli* and *Salmonella typhimurium*. *Journal of Bacteriology*, 103:513-516.

Zor, U., Kaneko, T., Schneider, H. P. G., McCann, S. M., Lowe, I. P., Bloom, G., Borland, B., and Field, J. B. (1969): Stimulation of anterior pituitary adenyl cyclase activity and adenosine $3',5'$-cyclic phosphate by hypothalamic extract and prostaglandin E_1. *Proceedings of the National Academy of Sciences*, 63:918-925.

DISCUSSION

RÄIHÄ: Did you try the effect of any other hormones on the pineal gland adenyl cyclase activity during development?

WEISS: One of the interesting properties of adenylate cyclase is the selectivity with which the enzyme responds to hormones. For example, adenylate cyclase of liver is activated by glucagon but not by ACTH; the enzyme from adrenal cortex is activated by ACTH but not by glucagon; and the enzyme from the corpus luteum is activated specifically by LH. We have found that adenylate cyclase of the adult pineal gland is activated specifically by the pharmacologically active catecholamines, norepinephrine, epinephrine, and isoproterenol, but not by ACTH, glucagon, or LH. Therefore, in these studies of the ontogenetic development of pineal adenylate cyclase, we have investigated only the acquisition of the sensitivity of adenylate cyclase to norepinephrine.

RÄIHÄ: The increase which you found in the activity of adenyl cyclase in the pineal gland after administration of norepinephrine, was it due to an actual increase in enzyme protein or to some other effect such as activation of preexisting enzyme?

WEISS: The increase in adenylate cyclase activity caused by the *in vitro* addition of norepinephrine probably is due to the activation of preexisting enzyme, since the effects are immediate. However, several of our studies suggested that the actual quantity of enzyme can be changed. Thus, alteration of sympathetic activity, sex hormones, environmental lighting, and, as shown in the present chapter, the age and development of the organ can influence the extent to which the hormone-sensitive adenylate cyclase system can be activated. By studying the pineal gland maintained in organ culture, perhaps we can obtain more definite evidence that the increased responsiveness of adenylate cyclase is caused by an actual change in the synthesis of protein.

BRØNDSTED: Is it possible to compare the maturity of brains from different animals on the basis of the kind of results you have presented?

WEISS: Not directly, but if one compares the results of these studies on the rat with those of others on the guinea pig, for example—whose brain is more developed at birth compared with the rat—then one can conclude that there is a relationship between the development of the structure and adenylate cyclase activity and, in particular, in the acquisition of hormonal responsiveness of the enzyme.

MIRKIN: How do you exclude the influence of norepinephrine uptake on its stimulatory influence upon adenyl cyclase?

WEISS: On our studies of the pineal gland maintained in tissue culture, we cannot rule out the possibility that the enhanced effect of norepinephrine on the concentration of cyclic AMP may be due to an altered uptake of the catecholamine. However, we have shown in other experiments that norepinephrine also increases adenylate cyclase activity in homogenates of pineal gland and that this activation is much greater in pineal glands that have been sympathetically denervated. I think that these experiments with homogenates and the fact that concentration-response studies showed an increase in the maximum response eliminates the possibility that the effect we observe is due to a change in the uptake of the catecholamine.

MIRKIN: Are dose-response curves shifted to the left?

WEISS: There is a small shift to the left of the concentration-response curve but a greater change in the maximum response.

MANN: An absolute requirement for the assay method which you described is that *all* of the adenylic acid originating from cyclic AMP by phosphodiesterase must be available for the subsequent step in the assay, namely, the conversion of adenylic acid by myokinase to ADP. How far is that requirement satisfied? Can one really rule out completely the possibility that some of the adenylic acid is eliminated from the assay by, for example, the action of 5-nucleotidase?

WEISS: The question you raise is certainly pertinent since the assay depends on the stoichiometric conversion of $5'$-AMP to ATP. Under the conditions of our assay, there is a rapid and complete conversion of $5'$-AMP to ATP. I can think of at least two reasons why we have not experienced any problem with $5'$-nucleotidase activity. One is the extreme sensitivity of the assay. The samples can be diluted to such a great degree that the activity of other interfering enzymes is greatly reduced. Moreover, we add large amounts of myokinase and pyruvate kinase so that as soon as $5'$-AMP is formed from the hydrolysis of cyclic AMP, it is converted immediately to ADP and then to ATP. We have added varying amounts of $5'$-AMP to several tissue homogenates in our assay and have found complete conversion of $5'$-AMP to ATP and no evidence that nucleotidase or any other enzymes interfere with the assay. However, I think this should be checked for each new tissue studied.

OWMAN: There has been some discussion about what is the functional sympathetic transmitter in the rat pineal since its sympathetic nerves contain both noradrenaline and serotonin. Have you tested activation of adenyl cyclase in rat pineal with serotonin and with sympathetic nerve stimulation?

WEISS: We have examined the influence of serotonin on pineal adenylate cyclase activity and have found that the indole does not activate enzyme activity. In fact, serotonin inhibits the activation of adenylate cyclase induced by norepinephrine.

I think it will be difficult to demonstrate an activation of adenylate cyclase after stimulating sympathetic nerves since the enzyme activity would have to be determined after the tissue was homogenized and this may mask any activation of the enzyme. We are currently studying the effects of sympathetic nerve stimulation on the concentration of cyclic AMP in the pineal gland. We hope to have more success with this approach.

PAOLETTI: Brain cortical adenyl cyclase is activated by different hormones in different animal species. Does pineal gland adenyl cyclase follow similar patterns?

WEISS: We have studied pineal adenylate cyclase activity of the rat and the steer. The enzyme from rat responded very well to the catecholamines, whereas that from the steer did not. We have not examined the effects of any other hormones in other species.

PAOLETTI: Have you any information about whether cyclic GMP is present during the prenatal life in the cerebellum?

WEISS: As far as I know, no data have been published on the concentration of cyclic GMP in any fetal tissue.

KARCZMAR: In view of certain statements that you made, one may expect some similarity between ontogenesis of the cyclic AMP system and of the norepinephrine system. Is there any such resemblance—in kinetics, time of appearance, accumulation? If not, to what do you relate the ontogenesis of cyclic AMP?

WEISS: In studying complex structures such as the brain, I see no reason to expect to find a correlation between the ontogenetic development of the cyclic AMP system and norepinephrine. After all, cyclic AMP is involved in the actions of such a multiplicity of hormones and has such a fundamental role in biology that I would be surprised to find a correlation between the ontogenetic development of adenylate cyclase and any hormone. On the other hand, in certain selective structures it may be possible to relate the development of a hormone-sensitive adenylate cyclase system with the appearance of specific hormone activators. This we can do in the pineal gland, for example, where the acquistion of hormonal sensitivity to norepinephrine coincides approximately with the invasion of sympathetic fibers into the gland. However, it is important to note that, at least in the pineal gland, a norepinephrine-sensitive adenylate cyclase system can develop even in the absence of an adrenergic innervation. Apparently, the message that a cell must receive to form a hormone-sensitive adenylate cyclase is genetically coded in the cell itself, and no exogenous stimulus is required.

Fetal Pharmacology, edited by L. Boréus
Raven Press, New York © 1973

Serotoninergic Mechanisms in Ontogenesis

Anja H. Tissari

Department of Pharmacology, University of Helsinki, Helsinki 17, Finland

The prime physiological importance of serotonin (5-hydroxytryptamine, 5-HT) is attributed to its assumed function as a neurotransmitter at CNS synapses controlling the induction of sleep, repression of sexually active behavior, and central regulation of body temperature. Sleep is no longer regarded as a passive resting state of the brain, but as being due to active mechanisms maintained by hypnogenic structures. Jouvet (1969) has provided evidence that the raphe system, which contains the bulk of the 5-HT neurons, may be the sleep-inducing structure, and that both states of sleep— slow-wave and paradoxical sleep—may be regulated by 5-HT. The part played by 5-HT in the hypothalamic control of temperature is less well understood. A rise in body temperature is followed by an increased turnover of brain 5-HT, suggesting that 5-HT neurons may be involved in cooling mechanisms (Reid, Volicer, Smookler, Beaven, and Brodie, 1968*b*; Weiss and Aghajanian, 1971). A contrary role for 5-HT neurons in the anterior hypothalamus has also been suggested (Feldberg, 1968; Myers and Beleslin, 1971). 5-HT administered intraventricularly may cause a rise or fall of body temperature depending on the species and dose (Feldberg, 1968). Meyerson (1964) was the first to suggest that a cerebral serotoninergic pathway may mediate heat-reaction inhibition in female rats. A similar conclusion was reached later with regard to male rodents by Tagliamonte, Tagliamonte, Gessa, and Brodie (1969), who observed activation of sexual behavior after a depletion of brain 5-HT.

The physiological role of 5-HT in peripheral structures is still largely unknown. In the intestine, 5-HT may occur in neurons as well as in entero-chromaffin cells and may participate in a transmitter function (Bülbring and Gershon, 1968).

Apart from its assumed functions as a neurotransmitter, 5-HT may have an important role in the biochemical mechanisms of cellular differ-entiation during early embryogenesis, as has been observed in invertebrates and amphibians and in a species of fish. Baker and Quay (1969) have re-viewed the present information on these mechanisms.

In the light of the basic physiological implications of the brain 5-HT neurons and pharmacological correlations involved, knowledge of their func-tional state during ontogenesis would be of great significance. The data ob-tained in studies on 5-HT metabolism in developing brain have recently been reviewed by Baker and Quay (1969) and by Renson (1971). This chapter summarizes our recent work on the maturation of various factors of brain 5-HT neurons, the results of which have previously appeared as abstracts and are now in press.

LEVELS OF 5-HYDROXYINDOLEACETIC ACID IN DEVELOPING BRAIN

Attempts have been made to correlate differences in behavioral matur-ity between species with the maturity of brain 5-HT and norepinephrine (NE) neurons based mainly on levels of amines and immediately related en-zymes (Kärki, Kunztman, and Brodie, 1962). No clear-cut differences be-tween species in amine levels have been revealed by these studies (Tissari, 1966; Baker and Quay, 1969). Changes in the impulse flow and turnover of transmitter amines (Sheard and Aghajanian, 1968) are reflected more sen-sitively by changes in the levels of acid metabolites of amines in the brain. This has been demonstrated for brain 5-HT neurons by means of electrical stimulation of a nerve (Aghajanian, Rosecrans, and Sheard, 1967; Sheard and Aghajanian, 1968), by thermal stress (Reid et al., 1968b; Weiss and Agha-janian, 1971) and by certain drug effects (Diaz, Ngai, and Costa, 1968).

The 5-hydroxyindoleacetic acid (5-HIAA) level of rat brain during on-togenesis has been measured by Tyce, Flock, and Owen (1964), by Tissari and Raunu (1972a) and by Tissari and Pekkarinen (1966) (Fig. 1, Table 1). These studies revealed an adult or near-adult 5-HIAA content at birth, whereas the 5-HT content was fragmentary. The strong increase of the 5-HIAA content of the brainstem on the day of birth might reflect an increase of 5-HT synthesis (Fig. 1). A clear caudal-rostral maturation gradient for

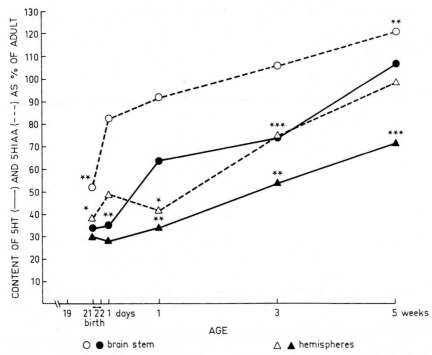

FIG. 1. Contents of 5-HT and 5-HIAA in the brainstem and hemispheres of developing rats. Rats of a laboratory inbred Sprague-Dawley strain were used. From the age of 1 week on, the pooled brain samples of developing rats were combined equally of males and females. Adult controls were about 75-day-old males. Results are expressed as a percentage of the adult values and are averages of five to seven measurements. *One star,* $p < 0.05$; *two stars,* $p < 0.01$; *three stars,* $p < 0.001$ when compared with the value of the next older age group.

5-HT and 5-HIAA contents was demonstrated by our data. The 5-HT content of the brainstem differed significantly from the adult at the age of only 1 week, whereas that of the hemispheres was still only 72% of the adult level at 5 weeks. A similar progression of brain 5-HT and NE levels has been found by Loizou and Salt (1970), and this was due to axons and terminals from cell bodies in the brainstem propagating rostrally for 3 and 5 weeks after birth, respectively (Loizou, 1969). Thus the 5-HIAA/5-HT ratio in the postnatal rat brain was higher than in the adult and was down to the adult level at 5 weeks in the brainstem (Table 1). The high 5-HIAA content of newborn rat brain coincides with the higher-than-adult plasma and brain tryptophan concentration (Tyce et al., 1964), and near-adult

TABLE 1. *Ratio of 5-HIAA to 5-HT in the brainstem of developing rats and rabbits.*

Age	Rat	Rabbit
Fetus	1.9 ± 0.3	1.2 ± 0.2
1 day	3.0 ± 0.4	2.5 ± 0.2
1 week	2.0 ± 0.3	1.7 ± 0.2
3 weeks	1.9 ± 0.1	1.8 ± 0.2
5 weeks	1.5 ± 0.1	—
Adult	1.3 ± 0.1	1.7 ± 0.1

The mean ratios ± SE of 5-HIAA/5-HT concentrations in nmoles per g of brainstem calculated from the same experiments as data presented in Figs. 1 and 2.

brain tryptophan hydroxylase (Renson 1971) and 5-hydroxytryptophan (5-HTP) decarboxylase activity (Kärki et al., 1962; Smith, Stacey, and Young, 1962). This may be due to a higher 5-HT and 5-HIAA synthesis, lower 5-HT storage capacity, or insufficient 5-HIAA elimination compared to that in the adult brain. The development of these mechanisms will be examined more closely in the following sections.

The rabbit is immature at birth, like the rat, and similarly it has a brain 5-HT content less than half of the adult (Kärki et al., 1962; Pscheidt, Schweigerdt, and Himwich, 1965). Tissari and Raunu (1972a) and Tissari and Pekkarinen (1966) have reported on the development of the brain 5-HIAA level in rabbit (Fig. 2, Table 1). Starting from the fetus stage, the increase of the brainstem 5-HIAA content differed from that in the rat, closely paralleling the 5-HT increase. From 1 week on, the 5-HIAA/5-HT ratio resembled the adult one. A small caudal-rostral maturation gradient of 5-HT content was apparent, as was noted by Pscheidt et al. (1965) for 5-HT content and by McCaman and Aprison (1964) for 5-HTP decarboxylase and monoamine oxidase (MAO) activity. Increases of 5-HT, 5-HIAA, and 5-HTP decarboxylase contents run parallel, whereas the MAO activity is adult or higher postnatally. No more data are yet available on the 5-HT mechanisms in the developing rabbit brain. No explanation has been found for the adult 5-HIAA/5-HT ratio observed, but it is interesting to note that it has not been possible to demonstrate any probenecid-sensitive acid transport in the rabbit brain (Werdinius, 1967; Roos quoted by Ashcroft, Dow, and Moir, 1968). Contrary to the two species mentioned above, the guinea pig is born mature. However, its brain 5-HT and 5-HTP decarboxylase levels at birth are not markedly higher than those of the rabbit; they amount to about 60% of the adult levels (Smith et al., 1962; Tissari, 1966). The brain of an adult or developing guinea pig has only a fragmentary 5-HIAA content, compared to its simultaneous 5-HT content (Tissari and Pekkarinen, 1966; Tissari and Raunu, 1972a), and 5-HIAA accumulates at a low rate after probenecid

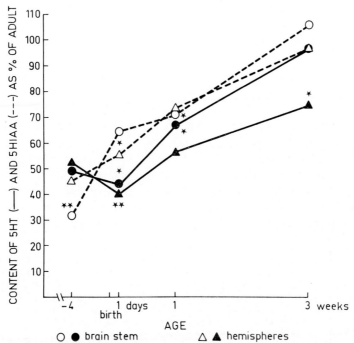

FIG. 2. Contents of 5-HT and 5-HIAA in the brainstem and hemispheres of developing rabbits. Albino rabbits were used, and the material of young rabbits was combined equally from males and females. Adult controls were males weighing 3 to 4 kg. Results are expressed as a percentage of the adult values and are averages of six measurements. *One star, $p < 0.05$; two stars, $p < 0.01$* when compared with the value of the next older age group.

treatment (Tissari and Suurhasko, 1971a). The content and probenecid-sensitive transport of homovanillic acid in the guinea pig brain resembles that in the rat brain (Juorio, Sharman, and Trajkov, 1966). 5-HIAA is probably not a major metabolite of 5-HT in the guinea pig brain (Nakai, 1958). In fact, measurements of 5-HIAA levels have revealed little information on the activity of the 5-HT neurons in the developing brain.

ELIMINATION OF 5-HYDROXYINDOLEACETIC ACID IN DEVELOPING BRAIN

In most species, including the rat, 5-HIAA is removed from the brain by an active transport mechanism, which is inhibited by acid metabolites of other monoamines (Werdinius, 1966; Cserr and Van Dyke, 1971), by organic acids such as probenecid (Neff, Tozer, and Brodie, 1967; Werdinius,

1967), and by metabolic inhibitors (Reid et al., 1968a); also, it may become saturated by the increased formation of 5-HIAA (Juorio et al., 1966; Ashcroft, Moir, and Eccleston, 1968). Transport occurs mainly through the blood-brain barrier, and elimination by the cerebrospinal fluid (Guldberg, Ashcroft, and Crawford, 1966; Bowers and Gerbode, 1968) plays only a minor role (Neff et al., 1967; Cserr and Van Dyke, 1971). In steady-state conditions, 5-HT and 5-HIAA are formed, 5-HIAA is eliminated at the same rate, and, after transport-block, 5-HIAA accumulates at the same rate (Tozer, Neff, and Brodie, 1966; Neff et al., 1967).

Tissari and Raunu (1970a,b; Tissari, 1972) have studied the mechanisms of eliminating 5-HIAA from the developing rat brain. The accumulation of 5-HIAA in the brain was measured after applying a transport block by administering probenecid (Fig. 3). In 1-day-old rat brain, no accumulation of 5-HIAA occurred during the first 90 min. In the following 90 min,

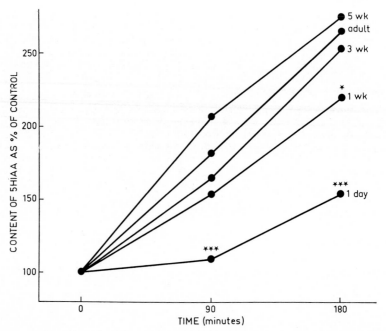

FIG. 3. Accumulation of 5-HIAA in the brain of developing and adult rats after the administration of probenecid (200 mg/kg i.p.) twice at 0 and 1 hr. At 3 hr, the probenecid concentration of 1-day-old rat brain was 250 μg/g and that of adult brain 135 μg/g; with only one probenecid dose, the concentrations were 80 and 25 μg/g, respectively. Results are expressed as a percentage of the control values and are averages of six experiments. One star, $p < 0.05$; three stars, $p < 0.001$ when compared with the adult value. Data from Tissari (1972).

TABLE 2. *Levels of brain 5-HIAA after the administration of pargyline and tranyl-cypromine to 1-day-old and adult rats.*

Hours after drug	5-HIAA (μg/g)			
	1-day-old		Adult	
	Pargyline	Tranylcypromine	Pargyline	Tranylcypromine
0	0.34 ± 0.03	0.42 ± 0.06	0.48 ± 0.03	0.59 ± 0.03
0.5	0.31 ± 0.03		0.35 ± 0.02	
1	0.22 ± 0.02		0.26 ± 0.03	
2	0.14 ± 0.01	0.17 ± 0.03	0.14 ± 0.02	0.20 ± 0.02
4	0.09 ± 0.01		0.07 ± 0.01	
6	0.10 ± 0.01	0.13 ± 0.01	0.09 ± 0.01	0.17 ± 0.01

Pargyline was administered 100 mg/kg at 0 hr and 50 mg/kg at 3 hr i.p. to 1-day-old and 100 mg/kg i.p. twice to adult rats. Tranylcypromine was administered 5 mg/kg i.p. Averages ± SE of six experiments. Data from Tissari (1972).

5-HIAA content rose to a level of 1.5 times the control, although the possibility of a rise due to an increase of plasma 5-HIAA was not excluded. From 3 weeks on, the adult rate of increase of the 5-HIAA content suggested a mature transport. The insufficient probenecid response of young rat brain was not caused by a failure of 5-HIAA formation; the turnover time of 5-HT in 1-day-old rats was approximately the same as that in adults (Tissari and Raunu, 1970*b*, 1972*c*).

After MAO block, the 5-HIAA content of the brain of the 1-day-old rats decreased fairly rapidly but not as completely as that of adult rat brain, which transports 5-HIAA at the same rate as 5-HT synthesis (Table 2). The decline of 5-HIAA in 1-day-old rat brain may have been caused by a passive diffusion. This view is supported by the high increase of brain 5-HIAA content found after i.p. administration, as compared to that in the adults (Table 3).

TABLE 3. *Levels of brain 5-HIAA after the administration of 5-HIAA to 1-day-old and adult rats.*

Age		5-HIAA (μg/g)		
		Min after 5-HIAA		
		0	30	60
1 day	Brainstem	0.9 ± 0.2	8.9 ± 0.9	9.5 ± 2.1
	Hemispheres	0.3 ± 0.1	7.5 ± 0.7	9.2 ± 1.7
Adult	Brainstem	1.1 ± 0.1	3.8 ± 0.8	2.1 ± 0.7
	Hemispheres	0.6 ± 0.0	3.0 ± 0.4	1.9 ± 0.3
	Blood	0.1 ± 0.0	1.2 ± 0.4	0.1 ± 0.0

5-HIAA was administered 100 mg/kg i.p. Averages ± SE of five experiments. Data from Tissari (1972).

There is a discrepancy between the adult 5-HIAA concentration of newborn rat brain and the low level and synthesis rate of 5-HT (Tissari and Raunu, 1970b, 1972c). This may arise from a combination of deficient 5-HIAA elimination and deficient 5-HT storage (Tissari and Raunu, 1970b, 1972b), part of the synthesized 5-HT being shunted directly to MAO. The lack of 5-HIAA transport indicates an immature blood-brain barrier in postnatal rat, as also suggested by the high permeability to monoamines (Loizou, 1970) and to 5-HIAA (Table 3). On the contrary, transport of 5-HT by nerve endings occurs in newborn rat (Tissari and Suurhasko, 1971b, 1972) and indicates that these two structures mature at different times.

TURNOVER OF SEROTONIN IN DEVELOPING BRAIN

The turnover rate of 5-HT in rat brain has been measured from the initial rate of 5-HT accumulation or 5-HIAA decline after a complete MAO block (Tozer et al., 1966) and from the accumulation of 5-HIAA after a transport block (Neff et al., 1967). All these methods have revealed a turnover time of 1.2 hr. The latter two methods depend on 5-HIAA transport, which does not yet seem to exist in the newborn rat brain (Tissari and Raunu, 1970a,b; Tissari 1972). Tissari and Raunu (1970b, 1972c) (Fig. 4) have measured the turnover rate of 5-HT in 1-day-old rat brain from the initial rate of 5-HT accumulation after an MAO block. A similar turnover time of about 1.5 hr was found in the young and adult brain. The turnover rate of 5-HT was about 0.3 μg/g/hr in the adults and 0.1 μg/g/hr in the 1-day-olds (i.e., 30% of the adult value, as also was the brain 5-HT content). Hyperactivity was observed in both age groups starting from 3.5 hr on, which possibly suggests a similar turnover time of brain 5-HT. The hyperactivity in these experiments may have been due to free 5-HT "spilling over" into the receptor sites (Grahame-Smith, 1971).

The results could be interpreted as demonstrating that the amount of serotoninergic nerve tissue per gram of whole brain is low in 1-day-old rats but that impulse flow exists as in adults. The low content of serotoninergic nerve tissue is in accord with the histochemically observed lack of 5-HT axons and terminals (Loizou, 1969). The importance of impulse flow for the turnover of the transmitter in 5-HT neurons is shown by the disappearance of 5-HIAA caudal to a transection of the spinal cord (Andén, Magnusson, Roos, and Werdinius, 1965) and by increased amine synthesis after electric stimulation of midbrain raphe 5-HT neurons (Sheard and Aghajanian, 1968). 5-HT turnover in the brain of newborn rats and guinea pigs is

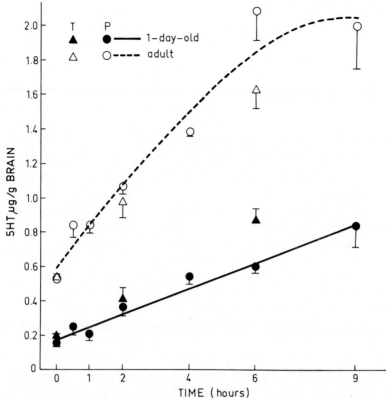

FIG. 4. Levels of brain 5-HT after the administration of pargyline (P) and tranylcypromine (T) to 1-day-old and adult rats. Pargyline was administered 100 mg/kg at 0 hr and 50 mg/kg at 3 hr i.p. to 1-day-old and 100 mg/kg i.p. twice to adult rats. Tranylcypromine was administered 5 mg/kg i.p. Averages ± SE of six experiments.

indicated by the results of Kärki et al. (1962).

Using NE synthesis block, Loizou (1971) found a normal turnover time of brain NE in newborn rats. A similar finding was reached by Kulkarni and Shideman (1968) in postnatal rats by means of an MAO block.

SUBCELLULAR DISTRIBUTION OF BRAIN SEROTONIN DURING DEVELOPMENT

In several laboratories it has repeatedly been found that, under standardized conditions, about 25% of the 5-HT content of a brain homogenate is recovered in the primary high-speed supernatant fraction (for references, see Michaelson, 1968). This percentage may be increased by technical factors, such as rougher homogenization (as demonstrated for brain acetylcholine by Whittaker and Dowe, 1965), insufficient cooling of the tissue [as found in the case of 5-HT by Haber, Kohl, and Pscheidt (1965) and of NE by Gutman and Weil-Malherbe, 1967] or repeated centrifugations (Giarman and Schanberg, 1958). The 5-HT in stored reserves and that in cytoplasm are evidently in a dynamic steady-state equilibrium and protected by MAO from excessive levels of a free, functionally active form. Soluble 5-HT may somehow be protected from becoming inactivated by MAO; in the case of brain-soluble NE, however, no linkage with a protein was detected (Gutman and Weil-Malherbe, 1967). This protection is perhaps removed by reserpine, which liberates amine first from the soluble fraction in the central 5-HT (Green and Sawyer, 1962; Giarman, Freedman, and Schanberg, 1964) and NE (Weil-Malherbe, Posner, and Bowles, 1961; Glowinski, Snyder, and Axelrod, 1966) and peripheral NE (Van Orden, Bensch, and Giarman, 1967) neurons. After an MAO block, the particulate and soluble fractions of brain 5-HT adjust to a new steady-state level without (Schanberg and Giarman, 1962; Levi and Maynert, 1964) or with only a slight increase (Green and Sawyer, 1962) of the percent of soluble 5-HT.

Bennett and Giarman (1965), Haber and Kamano (1966), and Tissari and Raunu (1970b, 1972b) have studied the subcellular distribution of 5-HT in the brain of rats aged from newborn to 5 weeks. All these data show an adult or less than adult proportion of supernatant 5-HT in the young rat brain. Our results (Table 4) indicated that up to the age of 3 weeks, the supernatant proportion of 5-HT was significantly lower, peaking in the 1-week-olds, than it was in the adults. A similar trend is found in the data of the other authors. We also studied the subcellular distribution of brain 5-HT after increasing its level by means of an MAO block or by administering 5-HTP (Table 4). After tranylcypromine treatment, soluble 5-HT in the adult rat brain increased from 25.1 to 29.2%. The 5-HT content reached in the 1-day-old rat brain was half of that in the adult, but the soluble 5-HT had risen from 18 to 29.4%. The changes in 5-HT distribution caused by administering 5-HTP were more marked. The increase of soluble 5-HT in the adult brain was similar to that reported by Schanberg and Giarman (1962). Adult 5-HT levels found in the young rat brain after 5-HTP administration could have been partly due to a low decarboxylation peripherally (Lundborg and Kellogg, 1971). The increase in the proportion of supernatant 5-HT up to the age of 3 weeks was several times higher than that in the adults. These results are in agreement with the findings of Palaic and

TABLE 4. *Subcellular distribution of 5-HT in the brain of developing and adult rats and the effect of tranylcypromine and 5-HTP.*

		Control		Experimental	
Age	Drug	5-HT (μg/g)	% in supernatant	5-HT (μg/g)	% in supernatant
1 day	Tranylcypromine	0.21 ± 0.01	18.0[a]± 1.7	0.8 ± 0.1	29.4 ± 2.2
Adult	"	0.58 ± 0.02	25.1 ± 2.0	1.5 ± 0.1	29.2 ± 1.1
1 day	5-HTP	0.20 ± 0.02	20.7[b]± 3.3	1.6 ± 0.2	51.4[c]± 1.5
1 week	"	0.35 ± 0.02	10.4[c]± 1.9	1.3 ± 0.3	40.2 ± 2.9
3 weeks	"	0.35 ± 0.01	17.3[c]± 0.8	2.0 ± 0.3	38.3 ± 2.4
5 weeks	"	0.43 ± 0.02	25.3 ± 1.0	1.2 ± 0.1	37.7 ± 0.9
Adult	"	0.56 ± 0.01	26.5 ± 1.2	1.6 ± 0.1	35.4 ± 1.9

About 1.5 g brain tissue was homogenized in nine volumes of 0.25 M sucrose containing 0.002 M disodium EDTA and 0.001 M tranylcypromine in a glass homogenizer with a Teflon pestle for 2 min. Homogenate was centrifuged at $100,000 \times g$ for 25 min. All procedures after decapitation were carried at 4°C. Tranylcypromine was administered 5 mg/kg i.p. 6 hr and 5-HTP 100 mg/kg i.p. 30 min before killing. Averages ± SE of four to six experiments.

[a] $p < 0.01$, [b] $p < 0.05$, [c] $p < 0.001$ when compared with the adult value.

Supek (1966), which suggest a difference between the binding of 5-HT and NE in the newborn and the adult rat brain owing to the earlier and stronger release of amines by irradiation in the newborn brain.

Despite the effect of technical factors on the proportion of 5-HT recovered in the supernatant fraction and despite high water content of newborn rat brain (Piccoli, Grynbaum, and Lajtha, 1971), it must be assumed that the low percentage of supernatant 5-HT found in the young rat brain normally is not an artifact. This is borne out by the different distribution of 5-HT under the experimental conditions and by the fact that the tissue water content matures more rapidly (Piccoli et al., 1971) than the subcellular distribution of 5-HT. The reason for the low percent of soluble 5-HT in the postnatal rat brain might be that, like the particulate storage pool, the soluble storage pool protected from MAO is immature.

TRANSPORT AND STORAGE OF SEROTONIN IN SYNAPTOSOMES OF DEVELOPING BRAIN

Brain 5-HT neurons take up 5-HT by a process similar to catecholamine uptake by brain NE and dopamine (DA) neurons and by peripheral adrenergic neurons. This uptake has been demonstrated by incubating brain slices (Blackburn, French, and Merrills, 1967; Ross and Renyi, 1967) and isolated nerve endings (synaptosomes) (Bogdanski, Tissari, and Brodie, 1968; Iversen, 1970) with 5-HT *in vitro* and by injecting 5-HT intraventricularly (Fuxe and Ungerstedt, 1967). Transport is mediated by a Na^+-dependent saturable carrier-mediated mechanism with a K_m of 0.07 μM for 5-HT (Bogdanski, Tissari, and Brodie, 1970b). Amine transport is blocked by ouabain or a K^+-free medium (Bogdanski et al., 1968; Colburn, Goodwin, Murphy, Bunney, and Davis, 1968) after a time delay (Tissari, Schönhöfer, Bogdanski, and Brodie, 1969; Bogdanski, Blaszkowski, and Tissari, 1970a) as against the immediate block of $(Na^+ + K^+)$-ATPase (Tissari et al., 1969), suggesting an indirect involvement of the enzyme. In synaptosomes, a minor part of the translocated 5-HT is stored intracellularly by a reserpine-sensitive mechanism; a major part is metabolized and returned to the incubation medium (Bogdanski et al., 1968; Tissari et al., 1969).

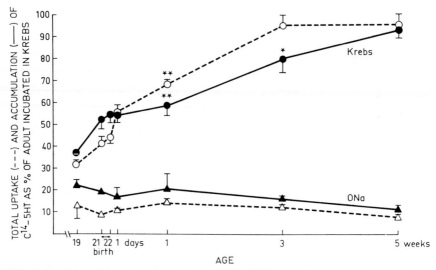

FIG. 5. Total uptake and accumulation of ^{14}C-5-HT by synaptosomes of developing rats incubated in Krebs-bicarbonate (KRB) and a Na^+-free solution. ^{14}C-5-HT (0.11 μM) was incubated 7 min at 37°C and 95% O_2–5% CO_2 with synaptosomes suspended in KRB or a Na^+-free solution (isotonicity maintained by sucrose) containing all other electrolytes normally present in KRB. Total uptake includes ^{14}C-5-HT accumulated by the synaptosomes plus total ^{14}C-deaminated metabolites in the suspension, expressed as a percentage of the amine originally present. Accumulation is expressed as the concentration ratio of intracellular to extracellular amine. Results are given as a percentage of the simultaneous adult value incubated in KRB. Averages ± SE of four to six experiments run in duplicate. *One star, p < 0.05; two stars, p < 0.01* when compared with the next older age group.

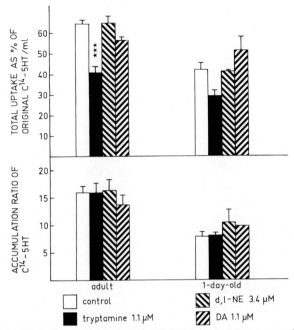

FIG. 6. Total uptake and accumulation of ¹⁴C-5-HT by synaptosomes of 1-day-old and adult rats in the presence of tryptamine and catecholamines. ¹⁴C-5-HT was incubated 7 min with synaptosomes in KRB with or without the simultaneous presence of nonradioactive tryptamine (1.1 μM), D,L-NE (3.4 μM), or DA (1.1 μM). Total uptake and accumulation defined as in Fig. 5. Averages $\pm$ SE of four experiments. *Three stars, p <* 0.001 when compared with the control value.

Properties of synaptosomes and the transport mechanism have recently been reviewed by Tissari and Bogdanski (1971).

Tissari and Suurhasko (1971*b*, 1972) have recently reported a study of the transport and storage of 5-HT in synaptosomes of the developing rat brain, from which the data in Figs. 5 and 6 are taken. Uptake and accumulation of 5-HT were detected in the fetal synaptosomes, and they were diminished by incubating at 0°C temperature or in the absence of Na⁺ or, in the case of accumulation, by the presence of 10⁻⁶M reserpine. Uptake and accumulation increased steadily at birth. The uptake then increased more rapidly, reaching the adult level at 3 weeks, parallel with the increase of synaptosome protein. The accumulation increased later and reached the adult level at 5 weeks—a finding similar to that made in studies on the subcellular distribution of 5-HT (Tissari and Raunu, 1970*b*, 1972*b*). Uptake and accumulation in samples containing ouabain or a K+-free medium were considered to be due to passive diffusion. A small, ouabain-sensitive uptake was found in the fetal samples. In the synaptosomes of 1-day-old rats, the ouabain and K+-lack-sensitive uptake and accumulation amounted to 35% and 43% of the adult values, respectively. The insensitive components remained similar in older age groups, so the increases observed were due to the increase of active transport. In the rat brain, the Na+ and K+ gradients across the cell membrane are established only on the day of birth (Piccoli et al., 1971), coinciding with the rapid increase of (Na+ + K+)-ATPase activity (Abdel-Latif, Brody, and Ramahi, 1967). The brain ATP content remains similar from the fetus to the adult stage (Piccoli et al., 1971), but its level does not affect amino acid transport in brain slices clearly either (Banay-Schwartz, Piro, and Lajtha, 1971). From the fetal stage to the age of 1 day, rat synaptosomes also undergo a distinct morphological maturation from a fragile and disorganized state to a near-adult one (Abdel-Latif et al., 1967). Our data suggest a marked development of 5-HT uptake and storage functions simultaneously.

Vernadakis and Kellog (1971) have reported a temperature-dependent, cocaine-sensitive uptake of NE by brain slices of chicken embryo at stages at which (Na+ + K+)-ATPase is still barely detectable (Bignami, Palladini, and Venturini, 1966). Using intraperitoneal administration of amines and histochemical detection, Loizou (1970) has found uptake of 5-HT and catecholamines in the central monoamine neurons in the newborn rat brain. The synaptosomes of the developing rat brain from birth on may have properties that qualitatively do not differ much from those of the adult; this is suggested by the similar stability of the 5-HT in the Na+-free incubating mixtures (Fig. 5), by the retention of 5-HIAA formed in the synaptosomes, and by the similar intracellular fate of translocated 5-HT (the total uptake/accumulation ratio of the 5-HT was about 10 in the synaptosomes of 1-day- and 1-week-old rats under the same test conditions as those in which it was 6.5 in the adults) (Tissari and Suurhasko, 1972). The similarity was also borne out by a similarity in the substrate specificity of 5-HT uptake by 1-day-old and adult rat synaptosomes (Fig. 6). 5-HT transport by synaptosomes at low substrate concentrations is not affected by catecholamines (Iversen, 1970; Tissari, 1971), but it is affected by tryptamine and derivatives (Tissari, 1971). By histochemical methods, Loizou (1970) found an accumulation of catecholamines in 5-HT neurons of the newborn rat brain, but similar results have also been obtained histochemically in the adult rat brain (Fuxe and Ungerstedt, 1966).

CONCLUDING REMARKS

From the data reviewed in the preceding sections, a picture can be formed of the maturation of 5-HT neurons in the rat brain. On the day of birth, a marked maturation of these neurons occurs, as implied by the increase of 5-HT synthesis and transport which coincides with the rapid increase of brain $(Na^+ + K^+)$-ATPase activity and the establishment of Na^+ and K^+ gradients across the cell membrane (Abdel-Latif et al., 1967). All the factors needed for impulse conduction in 5-HT neurons are present in the 1-day-old rat brain, although to a smaller extent than in the adult: the content (Nachmias, 1960; Bennett and Giarman, 1965), turnover rate (Tissari and Raunu, 1972c), transport and storage of 5-HT (Tissari and Suurhasko, 1972; Tissari and Raunu, 1972b), and the activity of the MAO (Nachmias, 1960; Kärki et al., 1962) are all about one-third of the corresponding adult value. The existence of impulse flow is indicated by the adult turnover time of the brain 5-HT (Tissari and Raunu, 1972c). In NE neurons of newborn rat brain, Loizou (1970, 1971) has histochemically discovered turnover and uptake of the amine which suggest impulse conduction.

Various biochemical and morphological components of brain 5-HT neurons reach the adult level at different times. 5-HT transport (Tissari and Suurhasko, 1972) and MAO activity (Nachmias, 1960; Bennett and Giarman, 1965) mature at 3 weeks. By that time, the histochemically observed distribution of axons and terminals originating in 5-HT cell bodies in the brainstem attain their adult form (Loizou, 1969). The last parameters to mature are the 5-HT content (Nachmias, 1960; Tyce et al., 1964; Bennett and Giarman, 1965) and storage capacity (Tissari and Raunu, 1972b; Tissari and Suurhasko, 1972) and the ratio of 5-HIAA/5-HT (Tissari and Raunu, 1972a), which reach the adult level at 5 weeks.

Continuous electrical activity in the rat brain begins on the day of birth (Abdel-Latif et al., 1967). As in other species, when the EEG starts, the brain 5-HT content is low. The relationship between the maturation of the EEG and brain 5-HT content is not uniform: in the cat, rat, and guinea pig, for example, EEG maturation occurs while the brain 5-HT content is still low and in the rabbit when it is adult (Pscheidt and Himwich, 1966; cf. Tissari, 1966).

Two states of sleep can already be detected in newborn rats: paradoxical sleep accounting for 80 to 90%, and fragmentary slow-wave sleep (Jouvet, 1967). In ontogenesis, the dissociated appearance of paradoxical sleep, waking reaction, and slow-wave sleep probably coincides with the caudal-rostral maturation of the structures and mechanisms responsible (Valatx, Jouvet, and Jouvet, 1964). In postnatal rats, sleeping and waking phases occur irregularly throughout the day. Asano (1971) has found that a daily adult sleep-activity rhythm starts simultaneously with the circadian rhythm of brain 5-HT content in rats at the age of 5 weeks. At that time, the brain 5-HT neurons reach full maturity. In these circadian rhythms, a high brain 5-HT content and sleep coincide in the light period and a low content and motor activity in the dark period (Albrecht, Visscher, Bittner, and Halberg, 1956; Scheving, Harrison, Gordon, and Pauly, 1968). The mechanisms regulating the circadian rhythm of brain 5-HT content and its significance are scarcely known. Plasma and brain tryptophan concentration have a circadian rhythm differing by 180° from that of brain 5-HT (Fernstrom and Wurtman, 1971). In the rat brain, the maturation of the circadian rhythm of 5-HT content coincides with the maturation of 5-HT storage capacity. Consistent with this, Grahame-Smith (1971) has suggested that the level of functionally active amine in 5-HT neurons may be regulated by the storage capacity and not by the rate of synthesis.

From birth on, the rat shows signs of thermoregulation; adult efficiency and homeothermia are reached at 2 weeks (Taylor, 1960). 5-HT administered intraventricularly causes hypothermia in rats (Feldberg and Lotti, 1967). Tirri (1971) has found that 2-day-old rats already respond to intraventricular 5-HT by hypothermia; from the 5th day on, the response is similar to that of the adult. Evidently, the 5-HT receptors in the anterior hypothalamus involved in temperature regulation are present at that time.

The circadian rhythm of the plasma corticosterone level has been correlated with that of brain 5-HT content (Krieger and Rizzo, 1969). Okada (1971) found that the circadian rhythm of brain 5-HT content was clearly slower to mature than that of plasma corticosterone level, so any functional correlation between them was improbable.

ACKNOWLEDGMENTS

This work was supported by grants from the National Research Council for Medical Sciences, Finland, the Finnish Medical Society "Duodecim," and the Yrjö Jahnsson Foundation.

REFERENCES

Abdel-Latif, A. A., Brody, J., and Ramahi, H. (1967): Studies on sodium-potassium adenosine triphosphatase of the nerve endings and appearance of electrical activity in developing rat brain. *Journal of Neurochemistry*, 14:1133-1141.

Aghajanian, G. K., Rosecrans, J. A., and Sheard, M. H. (1967): Serotonin: Release in the forebrain by stimulation of midbrain raphé. *Science*, 156:402-403.

Albrecht, P., Visscher, M. B., Bittner, J. J., and Halberg, F. (1956): Daily changes in 5-hydroxytryptamine concentration in mouse brain. *Proceedings of the Society for Experimental Biology and Medicine*, 92:703-706.

Andén, N.-E., Magnusson, T., Roos, B.-E., and Werdinius, B. (1965): 5-Hydroxyindoleacetic acid of rabbit spinal cord normally and after transection. *Acta Physiologica Scandinavica*, 64:193-196.

Asano, Y. (1971): The maturation of the circadian rhythm of brain norepinephrine and serotonin in the rat. *Life Sciences*, 10:883-894.

Ashcroft, G. W., Dow, R. C., and Moir, A. T. B. (1968): The active transport of 5-hydroxyindol-3-ylacetic acid and 3-methoxy-4-hydroxyphenylacetic acid from a recirculatory perfusion system of the cerebral ventricles of the unanaesthetized dog. *Journal of Physiology*, 199:397-425.

Ashcroft, G. W., Moir, A. T. B., and Eccleston, D. (1968): Discussion of *in vivo* measurement of brain serotonin turnover. *Advances in Pharmacology*, 6A:110-112.

Baker, P. C., and Quay, W. B. (1969): 5-Hydroxytryptamine metabolism in early embryogenesis, and the development of brain and retinal tissues. A review. *Brain Research*, 12:273-295.

Banay-Schwartz, M., Piro, L., and Lajtha, A. (1971): Relationship of ATP levels to amino acid transport in slices of mouse brain. *Archives of Biochemistry and Biophysics*, 145:199-210.

Bennett, D. S., and Giarman, N. J. (1965): Schedule of appearance of 5-hydroxytryptamine (serotonin) and associated enzymes in the developing rat brain. *Journal of Neurochemistry*, 12:911-918.

Bignami, A., Palladini, G., and Venturini, G. (1966): Sodium-potassium adenosine triphosphatase in the developing chick brain. *Brain Research*, 3:207-209.

Blackburn, K. J., French, P. C., and Merrills, R. J. (1967): 5-Hydroxytryptamine uptake by rat brain *in vitro*. *Life Sciences*, 6:1653-1663.

Bogdanski, D. F., Blaszkowski, T. P., and Tissari, A. H. (1970a): Mechanisms of biogenic amine transport and storage. IV. Relationship between K+ and the Na+ requirement for transport and storage of 5-hydroxytryptamine and norepinephrine in synaptosomes. *Biochimica et Biophysica Acta*, 211:521-532.

Bogdanski, D. F., Tissari, A. and Brodie, B. B. (1968): Role of sodium, potassium, ouabain and reserpine in uptake, storage and metabolism of biogenic amines in synaptosomes. *Life Sciences*, 7:419-428.

Bogdanski, D. F., Tissari, A. H., and Brodie, B. B. (1970b): Mechanism of transport and storage of biogenic amines. III. Effects of sodium and potassium on kinetics of 5-hydroxytryptamine and norepinephrine transport by rabbit synaptosomes. *Biochimica et Biophysica Acta*, 219:189-199.

Bowers, M. B., Jr., and Gerbode, F. (1968): CSF 5HIAA: Effects of probenecid and parachlorophenylalanine. *Life Sciences*, 7:773-776.

Bülbring, E., and Gershon, M. D. (1968): Serotonin participation in the vagal inhibitory pathway to the stomach. *Advances in Pharmacology*, 6A:323-333.

Colburn, R. W., Goodwin, F. K., Murphy, D. L., Bunney, W. E., Jr., and Davis, J. M. (1968): Quantitative studies of norepinephrine uptake by synaptosomes. *Biochemical Pharmacology*, 17:957-964.

Cserr, H. F., and Van Dyke, D. H. (1971): 5-Hydroxyindoleacetic acid accumulation by isolated choroid plexus. *American Journal of Physiology*, 220:718-723.

Diaz, P. M., Ngai, S. H., and Costa, E. (1968): Factors modulating brain serotonin turnover. *Advances in Pharmacology*, 6B:75-92.

Feldberg, W. (1968): The monoamines of the hypothalamus as mediators of temperature responses. In: *Recent Advances in Pharmacology*, edited by J. M. Robson and R. S. Stacey. J. & A. Churchill Ltd., London, pp. 349-397.

Feldberg, W., and Lotti, V. J. (1967): Temperature responses to monoamines and an inhibitor of MAO injected into the cerebral ventricles of rats. *British Journal of Pharmacology and Chemotherapy,* 31:152-161.

Fernstrom, J. D., and Wurtman, R. J. (1971): Brain serotonin content: Physiological dependence on plasma tryptophan levels. *Science,* 173:149-152.

Fuxe, K., and Ungerstedt, U. (1966): Localization of catecholamine uptake in rat after intraventricular injection. *Life Sciences,* 5:1817-1824.

Fuxe, K., and Ungerstedt, U. (1967): Localization of 5-hydroxytryptamine uptake in rat brain after intraventricular injection. *Journal of Pharmacy and Pharmacology,* 19:335-337.

Giarman, N. J., Freedman, D. X., and Schanberg, S. M. (1964): Drug-induced changes in the subcellular distribution of serotonin in rat brain with special reference to the action of reserpine. *Progress in Brain Research,* 8:72-80.

Giarman, N. J., and Schanberg, S. (1958): The intracellular distribution of 5-hydroxytryptamine (HT, serotonin) in the rat's brain. *Biochemical Pharmacology,* 1:301-306.

Glowinski, J., Snyder, S. H., and Axelrod, J. (1966): Subcellular localization of H^3-norepinephrine in the rat brain and the effect of drugs. *Journal of Pharmacology and Experimental Therapeutics,* 152:282-292.

Grahame-Smith, D. G. (1971): Studies *in vivo* on the relationship between brain tryptophan, brain 5-HT synthesis and hyperactivity in rats treated with a monoamine oxidase inhibitor and L-tryptophan. *Journal of Neurochemistry,* 18:1053-1066.

Green, H., and Sawyer, J. L. (1962): Intracellular distribution of serotonin in rat brain. 1. Effect of reserpine and monoamine oxidase inhibitors, tranylcypromine and iproniazid. *Archives Internationales de Pharmacodynamie et de Thérapie,* 135:426-441.

Guldberg, H. C., Ashcroft, G. W., and Crawford, T. B. B. (1966): Concentrations of 5-hydroxyindoleacetic acid and homovanillic acid in the cerebrospinal fluid of the dog before and during treatment with probenecid. *Life Sciences,* 5:1571-1575.

Gutman, Y., and Weil-Malherbe, H. (1967): The intracellular distribution of brain catecholamines. *Journal of Neurochemistry,* 14:619-625.

Haber, B., and Kamano, A. (1966): Sub-cellular distribution of serotonin in the developing rat brain. *Nature,* 209:404.

Haber, B., Kohl, H., and Pscheidt, G. R. (1965): Supernatant-particulate distribution of exogenous serotonin in rat brain homogenates. *Biochemical Pharmacology,* 14:1-6.

Iversen, L. L. (1970): Neuronal uptake processes for amines and amino acids. *Advances in Biochemical Psychopharmacology,* 2:109-132.

Jouvet, M. (1967): Neurophysiology of the states of sleep. *Physiological Reviews,* 47:117-177.

Jouvet, M. (1969): Biogenic amines and the states of sleep. *Science,* 163:32-41.

Juorio, A. V., Sharman, D. F., and Trajkov. T. (1966): The effect of drugs on the homovanillic acid content of the corpus striatum of some rodents. *British Journal of Pharmacology and Chemotherapy,* 26:385-392.

Kärki, N., Kuntzman, R., and Brodie, B. B. (1962): Storage, synthesis, and metabolism of monoamines in the developing brain. *Journal of Neurochemistry,* 9:53-58.

Krieger, D. T., and Rizzo, F. (1969): Serotonin mediation of circadian periodicity of plasma 17-hydroxycorticosteroids. *American Journal of Physiology,* 217:1703-1707.

Kulkarni, A. S., and Shideman, F. E. (1968): Catecholamine accumulation in the brains of infant and adult rats after monoamine oxidase inhibition. *European Journal of Pharmacology,* 3:269-271.

Levi, R., and Maynert, E. W. (1964): The subcellular localization of brain-stem norepinephrine and 5-hydroxytryptamine in stressed rats. *Biochemical Pharmacology,* 13:615-621.

Loizou, L. A. (1969): The development of monoamine-containing neurones in the brain of the albino rat. *Journal of Anatomy,* 104:588.

Loizou, L. A. (1970): Uptake of monoamines into central neurones and the blood-brain barrier in the infant rat. *British Journal of Pharmacology*, 40:800-813.

Loizou, L. A. (1971): Effect of inhibition catecholamine synthesis on central catecholamine-containing neurones in the developing albino rat. *British Journal of Pharmacology*, 41:41-48.

Loizou, L. A., and Salt, P. (1970): Regional changes in monoamines of the rat brain during postnatal development. *Brain Research*, 20:467-470.

Lundborg, P., and Kellogg, C. (1971): Formation of (^{3}H) noradrenaline and (^{3}H) dopamine in the brain and heart of the rat foetus. *Brain Research*, 29:387-389.

McCaman, R. E., and Aprison, M. H. (1964): The synthetic and catabolic enzyme systems for acetylcholine and serotonin in several discrete areas of the developing rabbit brain. *Progress in Brain Research*, 9:220-233.

Meyerson, B. J. (1964): Central nervous monoamines and hormone induced estrus behaviour in the spayed rat. *Acta Physiologica Scandinavica*, 63, Suppl. 241:1-32.

Michaelson, I. A. (1968): Discussion of the neuronal compartmentation of 5-hydroxytryptamine stores. *Advances in Pharmacology*, 6A:271-274.

Myers, R. D., and Beleslin, D. B., (1971): Changes in serotonin release in hypothalamus during cooling or warming of the monkey. *American Journal of Physiology*, 220:1746-1754.

Nachmias, V. T. (1960): Amine oxidase and 5-hydroxytryptamine in developing rat brain. *Journal of Neurochemistry*, 6:99-104.

Nakai, K. (1958): 5-Hydroxytryptamine metabolism in rabbits and guinea pigs. *Japanese Journal of Pharmacology*, 8:63-69.

Neff, N. H., Tozer, T. N., and Brodie, B. B. (1967): Application of steady-state kinetics to studies of the transfer of 5-hydroxyindoleacetic acid from brain to plasma. *Journal of Pharmacology and Experimental Therapeutics*, 158:214-218.

Okada, F. (1971): The maturation of the circadian rhythm of brain serotonin in the rat. *Life Sciences*, 10:77-86.

Palaic, D. J., and Supek, Z. (1966): Liberation of brain 5-hydroxytryptamine and noradrenaline by X-ray treatment in the new-born and adult rat. *Journal of Neurochemistry*, 13:705-709.

Piccoli, F., Grynbaum, A., and Lajtha, A. (1971): Developmental changes in Na$^+$, K$^+$ and ATP and in the levels and transport of amino acids in incubated slices of rat brain. *Journal of Neurochemistry*, 18:1135-1148.

Pscheidt, G. R., and Himwich, H. E. (1966): Biogenic amines in various brain regions of growing cats. *Brain Research*, 1:363-368.

Pscheidt, G. R., Schweigerdt, A., and Himwich, H. E. (1965): Effects of some psychoactive drugs on electroencephalogram and brain amines of immature rabbits. *Life Sciences*, 4:1333-1343.

Reid, W. D., Volicer, L., and Brodie, B. B. (1968a): Inhibition of 5-hydroxyindoleacetic acid transport from the brain by 2,4-dinitrophenol. *Life Sciences*, 7:577-581.

Reid, W. D., Volicer, L., Smookler, H., Beaven, M. A., and Brodie, B. B. (1968b): Brain amines and temperature regulation. *Pharmacology*, 1:329-344.

Renson, J. (1971): Development of monoaminergic transmissions in the rat brain. *Advances in Experimental Medicine and Biology*, 13:175-184.

Ross, S. B., and Renyi, A. L. (1967): Accumulation of tritiated 5-hydroxytryptamine in brain slices. *Life Sciences*, 6:1407-1415.

Schanberg, S. M., and Giarman, N. J. (1962): Drug-induced alterations in the subcellular distribution of 5-hydroxytryptamine in rat's brain. *Biochemical Pharmacology*, 11:187-194.

Scheving, L. E., Harrison, W. H., Gordon, P., and Pauly, J. E. (1968): Daily fluctuation (circadian and ultradian) in biogenic amines of the rat brain. *American Journal of Physiology*, 214:166-173.

Sheard, M. H., and Aghajanian, G. K. (1968): Stimulation of the midbrain raphe: effect on serotonin metabolism. *Journal of Pharmacology and Experimental Therapeutics*, 163:425-430.

Smith, S. E., Stacey, R. S., and Young, I. M. (1962): 5-Hydroxytryptamine and 5-hydroxytryptophan decarboxylase activity in the developing nervous system of rats and guinea-pigs. *Proceedings of the First International Pharmacological Meeting*, 8:101-105.

Tagliamonte, A., Tagliamonte, P., Gessa, G. L., and Brodie, B. B. (1969): Compulsive sexual activity induced by p-chlorophenylalanine in normal and pinealectomized male rats. *Science*, 166:1433-1435.

Taylor, P. M. (1960): Oxygen consumption in new-born rats. *Journal of Physiology*, 154:153-168.

Tirri, R. (1971): Central effects of 5-hydroxytryptamine and noradrenaline on body temperature and oxygen consumption in infant rats. *Experientia*, 27:274-276.

Tissari, A. (1966): 5-Hydroxytryptamine, 5-hydroxytryptophan decarboxylase and monoamine oxidase during foetal and postnatal development in the guinea-pig. *Acta Physiologica Scandinavica*, 67, Suppl. 265:1-80.

Tissari, A. H. (1971): Selectivity of amine transport in synaptosomes for substrates and drugs. *Scandinavian Journal of Clinical and Laboratory Investigation*, 27, Suppl. 116:78.

Tissari, A. H. (1972): Elimination of 5-hydroxyindoleacetic acid in postnatal rodent brain (*in press*).

Tissari, A. H., and Bogdanski, D. F. (1971): Effects of inorganic electrolytes on the membrane transport and metabolism of serotonin and norepinephrine by synaptosomes. *Progress in Brain Research*, 34:291-302.

Tissari, A. H., and Pekkarinen, E. M. (1966): 5-Hydroxyindoleacetic acid in the developing brain. *Acta Physiologica Scandinavica*, 68, Suppl. 277:201.

Tissari, A. H., and Raunu, E. M. (1970a): Factors regulating the brain 5HIAA level in developing mammals. *Scandinavian Journal of Clinical and Laboratory Investigation*, 25, Suppl. 113:19.

Tissari, A. H., and Raunu, E. M. (1970b): Formation and elimination of 5HIAA in developing brain. *Acta Pharmacologica et Toxicologica*, 28, Suppl. 1:86.

Tissari, A. H., and Raunu, E. M. (1972a): 5-Hydroxyindoleacetic acid in developing mammalian brain (*in press*).

Tissari, A. H., and Raunu, E. M. (1972b): Subcellular distribution of 5-hydroxytryptamine during development in rat brain: Effect of tranylcypromine and 5-hydroxytryptophan (*in press*).

Tissari, A. H., and Raunu, E. M. (1972c): Turnover of 5-hydroxytryptamine in developing rat brain (*in preparation*).

Tissari, A. H., Schönhöfer, P. S., Bogdanski, D. F., and Brodie, B. B. (1969): Mechanism of biogenic amine transport. II. Relationship between sodium and the mechanism of ouabain blockade of the accumulation of serotonin and norepinephrine by synaptosomes. *Molecular Pharmacology*, 5:593-604.

Tissari, A. H., and Suurhasko, B. V. A. (1971a): Sedation by probenecid treatment in rats. *Scandinavian Journal of Clinical and Laboratory Investigation*, 27, Suppl. 116:78.

Tissari, A. H., and Suurhasko, B. V. A. (1971b): Transport of 5HT in synaptosomes of developing rat brain. *Acta Pharmacologica et Toxicologica*, 29, Suppl. 4:59.

Tissari, A. H., and Suurhasko, B. V. A. (1972): Uptake of 5-hydroxytryptamine by synaptosomes during development. *Fifth International Congress of Pharmacology, Abstracts of Volunteer Papers*, p. 234.

Tozer, T. N., Neff, N. H., and Brodie, B. B. (1966): Application of steady state kinetics to the synthesis rate and turnover time of serotonin in the brain of normal and reserpine-treated rats. *Journal of Pharmacology and Experimental Therapeutics*, 153:177-182.

Tyce, G. M., Flock, E. V., and Owen, C. A., Jr., (1964): Tryptophan metabolism in the brain of the developing rat. *Progress in Brain Research,* 9:198-203.

Valatx, J. L., Jouvet, D., and Jouvet, M. (1964): Évolution électroencéphalographique des différents états de sommeil chez le chaton. *Electroencephalography and Clinical Neurophysiology,* 17:218-233.

Van Orden, L. S., III, Bensch, K. G., and Giarman, N. J. (1967): Histochemical and functional relationships of catecholamines in adrenergic nerve endings. II. Extravesicular norepinephrine. *Journal of Pharmacology and Experimental Therapeutics,* 155:428-439.

Vernadakis, A., and Kellogg, C. (1971): Development of neurotransmission mechanisms in chick embryos. *Proceedings of the International Union of Physiological Sciences,* 9:585.

Weil-Malherbe, H., Posner, H. S., and Bowles, G. R. (1961): Changes in the concentration and intracellular distribution of brain catecholamines: the effects of reserpine, β-phenylisopropylhydrazine, pyrogallol and 3,4-dihydroxyphenylalanine, alone and in combination. *Journal of Pharmacology and Experimental Therapeutics,* 132:278-286.

Weiss, B. L., and Aghajanian, G. K. (1971): Activation of brain serotonin metabolism by heat: Role of midbrain raphe neurons. *Brain Research,* 26:37-48.

Werdinius, B. (1966): Effect of probenecid on the level of homovanillic acid in the corpus striatum. *Journal of Pharmacy and Pharmacology,* 18:546-547.

Werdinius, B. (1967): Effect of probenecid on the levels of monoamine metabolites in the rat brain. *Acta Pharmacologica et Toxicologica,* 25:18-23.

Whittaker, V. P., and Dowe, G. H. (1965): The effect of homogenization conditions on sub-cellular distribution in brain. *Biochemical Pharmacology,* 14:194-196.

DISCUSSION

KELLOGG: Is the high concentration of 5-HIAA in the newborn rat primarily a function of low 5-HT storage and poor out-transport of 5-HIAA, or could it also represent a form of extraparenchymal decarboxylation of 5-HT?

TISSARI: I suppose that the high 5-HIAA concentration may be partly due to the lack of active 5-HIAA transport and partly to poor 5-HT storage, part of the 5-HT synthetized being shunted directly to MAO. I don't know if there is available extraneuronal 5-HTP for decarboxylase.

KELLOGG: Can the turnover of 5-HT measured in the newborn rat be decreased by 5-HT receptor stimulation?

TISSARI: At least it cannot be decreased by tricyclic antidepressants as in adult rats.

Fetal Pharmacology, edited by L. Boréus
Raven Press, New York © 1973

Effects of Atropine and Beta-Adrenergic Drugs on the Heart Rate of the Human Fetus

Pierre-Yves Schifferli* and Roberto Caldeyro-Barcia

Centro Latinoamericano de Perinatologia, y Desarrollo Humano, Hospital de Clinicas, Montevideo, Uruguay

The purpose of the present work is to explore the role played by the autonomic innervation in the control of fetal heart rate (FHR). These studies have been made at different stages of pregnancy and also during labor, both in normal conditions and in intrapartum fetal asphyxia.

The first section of this chapter presents the studies made with atropine and neostigmine. The second section shows the results obtained using drugs which stimulate or block the beta-adrenergic receptors.

EFFECTS OF ATROPINE ON FETAL HEART RATE

The effects of atropine on FHR were studied throughout pregnancy and also during labor, using different methods for administration of atropine and for recording its effects. Therefore both studies will be described separately.

---

* Present address: Clinique de Gynécologie et d'Obstétrique, Maternité, 1205 Geneve 4, Suisse

Studies made during pregnancy

Material and methods

Subjects studied. Thirty-six atropine tests were performed in 14 pregnant women at different gestational ages ranging from the 14th to the 40th week of pregnancy. In five patients, the atropine test was repeated five or six times during the same pregnancy at intervals of 1 or 2 weeks. All patients were delivered at term in our Service, and all fetuses were in good condition at birth. The follow-up of the infants showed no abnormalities in their development.

Dose of atropine. Two mg of atropine sulfate dissolved in 10 ml saline was slowly injected i.v. to the mother in a 2- to 4-min period. The dose of 2 mg was selected for the test because of the following reasons:

(1) From previous work (Hellman, Johnson, Tolles, and Jones, 1961; Hellman, Morton, Wallach, Tolles, and Fillisti, 1963) it is known that a dose of 1 mg atropine sulfate given i.v. to the mother failed to produce vagal blockade in 2 out of 13 fetuses.

(2) The dose of 2 mg has been employed in human subjects by several groups of investigators (Elisberg, Miller, Weinberg, and Katz, 1953; Cullumbine, McKee, and Creasy, 1955; Berry, Thompson, and Miller, 1959). The effects observed were tachycardia, palpitation, dryness of mouth, thirst, dilated pupils, and some blurring of near vision.

(3) A larger dose (5 mg) is needed to produce restlessness, fatigue, and disturbances in swallowing and in micturition (Innes and Nickerson, 1965).

Methods for recording fetal and maternal heart rates. FHR was graphically recorded by a beat-to-beat cardiotachometer which is triggered by an ultrasound emit-receive system, applied on the abdominal wall of the mother and directed to the fetal heart. This system was activated by each heart beat by means of the Doppler effect (Pose, Castillo, Mora-Rojas, Soto-Yances, and Caldeyro-Barcia, 1969). The FHR tracings obtained with this method (Fig. 1) had more artifacts and were less neat than when the tachometer is triggered with the fetal EKG (see Figs. 8–13).

Maternal heart rate (MHR) was recorded with a beat-to-beat cardiotachometer triggered by the R wave of the maternal ECG. MHR and FHR tracings appear in two different channels of the same recorder (Fig. 1).

In each atropine test, the recording of FHR and MHR was started at least 30 min before the injection of the drug and lasted for 2 or 3 hrs.

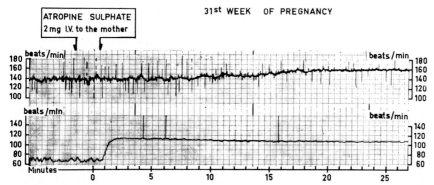

FIG. 1. Effects of atropine on maternal and fetal heart rate. Record obtained at the 31st week of pregnancy.

Effects of atropine on the mother

Atropine caused a marked and rapid rise in MHR of 30 to 50 beats/min amplitude and reduced the irregularities in the MHR record (Fig. 1). Maternal tachycardia was long-lasting; 30 min after the end of the injection, it was still present at 80% of its maximum value. The effect of atropine on MHR does not bear any significant relation to the gestational age. No consistent or significant changes occurred in maternal arterial pressure which was periodically measured during the test.

As mentioned before, palpitation, dryness of mouth, thirst, and some blurring of near vision were reported by the patients. The spontaneous disappearance of these effects is slow. A rapid correction of the effects of atropine on the mother was obtained with the i.v. injection of 0.5 mg neostigmine (Prostigmine®, Roche) as described later in this chapter (see Fig. 6).

Effects of atropine on FHR

In 33 of the 36 cases studied, atropine produced a significant rise in FHR. This was much smaller and slower than that produced in the heart rate of the mother (Fig. 1). Atropine also reduced irregularities in the FHR recording.

The full development of the effect of atropine on FHR takes 15 to 20 min after the end of the injection. The duration of this lag time does not bear any significant correlation with the gestational age, a finding which agrees with previous reports (Hellman et al., 1963).

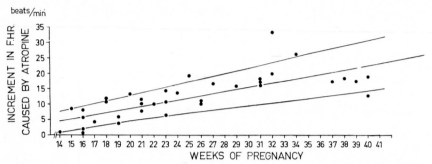

FIG. 2. The rise in FHR caused by atropine increases with gestational age. Each point corresponds to one atropine test. The best fitted line and 95% limits for regression coefficient are shown. The regression equation is $[Y = (-4.9 + 0.7\ (x)]$ (from Schifferli, 1968).

The increment in FHR produced by atropine is measured as the difference between the mean values of FHR before and after the injection of the drug. To calculate each mean value of FHR, 20 to 40 consecutive readings were made in the FHR tracing (one reading every 30 sec). For the determination of the post-atropine mean value, the 15-min interval following the injection was not considered since the effect of atropine develops during this interval.

Figure 2 shows the results obtained in the 36 tests. The best-fitted line shows that the post-atropine increment of FHR augments with gestational age. The regression coefficient ($b = 0.7$) indicates that the effect of atropine increases approximately 0.7 beats/min every week. This regression coefficient is significantly different from zero ($p < 0.001$). According to the regression equation $[Y = (-4.9) + 0.7\ (x)]$, the amplitude of the post-atropine rise in FHR is 5 beats/min at 15 weeks and 19 beats/min at 35 weeks (Schifferli, 1968).

The correlation coefficient between the effect of atropine and the gestational age is ($r = 0.74$); this correlation is significant ($p < 0.001$). The determination coefficient ($r^2 = 0.55$) indicates that 55% of the changes in the post-atropine increment in FHR are due to variations in gestational age.

The correlation reported in this paper between the gestational age and the atropine effect on FHR was not noticed by Hellman et al., (1963), probably because gestational age in most of their patients was greater than 25 weeks.

Figure 3 shows the mean value of the post-atropine FHR in each of the 36 tests plotted against the corresponding gestational age. The average

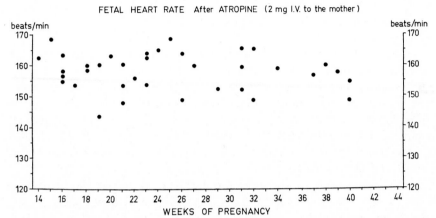

FIG. 3. Post-atropine FHR is not influenced by gestational age. Mean values of FHR in the post-atropine period for each of the 36 atropine tests.

post-atropine FHR is close to 160 beats/min, and there is no clear trend to fall or increase as gestation progresses.

Fall of normal FHR throughout pregnancy

Figure 4 shows 76 values of FHR of nonmedicated fetuses plotted against the corresponding gestational age. Each value plotted is the mean

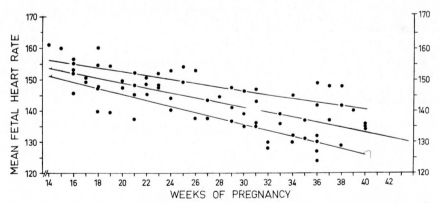

FIG. 4. FHR (in the nonmedicated fetus) falls throughout pregnancy. Each point indicates the mean value of FHR of a given fetus measured before any drug was given to the mother. The best fitted line and the 95% confidence interval for the regression coefficient are shown. The regression equation is $[Y = 164.7 - 0.8(x)]$ (from Schifferli, 1968).

of 20 or more readings made in the record of FHR. Thirty-six of the 73 values correspond to the pre-atropine period of the atropine tests, reported in this paper.

The results in Fig. 4 indicate that FHR diminishes as gestational age increases. According to the regression coefficient there is a fall of 0.8 beats/min for every week of increment in gestational age. The regression coefficient is significantly different from zero ($p < 0.001$). The correlation coefficient between FHR and gestational age is ($r = -0.7$) and is statistically significant ($p < 0.001$) (Schifferli, 1968). A similar fall in FHR throughout pregnancy has been found by Ibarra-Polo, Guiloff, and Gómez-Rogers (1972) and also by Kubli (1971).

The fall in FHR as gestation advances may be largely due to increase in the cardiomoderator tone of the vagus. The rationale for such a statement is discussed below.

Increase in vagal tone with fetal maturation

The findings reported in Figs. 2–4 are diagrammatically summarized in Fig. 5. For each gestational age, the difference in FHR between the non-

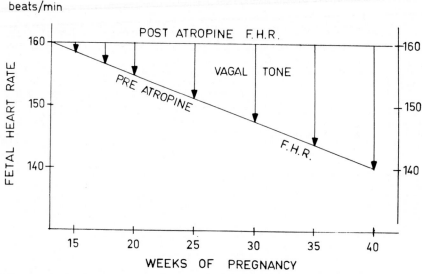

FIG. 5. Increase in vagal tone with fetal maturation. Diagrammatic interpretation of the results. Post-atropine FHR shows no changes with gestational age (see Fig. 3). Pre-atropine FHR (i.e., the heart rate of a nonmedicated fetus) falls as gestational age increases (Fig. 4). The difference between pre- and post-atropine FHR is attributed to the cardiomoderator influence of the vagal tone.

medicated and the atropinized fetuses is attributed to the presence of a cardiomoderator vagal tone. Assuming that atropine blocks the vagal effect on FHR, the amplitude of the post-atropine rise in FHR is taken as a measure of the preexisting vagal tone. According to the results reported in the preceding paragraphs, in the human fetus the cardiomoderator vagal tone, although small, is already detectable at 15 weeks of pregnancy and increases significantly as gestation advances.

Antagonization of atropine effects with neostigmine

Neostigmine was injected to the mother 40 min after the administration of 2 mg of atropine, in 19 of the 36 atropine tests described above.

Neostigmine was administered to the mother by slow (3 to 6 min) i.v. injection in doses of 0.5 to 1.0 mg.

Effects of neostigmine on the atropinized mother. In all 19 tests, neostigmine rapidly antagonized the effects of atropine on the mother and

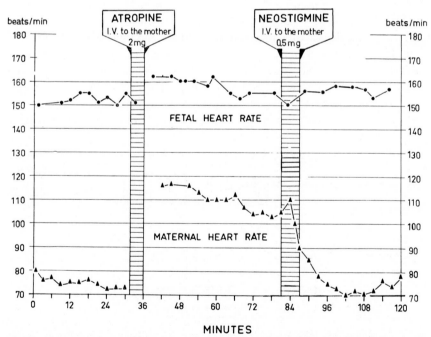

MINUTES

FIG. 6. Neostigmine antagonizes atropine effect on MHR. Plotting based on values of FHR and MHR read periodically on one analog record similar to that shown in Fig. 1. Recording was made at the 16th week of pregnancy (from P. Y. Schifferli, *unpublished data*).

caused a fall of MHR to the pre-atropine level in 12 to 16 min after the end of the neostigmine injection (Fig. 6).

Neostigmine also corrected other maternal effects of atropine such as dryness of the mouth, thirst, blurring of near vision, and dilated pupils.

Effects of neostigmine on the atropinized fetus. Neostigmine had no clear effect on FHR, which could be explained by the slow transfer of this drug across the placental barrier, in keeping with its quaternary ammonium nature.

This interpretation is supported by a preliminary study during which neostigmine was injected directly into the peritoneum of an anencephalic human fetus at term, to avoid the placental barrier. A dose of 200 μg of neostigmine could antagonize the rise in FHR caused by 150 μg of atropine which had been injected by the same route 25 min earlier.

Studies made during labor

Variables recorded during labor

FHR is recorded during labor with a beat-to-beat cardiotachometer triggered by the R wave of the fetal EKG. This is obtained by means of an electrode inserted subcutaneously under the fetal scalp (after rupture of membranes) or in the fetal buttock (Méndez-Bauer, Poseiro, Arellano-Hernández, Zambrana, and Caldeyro-Barcia, 1963). MHR was recorded by the method described for the pregnancy tests. Amniotic (intrauterine) pressure was recorded with a catheter introduced into the amniotic cavity

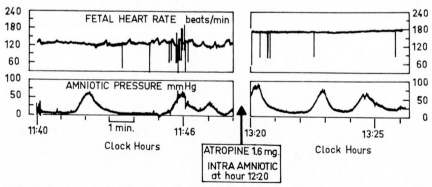

FIG. 7. Intra-amniotic injection of 1.6 mg of atropine sulfate in a parturient woman. One hour after the injection, the FHR tracing indicates that the fetus is atropinized (from Méndez-Bauer et al., 1970).

through the cervix (when membranes were ruptured) or by transabdominal amniocentesis. In some cases maternal arterial pressure was recorded through a catheter introduced in one femoral artery. Amniotic and arterial catheters were connected to pressure transducers.

Routes for atropine administration

Two routes have been employed during labor for the administration of atropine to the fetus avoiding the maternal compartment: intra-amniotic and directly to the fetus.

Intra-amniotic injection of atropine. In 12 women during labor, Méndez-Bauer, Poseiro, Escarcena, Hill, Smeeby, and Freeman (1970) injected 1.6 mg of atropine sulfate into the amniotic cavity via the catheter which was being used for recording amniotic pressure. This catheter had been introduced through the uterine cervix after rupture of the ovular membranes. After a lag time which ranged from 14 to 55 min, the FHR tracing showed the typical signs of atropinization, namely a rise of base-line FHR of approximately 20 beats/min and concomitant disappearance of the irregularities in the FHR tracing (Fig. 7). These effects lasted for several hours. The mother showed no sign of atropinization (tachycardia, dry mouth, blurring of near vision).

Intramuscular injection in the fetal buttock. Atropine has been admin-

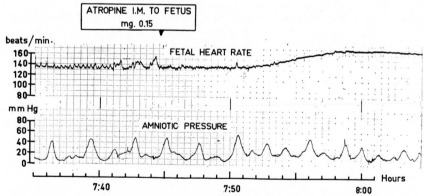

FIG. 8. Effect of intrafetal injection of atropine on FHR in a normal fetus during labor. Injection of atropine sulfate into the muscles of the fetal buttock. Term pregnancy, in the early stage of spontaneous labor. Intact membranes, cervical dilation 4 cm, fetal head in —3 station. Before atropine the tracing of FHR shows that the fetal condition was good. A healthy and vigorous newborn was delivered 6 hr later (Apgar score 10 at 1 min) (from Méndez-Bauer et al., 1963).

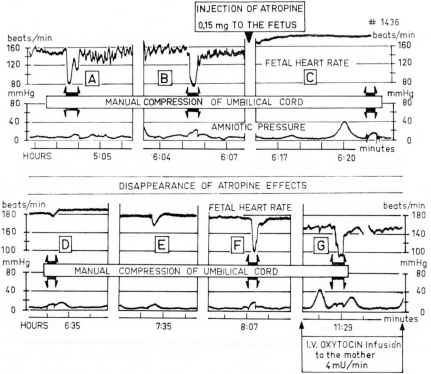

FIG. 9. Effects of atropine on FHR response to manual compression of umbilical cord. Atropine was injected in the fetal buttock. Record obtained at 37 weeks of pregnancy in an Rh negative mother before starting the induction of labor with oxytocin. Spontaneous uterine contractions were weak. Induction of labor with oxytocin infusion started at hour 9:10, and natural delivery occurred at hour 16:25. The cord was tightly wound around the fetal neck, which confirms the diagnosis based on the response of FHR to compression in the area of the fetal neck.

istered directly to the human fetus during labor (Méndez-Bauer et al., 1963). When the fetus has its back against the anterior wall of the uterus and the placenta is not inserted in that wall, it is possible to recognize the fetal buttock by palpation. Using a 6-cm long, 20-gauge needle, the injection can be made into the muscles of the fetal buttock. The place where the fetus was punctured was carefully checked after delivery.

The dose of atropine used was 0.15 (i.e., 0.05 mg/kg for a 3-kg fetus). This dose completely blocked the cardiac effect of the fetal vagus and had no detectable effect on the mother.

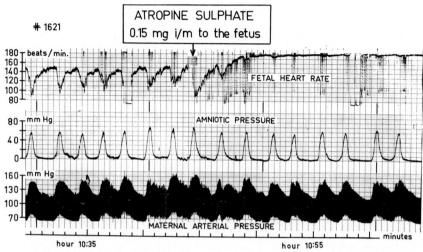

FIG. 10. Effects of atropine on FHR in a fetus with type I dips. Atropine was injected in the fetal buttock. Record obtained during induced labor after the membranes were ruptured, cervical dilatation 7 cm. At birth, a loop of cord was found around the fetal neck. The newborn was depressed (Apgar score: 3 at 1 min) (from Caldeyro-Barcia et al., 1966).

When given directly to the fetus, the effects of atropine on FHR appeared after a lag time of 3 to 7 min. Maximum effects were developed in 10 to 20 min after the injection. Then the effects disappeared slowly in 1 to 3 hr. In all the studies described in the following paragraphs, atropine was injected in the fetal buttock.

Effects of atropine on normal FHR

Figure 8 illustrates a typical example of the effects of atropine injection. Seven minutes after the intrafetal injection of atropine, FHR started to rise and reached a plateau 7 min later (Fig. 8), where it remained for 25 min. Then FHR fell slowly, returning to the original base-line level in 2 hr. The amplitude of the FHR rise was 30 beats/min. Atropine also caused a marked reduction in the irregularities of FHR tracing. These effects are interpreted as an indication that under normal conditions during labor, the fetal vagus exerts a tonic moderator effect on FHR, and that small rapid changes in vagal tone are responsible for the irregularities in the FHR tracing (Méndez-Bauer et al., 1963).

Effect of atropine on FHR response to cord compression

When a loop of the umbilical cord is around the fetal neck, it is possible to compress the cord by exerting pressure on the abdominal wall with the fingers of both hands, between the fetal head and shoulders (Hon, Bradfield, and Hess, 1961). Each manual compression of the cord causes an abrupt fall in FHR (Fig. 9*A, B*). This maneuver is employed for the diagnosis of a nuchal cord. Nine minutes after the injection of 0.15 mg of atropine sulfate to the fetus, manual compression of the umbilical cord no longer had any efect on FHR (Fig. 9*C*). This result indicates that compression of the cord increased vagal fetal tone which was the only factor responsible for the FHR fall. As the effects of atropine faded away (Fig. 9*D, E, F*), the response of FHR to cord compression reappeared progressively. Three hours later, the effect of atropine on FHR had disappeared completely (Fig. 9*G*).

Effect of atropine on type I dips (*early dips*)

A dip is a transient fall in FHR caused by one uterine contraction. In type I dips, the fall of FHR occurs early, during the ascending phase of the

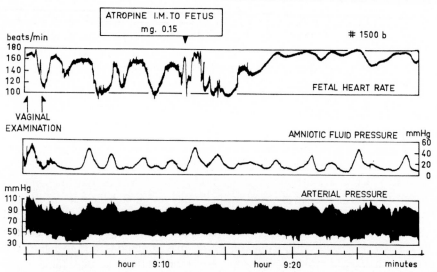

FIG. 11. Effect of atropine on FHR in a fetus with type II dips. Atropine was injected in the fetal buttock. Record obtained at the beginning of the induction of labor with infusion of oxytocin. Cervical dilatation 3 cm, head in station −4. The fetus was delivered 10 hr later. The newborn was depressed (Apgar score 3) (from Méndez-Bauer et al., 1963).

uterine contraction (early dip). The bottom of the dip is recorded at the same time as the peak of the contraction (Fig. 10).

Uterine contractions may produce type I dips by compressing the umbilical cord or the fetal head or both (Caldeyro-Barcia, Méndez-Bauer, Poseiro, Escarcena, Pose, Bieniarz, Arnt, Gulin, and Althabe, 1966). The artificial rupture of membranes greatly facilitates the production of type I dips (Althabe, Aramburú, Schwarcz, and Caldeyro-Barcia, 1969).

Figure 10 shows a record with type I dips, in a case with a loop of cord around the fetal neck. Membranes were ruptured and cervical dilatation was 7 cm. The fetal head was in station 0. Eight min after the injection of atropine to the fetus, type I dips disappeared completely from the FHR tracing showing that the increased vagal tone was the only mechanism involved in their production.

Effect of atropine on type II dips (late dips)

In type II dips the fall in FHR occurs late in the contraction. The descending limb of the dip is simultaneous with the phase of uterine decontraction (Fig. 11). The bottom of the dip is recorded 40 to 60 sec after the peak of the contraction (Caldeyro-Barcia et al., 1966). Uterine contractions produce type II dips when the fetus is suffering from intrapartum asphyxia because of insufficient flow of maternal blood through the placenta. Each uterine contraction further aggravates placental ischemia and fetal asphyxia (Caldeyro-Barcia, Ibarra-Polo, Gulin, Poseiro, and Méndez-Bauer, 1969).

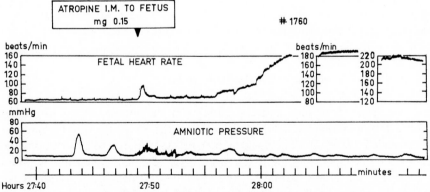

FIG. 12. Effect of atropine on the FHR of a fetus (anencephalic) suffering prolonged bradycardia. The severe asphyxia present in this anencephalus was produced by uterine hypercontractility induced with oxytocin which lasted several hours. Atropine was injected in the fetal buttock. The fetus died *in utero* at hour 29:00.

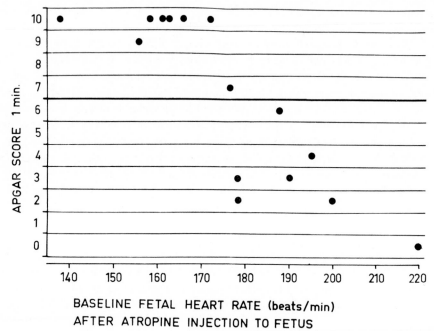

FIG. 13. Correlation between the value of post-atropine FHR and the Apgar score 1 min after delivery, in 15 fetuses who had received atropine during labor.

The administration of atropine to the fetus greatly reduces the amplitude of "late dips" but does not suppress them completely. This effect of atropine indicates that although a transient increase in vagal tone plays a major role in the genesis of each "late dip," there are other nonvagal factors involved which also contribute to the fall in FHR (Méndez-Bauer et al., 1963).

Effect of atropine on long-lasting bradycardia

In very severe fetal distress, usually in the terminal stage preceding fetal death, a continuous fetal bradycardia at the level of 60 beats/min may be recorded (Fig. 12). The vagal nature of such bradycardia is demonstrated by the effects of atropine. After a lag time of 7 min following the injection of atropine, FHR started to rise, reaching 220 beats/min 14 min later. After remaining at this very high level for 10 min, FHR fell slowly, and, 50

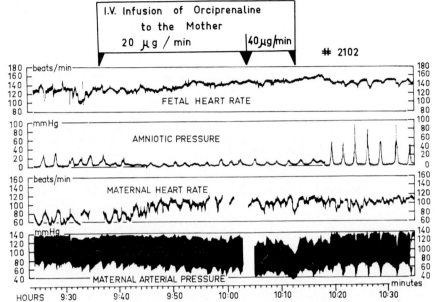

FIG. 14. Effect of orciprenaline (stimulant of beta adrenoceptors) on FHR during labor. In addition to causing a slow rise of FHR, orciprenaline produced inhibition of uterine contractions, maternal tachycardia, and a fall in arterial pressure.

min after atropine injection, was again down at 60 beats/min (the fetus died *in utero* within the next 20 min).

Diagnostic meaning of post-atropine FHR

When the fetuses were in good condition after the injection of atropine, FHR increased to 150 to 170 beats/min (Fig. 8). At birth the corresponding newborns had a normal Apgar score.

In fetuses which suffered from a more severe asphyxia, post-atropine FHR climbed to higher levels, 175 to 200 beats/min (Figs. 10 and 11). The corresponding newborns were depressed, their Apgar score being lower than 6 (Fig. 13). In the fetus which was in the worst condition of this series (Fig. 12), post-atropine FHR reached the highest value recorded (220 beats/min). These results, summarized in Fig. 13, suggest that the level of post-atropine FHR may be of diagnostic and prognostic value in cases of suspected intrapartum fetal distress.

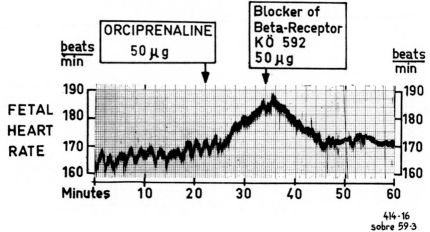

FIG. 15. Orciprenaline injection in the peritoneum of an anencephalic fetus caused an immediate rise in FHR. The effect was antagonized by the injection of a beta blocker, 1,3-methylphenoxy-3-isopropylaminopropanol-2-hydrochloride (Kö 592, Boehringer Ingelheim).

DRUGS ACTING ON BETA-ADRENERGIC RECEPTORS

Beta-adrenergic stimulation

Orciprenaline (Alupent®, Boehringer, Ingelheim), a stimulant of beta adrenoceptors, has a strong inhibitory effect on the contractions of the pregnant human uterus (Fig. 14) and is therefore employed in obstetrics. Two indications for its use are the treatment of threatened premature labor (Delard, Magaña, Belitzky, and Caldeyro-Barcia, 1969) and of acute intrapartum fetal asphyxia (Caldeyro-Barcia, Magaña, Castillo, Poseiro, Méndez-Bauer, Pose, Escarcena, Casacuberta, Bustos, and Giussi, 1969). Orciprenaline is administered by continuous i.v. infusion in doses of 20 to 40 μg/min. It produces a rapid rise in maternal heart rate (Fig. 14), of 20 to 40 beats/min above the preceding rate. It also causes a fall in maternal arterial pressure, more marked for the diastolic than for the systolic level. If ocriprenaline administration lasts more than 30 min, FHR shows a slow and steady rise (Fig. 14) which continues at a rate of 10 to 15 beats/min every hour until it reaches 160 to 175 beats/min. Fetal tachycardia is probably caused by the direct action of orciprenaline on the fetal heart, and it is not a sign of fetal asphyxia, as is seen by measuring the O_2, CO_2, and pH in fetal blood.

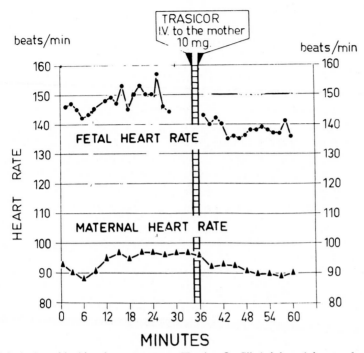

FIG. 16. A drug blocking beta receptors (Trasicor®, Ciba) injected i.v. to the mother caused small falls in maternal and fetal heart rate. Plotting built from data measured in an analog record of MHR and FHR obtained at 29 weeks of pregnancy (from P. Y. Schifferli, *unpublished data*).

The rise in FHR caused by orciprenaline lasts for 2 or 3 hr after the infusion of the drug has been discontinued. If the fetus is delivered within this period, the newborn will also be tachycardic.

Figure 15 shows the immediate rise in FHR produced by the injection of 50 µg of orciprenaline into the peritoneum of a human anencephalic fetus. The effect of orciprenaline was antagonized by subsequently injecting the fetus with a drug blocking the beta receptors, 1,3-methylphenoxy-3-isopropylaminopropanol-2-hydrochloride (Kö 592, Boehringer, Ingelheim).

Blockade of beta-adrenergic receptors

The beta-adrenergic receptor blocker employed, Trasicor® [1-(O-allyloxyphenoxy)-3-isopropylamino-2-propanol hydrochloride] (Ciba), is a derivative of isopropyl-aminopropane. The dose of 10 mg was injected i.v. to eight women in the fourth quarter of pregnancy. In all mothers the beta blocker caused a small fall in MHR (amplitude: 5 to 10 beats/min). Only in four of the eight fetuses did the beta blocker cause a significant fall in FHR (Fig. 16). The amplitude of the FHR fall ranged from 5 to 10 beats/min, and it occurred within the first 5 min following the injection. No relation was found between the gestational age and effect of the beta blocker on FHR.

In the four remaining fetuses, the beta blocker had no significant effect on FHR. Two of these patients were tested several times with a consistent absence of effect on FHR. These preliminary results suggest that, in the human fetus during the last quarter of pregnancy, the effects on FHR of the beta blocker employed in this study are smaller and less consistent than those of atropine.

SUMMARY

The i.v. injection of 2 mg of atropine to pregnant women caused a slow, small rise in fetal heart rate (FHR). The amplitude of the rise increased with gestational age as of the 15th week. During labor, atropine was injected in the amniotic cavity (1.6 mg) or directly into the fetal buttock (0.15 mg). When the fetus was in a normal condition, atropine caused a rise in the base line of FHR (20 to 30 beats/min) and a reduction of the irregularities in FHR tracing. Atropine canceled type I (early) dips which are transient falls of FHR due to compression of the fetal head or umbilical cord by uterine contractions. Atropine reduced the amplitude of type II dips (late dip) which are transient falls of FHR caused by uterine contractions in cases of intrapartum fetal asphyxia. Atropine suppressed the prolonged bradycardia present in very severe intrapartum fetal distress.

Drugs stimulating beta-adrenoceptors caused a rise in FHR. This effect is antagonized by beta-blocking drugs.

ACKNOWLEDGMENT

The authors acknowledge the advice received from Dr. Roberto Yabo, Consultant in Statistics of the Pan American Health Organization/World Health Organization, for the statistical analysis of the data.

REFERENCES

Althabe, O., Aramburú, G., Schwarcz, R. L., and Caldeyro-Barcia, R. (1969): Influence of the rupture of membranes on compression of the fetal head during labor. In: *Perinatal Factors Affecting Human Development*, edited by PAHO Advisory Committee on Medical Research. Pan American Health Organization, Washington, D.C., pp. 143-149.

Berry, J. N., Thompson, H. K., Jr., and Miller, D. E. (1959): Changes in cardiac output, stroke volume and central venous pressure induced by atropine in man. *American Heart Journal*, 58:204-213.

Caldeyro-Barcia, R., Ibarra-Polo, A. A., Gulin, L., Poseiro, J. J., and Méndez-Bauer, C. (1969): Diagnostic and prognostic significance of intrapartum fetal tachycardia and type II dips. In: *Prenatal Life*, edited by H. C. Mack. Wayne State University Press, Detroit, Michigan, pp. 129-153.

Caldeyro-Barcia, R., Magaña, J. M., Castillo, J. B., Poseiro, J. J., Méndez-Bauer, C., Pose, S. V., Escarcena, L., Casacuberta, C., Bustos, J. R., and Giussi, G. (1969): A new approach to the treatment of acute intrapartum fetal distress. In: *Perinatal Factors Affecting Human Development*, edited by PAHO Advisory Committee on Medical Research. Pan American Health Organization, Washington, D.C., pp. 248-253.

Caldeyro-Barcia, R., Méndez-Bauer, C., Poseiro, J. J., Escarcena, L. A., Pose, S. V., Bie-iarz, J., Arnt, I. C., Gulin, L., and Althabe, O., Jr. (1966): Control of human fetal heart rate during labor. In: *The Heart and Circulation in the Newborn and Infant*, edited by D. E. Cassels. Grune & Stratton, New York, pp. 7-36.

Cullumbine, H., McKee, W. H. E., and Creasy, N. H. (1955): The effects of atropine sulphate upon healthy male subjects. *Quarterly Journal Experimental Physiology*, 40:309-319.

Delard, G., Magaña, J. M., Belitzky, R., and Caldeyro-Barcia, R. (1969): Profilaxis y tratamiento de la amenaza de parto prematuro. Informe preliminar sobre dos casos. *Archivos de Ginecologia y Obstetricia* (Uruguay), 24:25-31.

Elisberg, E. I., Miller, G., Weinberg, S. L., and Katz, L. N. (1953): The effect of the Valsalva maneuver on the circulation. II. The role of the autonomic nervous system in the production of the overshoot. *American Heart Journal*, 45:227-236.

Hellman, L. M., Johnson, H. L., Tolles, W. E., and Jones, E. H. (1961): Some factors affecting the fetal heart rate. *American Journal of Obstetrics and Gynecology*, 82:1055-1063.

Hellman, L. M., Morton, G. W., Wallach, E. E., Tolles, W. E., and Fillisti, L. P. (1963): An analysis of the atropine test for placental transfer in 28 normal gravidas. *American Journal of Obstetrics and Gynecology*, 87:650-659.

Hon, E. H., Bradfield, A. H., and Hess, O. W. (1961): The electronic evaluation of the fetal heart rate. V. The vagal factor in fetal bradycardia. *American Journal of Obstetrics and Gynecology*, 82:291-300.

Ibarra-Polo, A. A., Guiloff, E., and Gómez-Rogers, C. (1972): Fetal heart rate patterns throughout pregnancy. *American Journal of Obstetrics and Gynecology* (*in press*)

Innes, I. R., and Nickerson, M. (1965): Drugs inhibiting the action of acetylcholine on structures innervated by postganglionic parasympathetic nerves (antimuscarinic or atropinic drugs). In: *The Pharmacological Basis of Therapeutics*, edited by L. S. Goodman and A. Gilman, third edition. Macmillan, New York, pp. 521-545.

Kubli, F. (1971): The heart rate of the human fetus. Presented at the International Conference on the Monitoring of the Fetal Heart, Newark, N.J. To be published in *International Journal of Gynaecology and Obstetrics*, 1972.

Méndez-Bauer, C., Poseiro, J. J., Arellano-Hernández, G., Zambrana, M. A., and

Caldeyro-Barcia, R. (1963): Effects of atropine on the heart rate of the human fetus during labor. *American Journal of Obstetrics and Gynecology,* 85:1033-1053.

Méndez-Bauer, C., Poseiro, J. J., Escarcena, L. A., Hill, D. L., Smeeby, L. A., and Freeman, D. W. (1970): Absorción fetal de sustancias inyectadas en el líquido amniótico. Posibles usos terapéuticos. In: *Fourth Meeting of the Latin American Association for Research in Human Reproduction,* Ixtapan de la Sal, México, April 5-9.

Pose, S. V., Castillo, J. B., Mora-Rojas, E. O., Soto-Yances, A., and Caldeyro-Barcia, R. (1969): Test of fetal tolerance to induced uterine contractions for the diagnosis of chronic distress. In: *Perinatal Factors Affecting Human Development,* edited by PAHO Advisory Committee on Medical Research. Pan American Health Organization, Washington, D.C., pp. 96-104.

Schifferli, P. Y. (1968): La frecuencia cardíaca fetal a lo largo del embarazo. Estudio de la influencia del sistema nervioso autónomo sobre el cronotropismo cardíaco fetal. *Archivos de Ginecología y Obstetricia* (Uruguay), 23:87-97.

DISCUSSION

HOLMSTEDT: Dr. Caldeyro-Barcia, what was your rationale for giving 2 mg of atropine i.v. to pregnant women? In Sweden such a dose would only be given to severe cases of intoxications with cholinesterase inhibitors.

CALDEYRO-BARCIA: The dose of 2 mg was selected because it was considered as the minimum required for blocking the vagal effects on fetal heart rate. Similar doses had been used in New York to evaluate placental transfer of atropine in pregnant women and the only untoward effects reported were tachycardia, dry mouth, and disturbances in visual accommodation.

The pregnant women who received atropine injections were previously informed about the side effects. Furthermore, several of these women returned voluntarily for repetition of the atropine test after having experienced the discomfort of the side effects.

KARCZMAR: Don't you get marked CNS (EEG) effects with 2 mg i.v. of atropine? Short-time amnesia? Hallucinations?

CALDEYRO-BARCIA: Short-time amnesia or hallucinations were not detected. EEG was not recorded in the mothers receiving atropine.

FUCHS: It should be mentioned that studies of this kind cannot be carried out in monkeys because it is almost impossible to observe and monitor spontaneous labor in monkeys.

DAWES: The normal dose required for full parasympathetic blockade in many animal species is 1 mg per kg body weight given intravenously, and this has the usual atropinic effect (dry mouth etc.) but is safe. This dose is some 30 times greater than that used by Caldeyro-Barcia.

INGELMAN-SUNDBERG: I have personally seen some of these experiments when 2 mg of atropine was given intravenously to the mother and I can assure that no other side effects than those described appeared.

I wonder if not the most common cause of deceleration of the fetal heart rate synchronous to the uterine contractions is increased intracranial pressure when the head is forced against the cervix after rupture of the membranes instead of compression of the umbilical cord.

Fetal Pharmacology, edited by L. Boréus
Raven Press, New York © 1973

Perinatal Risks of Paracervical Block

Kari Teramo

Department of Obstetrics, University of Helsinki, Helsinki 29, Finland

Paracervical block (PCB) is one of the most common obstetrical blockades mainly because it is technically easy to perform. A large number of reports emphasize that PCB is harmless for the mother, the fetus, and the newborn infant, although fetal bradycardia is a frequently observed side effect after PCB. Fetal bradycardia has been reported after PCB at least with procaine, lidocaine, mepivacaine, and bupivacaine. The incidence of fetal bradycardia after PCB varies from none to over 50% of the cases. In our studies in Helsinki, we have found a relationship between the incidence of fetal bradycardia and the dose of mepivacaine used for PCB (Table 1). This suggests that the local anesthetic agent is responsible for the fetal bradycardia after PCB. However, in the PCB groups with 50 and 100 mg of bupivacaine with epinephrine, the incidence of the fetal bradycardia was almost the same (Table 1).

We also found that when the fetal heart rate decreased below 120 beats per minute or when a late-deceleration heart-rate pattern occurred after PCB, the fetal pH decreased. Both the fetal bradycardia and the pH decrease were transient in the majority of the cases. The magnitude of the fetal heart-rate deceleration correlated with the degree of fetal pH decrease after PCB irrespective of the dose of bupivacaine used (Teramo, 1969). This suggests that the fetal bradycardia after PCB is at least partially a sign of fetal asphyxia,

TABLE 1. *Incidence of fetal bradycardia below 120 beats per minute or heart-rate pattern of late-deceleration type after paracervical block with mepivacaine and bupivacaine*

Local anesthetic	Amount (mg)	Total number of cases	Number of cases with fetal bradycardia	%
Mepivacaine	200	20	3	15
	400	16	12	75
Bupivacaine	50	14	8	57
Bupivacaine with epinephrine	50	12	6	50
	100	12	7	58

Several causes have been proposed as etiological factors for the fetal bradycardia or pH decrease after PCB (Table 2). Intravenous injection of mepivacaine (100 to 200 mg) to the mother during labor produced in two out of seven cases a heart-rate pattern similar to that after PCB (Teramo, *in press*). We also observed (K. Teramo, M. A. Heymann, A. M. Rudolph, N. Räihä, and C. Barrett, 1969, *unpublished*) fetal bradycardia and an immediate decrease in cartotid arterial pressure in a fetus at midgestation after intravenous injection of mepivacaine directly into the fetus. These observations support the hypothesis that it is the local anesthetic agent that causes the fetal bradycardia. Most probably the local anesthetic agent has a direct

TABLE 2. *Factors proposed to cause fetal bradycardia and/or pH decrease after obstetrical paracervical block*

1. Epinephrine in the anesthetic solution (Kobak and Sadove, 1961)
2. Supine hypotensive syndrome (Page, Kamm, and Chappel, 1961)
3. Over-strong uterine contractions and/or uterine hypertonicity (McGowan, 1962; Vasicka, Scheffs, Robertazzi, and Raji, 1970)
4. Paracervical manipulation (Davis, Frudenfeld, Frudenfeld, Frudenfeld, and Webb, 1964)
5. Vasovagal reflex in the fetus (Davis et al., 1964)
6. Amniotomy immediately before the block (Davis et al., 1964)
7. Direct depressant effect of the local anesthetic on the fetal myocardium or central nervous system or both (Nyirjesy, Hawks, Hebert, Hopwood, and Falls, 1963; Teramo and Widholm, 1967)
8. Compression of uterine vessels in the paracervical space (Stockhausen, 1967)
9. Altered carbohydrate metabolism in the fetus (Frangipani, Samaja, Tinti, Spandrio, and Tampalani, 1969)
10. Interference of the umbilical and placental circulations (Teramo and Widholm, 1967; Jung, Kopecky, and Klöck, 1969)
11. Inhibition of the fetal "oxygen conserving adaptation" (Obolensky, Kupferschmied, and Vullièmoz, 1969)

depressant effect on the fetal myocardium or the central nervous system or both.

Asling, Shnider, Margolis, Wilkinson, and Way (1970) reported higher fetal than maternal concentrations of mepivacaine in six out of seven fetal bradycardia cases after PCB. They concluded that the fetal bradycardia after PCB is caused by high fetal levels of the local anesthetic agent, which is a result of a direct absorption of the local anesthetic from the paracervical space to the placenta and the fetus. There is some experimental evidence in sheep that mepivacaine can diffuse rapidly through the wall of a major artery (Steffenson, Shnider, and deLorimier, 1970). On the other hand, our PCB studies showed that fetal bradycardia and acidosis occur also in cases in which the fetal concentration of the local anesthetic agent parallels or is clearly lower than the corresponding maternal concentration (Teramo and Rajamäki, 1971). The mothers did not show any signs of toxicity from the local anesthetic in these studies. It is possible that the fetal heart becomes depressed at a lower plasma level of a local anesthetic than the adult heart. However, further studies are needed to elucidate this.

In most fetuses the bradycardia and pH decrease after PCB is transient, and the majority of these fetuses are vigorous at birth. In 80 PCB cases with mepivacaine (200 to 400 mg) and bupivacaine (50 to 100 mg) there were 13 fetuses in which the pH decreased below 7.20 during 60 min following PCB (Teramo, in press). All of the fetuses had a pH of 7.25 or more before the application of the block. The consequences of fetal bradycardia below 100 beats per minute for up to 8 min and of fetal pH de-

TABLE 3. *References on perinatal deaths in which paracervical block is suspected to be the etiological factor*

Local anesthetic	Number of perinatal deaths	References
Bupivacaine	29	Whitehouse, 1968; Beck and Martin, 1969; Jung et al., 1969; Picton, 1969; Murphy, Wright, and Fitzgerald, 1970; Westholm, Magno, and Å-son Berg, 1970
Mepivacaine	8	Gad, 1967; Teramo and Widholm, 1967; Rosefsky and Petersiel, 1968; R. E. Rogers, *personal communication*, 1970
Prilocaine	5	Beck and Martin, 1969
Lidocaine	2	Nyirjesy et al., 1963; R. E. Rogers, *personal communication*, 1970
Hexylcaine	2	Freeman, Bellville, and Barno, 1956
Unknown	4	Sandmire and Austin, 1964; Taw, 1964; Beard, 1969; Meinrenken, 1969

crease below 7.20 for more than 30 min on the later development of the infant are unknown. If the fetus is already compromised before the application of PCB, the fetus may become even more depressed after the block. In the literature, at least 50 perinatal deaths have been reported, in which PCB is suspected to be the etiological factor (Table 3).

It is concluded that PCB should be used in obstetrics only when the condition of the fetus can be followed by continuous fetal heart-rate monitoring or by sampling fetal capillary blood for acid-base determinations. Bupivacaine (50 mg) with or without epinephrine cannot be recommended for a single-injection PCB because of the high frequency of fetal bradycardia (Table 1) and acidosis found with this dose (Teramo, 1969). Two-hundred mg of mepivacaine for PCB seem to be less toxic to the fetus than 50 mg of bupivacaine, but even with this dose of mepivacaine there is a slight but definite risk to the fetus.

REFERENCES

Asling, J. H., Shnider, S. M., Margolis, A. J., Wilkinson, G. L., and Way, E. L. (1970): Paracervical block anesthesia in obstetrics. II. Etiology of fetal bradycardia following paracervical block anesthesia. *American Journal of Obstetrics and Gynecology,* 107:626.

Beard, R. W. Cited by Obolensky, W., Kupferschmied, H., and Vullièmoz, P. (1969): Is paracervical anesthesia safe for the fetus? *Gynaecologia,* 168:234.

Beck, L., and Martin, K. Über das Risiko beim parazervikalem Block in der Geburtshilfe. *Geburtsh. Frauenheilk.,* 29:961.

Davis, J. E., Frudenfeld, J. C., Frudenfeld, K., Frudenfeld, J. H., and Webb, A. N. (1964): Combined paracervical-pudendal block anesthesia for labor and delivery. A review of 2100 private cases. *American Journal of Obstetrics and Gynecology,* 89:366.

Frangipani, G. C., Samaja, B. A., Tinti, A., Spandrio, L., and Tampalini, L. (1969): Lattacidemia, piruvicemia ed equilibrio acido-base materna-fetali in travaglio di parto. III. Durante blocco paracervicale. *Ann. Ostet. Ginec.,* 91:24.

Freeman, D. W., Bellville, T. P., and Barno, A. (1956): Paracervical block anesthesia in labor. *Obstetrics and Gynecology,* 8:270.

Gad, C. (1967): Paracervical block. A 30 months report. *Acta Obstet. Gynec. Scand.,* 46:7.

Jung, H., Kopecky, P., and Klöck, F. K. (1969): Die fetale Gefährdung durch die "Parazervikalblockaden". *Geburtsh. Fruenheilk.,* 29:519.

Kobak, A. J., and Sadove, M. S. (1961): Combined paracervical and pudendal nerve blocks. *American Journal of Obstetrics and Gynecology,* 81:72.

McGowan, G. W. (1962): Uterosacral or paracervical block for obstetrical anesthesia. *Western Journal of Surgery,* 70:307.

Meinrenken, H. (1969): Die Paracervicalanaesthesie in der Geburtshilfe. *Arch. Gynäk.,* 207:208.

Murphy, P. J., Wright, J. D., and Fitzgerald, T. B. (1970): Assessment of paracervical nerve block anaesthesia during labour. *British Medical Journal,* 1:526.

Nyirjesy, I., Hawks, B. L., Hebert, J. E., Hopwood, H. G., Jr., and Falls, H. C. (1963): Hazards of the use of paracervical block anesthesia in obstetrics. *American Journal of Obstetrics and Gynecology*, 87:231.

Obolensky, W., Kupferschmied, H., and Vullièmoz, P. (1969): Wirkung der Parazervikalanästhesie auf Mutter und Kind. *Gynaecologia*, 167:314.

Page, E. P., Kamm, M. L., and Chappel, C. C. (1961): Usefulness of paracervical block in obstetrics. *American Journal of Obstetrics and Gynecology*, 81:1094.

Picton, F. C. R. (1969): Paracervical nerve block in labour. *British Journal of Clinical Practice*, 23:162.

Rosefsky, J. B., and Petersiel, M. E. (1968): Perinatal deaths associated with mepivacaine paracervical-block anesthesia in labor. *New England Journal of Medicine*, 278:530.

Sandmire, H. F., and Austin, S. D. (1964): Paracervical block anesthesia in obstetrics. *Journal of the American Medical Association*, 187:775.

Steffenson, J. L., Shnider, S. M., and de Lorimier, A. A. (1970): Transarterial diffusion of mepivacaine. *Anesthesiology*, 32:459.

Stockhausen, H. (1967): Erfahrungen mit einem neuen Lokalanästhetikum bei der Parazervikalblockade. *Deutsche Med. Wschr.*, 92:2220.

Taw, R. L. In Discussion, Davis et al. (1964): The combined paracervical-pudendal block anesthesia for labor and delivery. *American Journal of Obstetrics and Gynecology*, 89:366.

Teramo, K. (1969): Foetal acid-base balance and heart rate during labour with bupivacaine paracervical block anaesthesia. *Journal of Obstetrics and Gynaecology of the British Commonwealth*, 76:881.

Teramo, K.: Obstetrical paracervical blockade with special reference to the aetiology of fetal bradycardia followed by paracervical blockade (*in press*).

Teramo, K., and Rajamäki, A. (1971): Foetal and maternal plasma levels of mepivacaine and foetal acid-base balance and heart rate after paracervical block during labour. *British Journal of Anaesthesiology*, 43:300.

Teramo, K., and Widholm, O. (1967): Studies of the effect of anaesthetics on foetus. I. The effect of paracervical block with mepivacaine upon foetal acid-base values. *Acta Obstet. Gynec. Scand.*, 46: suppl. 2.

Vasicka, A., Scheffs, J., Robertazzi, R., and Raji, M. (1970): Fetal bradycardia after paracervical block. Abstr. Scient. Exhib. 6th World Congr. Gynec. Obstet., New York, p. 1.

Westholm, H., Magro, R., and Å-son Berg, A. (1970): Experiences with paracervical block. *Acta Obstet. Gynec. Scand.*, 49:335.

Whitehouse, D. B. (1968): Paracervical block with bupivacaine. *British Medical Journal*, 2:764.

DISCUSSION

GENNSER: I would like to report some observations which add further information to our understanding of the mepivacaine effect on the human fetal heart. In perfused, spontaneously beating isolated hearts from human fetuses at midgestation, the active systolic pressure in the left ventricle was found to be decreased during perfusion with mepivacaine (Andersson et al., *Acta Physiol. Scand.*, Suppl. 353, 34, 1970). As the intraventricular excitation time was increased by mepivacaine, the negative inotropic effect observed might be due to a more asynchronous excitation and contraction of the myocardial cells. With another technique we were also able to demonstrate that mepivacaine exerts an effect directly on the myocardium. Isolated papillary muscles from human fetal heart were studied during multielectrode stimulation which led to a practically simultaneous activation of the whole preparation. With this arrangement, a dose-related reduction of the maximum isometric force of the muscle was obtained when mepivacaine was added to the bath (Gennser et al., to be published in *Acta Physiol. Scand.*). These results show that also on the cellular level, mepivacaine reduces the contractility of the human fetal myocardium.

McBride: We have found that fetal bradycardia is not produced if a slow infusion technique for PCB is used. If a single injection of the same dose is given, severe fetal bradycardia is produced.

Teramo: In our patients the PCB was performed as a single, short injection which was completed within 5 min on both sides. I agree with you that the prolongation of the administration time will decrease the incidence of fetal bradycardia and pH decrease because these changes are related to the dose of the local anesthetic used.

Drabkova: If you inject the same amount of the same local anesthetic for pudendal block, you never get these fetal side effects.

Shnider found that in all fetuses suffering from bradycardia and decrease of pH following PCB, the plasma concentration was approximately 3 μg/ml or higher. Therefore, he considered as the main factor for the adverse effects in the fetus not the amount of the drug but the region of administration. In the region of the uterine artery, its nutritional vessels can probably be responsible for a rapid absorption of anesthetic which is transferred directly to the intervillous space. Our results with ^{14}C-succinyldicholine support this. The transfer to the fetus after administration of the same dose either intravenously or intraaortally was significantly higher in the latter case.

Teramo: I do not have any data on the effects of pudendal block on the fetus or the newborn. Also I am not aware of any in the literature. In six out of seven cases of fetal bradycardia following PCB with 200 mg of mepivacaine, Shnider found higher levels of the drug in fetal than in maternal blood. On the other hand, in our PCB series (Teramo and Rajamäki, *Brit. J. Anaesth. 43*, 300, 1971), there was only one case out of six of fetal bradycardia after PCB with 300 to 400 mg mepivacaine in which the fetal plasma concentration was clearly higher than the corresponding maternal concentration. In the other five fetuses, the plasma concentration of mepivacaine paralleled the maternal concentration or was lower. It seems evident that fetal bradycardia and pH decrease can occur after PCB also in cases in which the drug reaches the fetus via the systemic circulation of the mother. Also this suggests that the fetus is more susceptible to toxic effects of local anesthetics than the mother at the same plasma level. This question should be studied further.

Fetal Pharmacology, edited by L. Boréus
Raven Press, New York © 1973

Drug Metabolism in the Human Fetus

Anders Rane, Christer von Bahr, Sten Orrenius, and Folke Sjöqvist

Departments of Pharmacology (Division of Clinical Pharmacology) and Forensic Medicine, Karolinska Institutet, S-104 01 Stockholm 60, Sweden

Drug metabolic processes during fetal life have previously been investigated in various species of animals, usually at the very end of gestation. Only negligible metabolism has been found, and the ability to metabolize drugs increases postnatally with rates depending on the species and drug substrate studied (Jondorf, Maickel, and Brodie, 1958; Fouts and Adamson, 1959; Done, 1964; Short and Davies, 1970; Feuer and Liscio, 1970).

Systematic studies of the development of drug metabolic processes in the human fetus and newborn cannot be performed since legal abortions are usually permitted only during the first 20 weeks of gestation. Thus, only scanty observations have been published on fetal drug metabolism during the second half of human gestation. In these studies, tissue specimens from, for example, stillborn babies have been utilized, but the relevance of such findings for the situation *in vivo* may be questioned.

The prevailing concept about drug metabolism in the human fetal liver has been that the metabolizing enzymes are absent or have negligible activities. This view is probably based on data obtained in animal studies which have been extrapolated to man.

This chapter challenges this concept and reports the presence of a liver microsomal drug-oxidizing enzyme system in the human fetus as early as the first half of gestation. *In vitro* observations of drug metabolism in the human fetal liver are reviewed. The possible pharmacological and toxicological importance of these findings is discussed.

BIOCHEMICAL BACKGROUND

The drug-metabolizing activity of liver microsomes[1] was first discovered by Brodie and associates (Brodie, Gillette, and La Du, 1958). They showed that in the presence of NADPH and molecular oxygen, liver microsomes catalyze the oxidation of a variety of drugs. Depending on the chemical nature of the drug, the reaction may lead to the oxidation of an aromatic ring or a hydrocarbon side-chain, an oxidative dealkylation or deamination, or the formation of a sulfoxide. The system was similar to that first described by Mueller and Miller (1948), who found that liver homogenates supplemented with NADH or NADPH in the presence of O_2 catalyzed the oxidative demethylation of the carcinogenic dye 4-dimethylaminoazobenzene to 4-aminoazobenzene and formaldehyde (Mueller and Miller, 1948, 1953). Later it was found that a similar system is involved in the hydroxylation of aliphatic hydrocarbons and the ω-oxidation of fatty acids (Robbins, 1961; Wakabayashi and Shimazono, 1961; Das, Orrenius and Ernster, 1968).

The hydroxylating enzyme system has been termed as a "mixed-function oxidase" (Mason, 1957) or "monooxygenase" (Hayaishi, 1962), since in the course of the reaction one of the oxygen atoms of O_2 is incorporated into the compound undergoing hydroxylation, and the other into H_2O. The process may be described by the general reaction:

$$RH + NADPH + H^+ + O_2 \rightarrow ROH + NADP^+ + H_2O$$

where RH is the substrate and ROH the product of the hydroxylation reaction.

It is now fairly well established that the microsomal oxidative system consists of at least two catalytic components (see Fig. 1): a cytochrome called P-450 (Omura and Sato, 1964a,b) and a flavoprotein catalyzing the reduction of this cytochrome by NADPH, suitably termed NADPH-cytochrome P-450 reductase. Cytochrome P-450 is characterized by a sensitivity to carbon monoxide, which binds to the reduced form of the cytochrome, giving rise to a characteristic absorption spectrum with a maximum of 450 nm (Klingenberg, 1958; Garfinkel, 1958).

The cytochrome is easily denatured and converted into a hemochromogen with a shift of the absorption maximum of its CO-complex to 420 nm (Omura and Sato, 1964a,b). Successful attempts have recently been reported toward extraction of cytochrome P-450 from microsomes in its native

[1] Microsomes are derived from the endoplasmic reticulum upon homogenization of the liver.

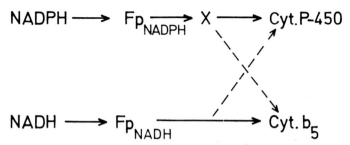

FIG. 1. Electron transport systems in liver microsomes. Fp, flavoprotein.

form, by a procedure that involves the use of glycerol and deoxycholate (Lu, Junk, and Coon, 1969). The "solubilized" cytochrome P-450 has been used for a reconstruction of the hydroxylating system with NADPH-cytochrome P-450 reductase and a phospholipid fraction as additional components. A cytochrome P-450 has been purified from *Pseudomonas putida*, where it is involved in the hydroxylation of camphor (Katagiri, Ganguli, and Gunsalus, 1968).

The flavoprotein NADPH-cytochrome P-450 reductase most probably is closely related to the enzyme known since 1950 as NADPH-cytochrome *c* reductase (Horecker, 1950), which in recent years has been purified and studied in great detail by several groups of investigators (Lang and Nason, 1959; Williams and Kamin, 1962; Phillips and Langdon, 1962). The purified enzyme has the interesting property of catalyzing a one-electron transfer from NADPH to cytochrome *c*, its prosthetic group flavin adenine dinucleotide (FAD) undergoing cyclic oxido-reductions between the half-reduced (free radical) and fully reduced states (Kamin, Masters, Gibson, and Williams, 1965). Cytochrome *c* appears to serve merely as an artificial electron acceptor for the enzyme.

Whether the flavoprotein interacts directly with cytochrome P-450 in the course of the hydroxylation process is not known. There are indications that this may not be the case. For example, some results have indicated that neotetrazolium chloride interacts with the system at a site intermediate between the flavoprotein and cytochrome P-450 (Ernster and Orrenius, 1965).

There is also evidence for an interaction of the NADPH-linked hydroxylating system with the NADH-cytochrome *c* reductase present in liver microsomes, consisting of the flavoprotein NADH-cytochrome b_5 reductase and cytochrome b_5 (see Fig. 1) (Strittmatter, 1965). Such an interaction is indicated by the fact that, in liver microsomes, NADH is capable of reducing cytochrome P-450 and, conversely, NADPH can serve as a reducing agent for cytochrome b_5, although the rates of these "cross-reactions" are lower than those of the NADPH-cytochrome P-450 reductase and NADH-cytochrome b_5 reductase, respectively (Cooper, Narasimhulu, Rosenthal, and Estabrook, 1965; Sato, Omura, and Nishibayashi, 1965). Recent evidence suggests that these cross-reactions are not due to a lack of specificity of the flavoproteins, with respect to the reduced nicotinamide nucleotides, but rather to an interaction between the two electron-transport chains in the flavin → cytochrome region, through intermediates that yet remain to be identified (Orrenius, Berg, and Ernster, 1969).

There is evidence that the reaction catalyzed by the hydroxylating system involves a binding of the substrate to cytochrome P-450. Such a binding has been inferred from spectral changes that occur when various substrates capable of undergoing hydroxylation are added to a suspension of microsomes (Remmer, Schenkman, Estabrook, Sasame, Gillette, Narasimhulu, Cooper, and Rosenthal, 1966; Imai and Sato, 1966; Schenkman, Remmer, and Estabrook, 1967b). The spectral changes obtained with various substrates can be divided into two classes, as illustrated in Fig. 2: a type I

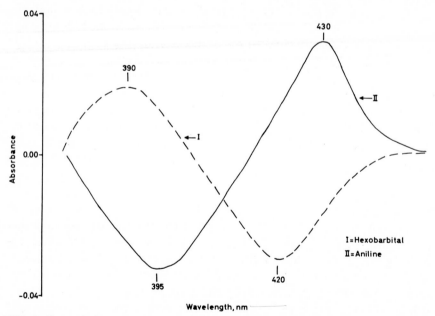

FIG. 2. Spectral changes produced by the addition of hexobarbital (I) and aniline (II) to suspensions of rat liver microsomes. Each cuvette contained, in a volume of 2.9 ml, 3 mg of microsomal protein and 50 mM Tris-Cl buffer, pH 7.5. Hexobarbital or aniline was added to the sample cuvette in a final concentration of 3.3 mM.

spectral change, characterized by a peak at about 390 nm and a trough at about 420 nm, and a type II spectral change, characterized by a trough in the 400-nm region and a peak in the 430-nm region of the difference spectrum of the microsomes. That these spectral changes reflect binding of the substrate to cytochrome P-450 is shown by the fact that they are also observed with solubilized microsomal cytochrome P-450 (Lu et al., 1969), as well as with the cytochrome P-450 purified from *Pseudomonas putida* (Gunsalus, 1968). The type I spectral change is generally believed to be due to a binding of the substrate to the apoprotein of the cytochrome, whereas Type II is due to an interaction between the substrate and the heme prosthetic group. It is the type I spectral change that appears to be related to the hydroxylating activity.

The reaction sequence catalyzed by the microsomal hydroxylating system may thus be visualized to consist of the following steps (Estabrook, Hildebrandt, Remmer, Schenkman, Rosenthal, and Cooper, 1968): (1) reduction of the flavoprotein by NADPH; (2) binding of substrate to the oxidized form of cytochrome P-450; (3) reduction of the cytochrome P-450-substrate complex by the reduced flavoprotein; (4) binding of O_2 to the reduced complex; and (5) dissociation of the oxidized cytochrome P-450 and the oxidized product.

ULTRASTRUCTURE OF HUMAN FETAL LIVER

Drug-metabolizing enzymes are located in the endoplasmic reticulum of the cell. In 1965, a thorough study of the ultrastructure of human fetal liver was published (Zamboni). The development of the hepatocytes was studied in fetuses between the 7th and 20th weeks of gestation. In the 7th and 9th weeks of gestation, the reticulum consists of a system of short tubules with ribosome-studded membranes. Around the 3rd month, a marked increase of agranular reticulum is seen. Concomitantly, deposits of glycogen and iron appear in the hepatocytes. Thus the morphological correlate to drug-metabolizing enzymes seems to be present early in human fetal life.

BIOCHEMICAL STUDIES WITH HUMAN FETAL LIVER MICROSOMES

Despite the early demonstration of endoplasmic reticulum in the human fetal liver, the drug-metabolizing enzymes localized in these structures were not demonstrated until 1970 (Yaffe, Rane, Sjöqvist, Boréus, and Orrenius,

1970). The livers from 13 fetuses were included in that study. The fetuses were obtained via hysterotomy during the interruption of pregnancy for socio-medical reasons. Microsomes were prepared accordng to Ernster, Sie-kevitz, and Palade (1962), with an additional wash in order to minimize the contamination of hemoglobin.

Cytochrome P-450 as well as the flavoprotein NADPH-cytochrome *c* reductase were detected in all livers investigated. The levels varied but were not correlated to gestational age. The concentration of cytochrome P-450 varied between 0.04 and 0.38 nmoles/mg microsomal protein (mean 0.15). NADPH-cytochrome *c* reductase ranged from 8 to 85 nmoles cytochrome *c* reduced/mg protein/min (mean 47). Significant activity of NADPH-cyto-chrome P-450 reductase was recorded.

Our figures on the level of cytochrome P-450 in human fetal liver are of the same order of magnitude as those reported previously for human adult microsomes obtained at surgical biopsy (Alvares, Shilling, Levin, Kuntzman, Brand, and Mark, 1969; Ackermann, 1970). However, the specific activity of NADPH-cytochrome *c* reductase seems to be about three times higher in adult liver microsomes (Ackermann, 1970).

During these studies, we found low yields of microsomes from human fetal livers compared to livers from human adults and animals. A combined biochemical and morphologic study of the different centrifugal fractions ob-

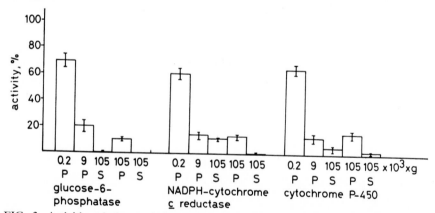

FIG. 3. Activities of glucose-6-phosphatase (n = 4) and NADPH-cytochrome *c* reductase (n = 7) and concentration of cytochrome P-450 (n = 4) expressed as percent of total, in the 200 × *g* pellet, the 9,000 × *g* pellet, the 105,000 × *g* supernatant, the 105,000 × *g* pellet, and supernatant (the last two fractions after wash) in the human fetal liver. ± SE is indicated in each bar (from Ackermann, Rane, and Ericsson, 1971).

tained from fetal liver was therefore initiated (Ackermann, Rane, and Ericsson, 1971).

Glucose-6-phosphatase, NADPH-cytochrome c reductase, and cytochrome P-450 were used as marker enzymes of the endoplasmic reticulum (microsomes). With the conventional technique for preparation of rat liver microsomes (Ernster et al., 1962), the microsomal recovery in the 105,000 $\times$ g pellet was about 10 to 15%. The mitochondrial fraction (9,000 $\times$ g pellet) contained about 85% of the total activity. Even when the procedure was initiated with a 200 $\times$ g centrifugation of the homogenate (with the purpose of spinning down hematopoietic cells which might interfere with the sedimentation of microsomes), the major part (60 to 70%) of the total microsomal enzyme activity was recovered in the 200 $\times$ g pellet (Fig. 3).

Electron-microscopic studies of the different fractions revealed that the endoplasmic reticulum was converted only partly to uniform microsomes during the homogenization. The rest formed long slender cisternae, which led to a loss of microsomal enzyme activity into low-speed fractions, which also contained unbroken hepatocytes with endoplasmic reticulum. The 105,-000 $\times$ g pellet was the most homogeneous one with respect to microsomes.

IN VITRO STUDIES OF DRUG METABOLISM

An interesting study of drug metabolism in human trophoblast tissue culture was published by Uher (1969). Various drugs were added in concentrations expected to occur in a therapeutic situation. Metabolism was detected of the following drugs: sulfamethoxypyrimidine (acetylation), ketophenylbutazone, benzopyrazone, and mebrophenhydramine (hydroxylation).

Most prenatal studies have been performed later in gestation. Pomp, Schnoor, and Netter (1969) were unable to find oxidation of either p-nitroanisol or N-monomethyl-p-nitroaniline in the 8,400 $\times$ g supernatant from human fetal liver. The age of the fetuses varied between the 3rd and the 10th months of gestation.

Demethylation of aminopyrine in human fetal liver microsomes was studied by Yaffe et al., (1970). A varying activity was found (between 0 and 5.9 nmoles formaldehyde formed/mg protein/min). There was also significant oxidation of laurate and testosterone.

Pelkonen, Vorne, Arvela, Jouppila, and Kärki (1971a) reported that benzpyrene was hydroxylated at a slow rate in human fetal liver (5 to 15%

of the activity in adult rat liver). Metabolism of N-methylaniline, chlorpromazine, and p-nitrobenzoic acid was also reported. Utilizing the 12,000 $\times$ g supernatant, Pelkonen, Vorne, Jouppila, and Kärki (1971b) demonstrated a slow rate of disappearance of chlorpromazine and formation of p-aminobenzoic from p-nitrobenzoic acid in human fetal liver and intestine.

Rane and Ackermann (1971a,b) studied the oxidative metabolism of ethylmorphine and aniline in various subcellular fractions of human fetal liver. The formation of formaldehyde and p-aminophenol was measured. In the 105,000 $\times$ g pellet, about 1.4 nmoles of formaldehyde and about 0.22 nmoles of p-aminophenol were formed per mg protein/min. These values are 35 and 40%, respectively, of those reported in microsomes from human adult liver, obtained by surgical biopsy (Ackermann, 1971). As seen in Fig. 4, the relative distribution of drug metabolic activity in the different fractions is similar to the distribution of microsomal marker enzymes (cf. Fig. 3). Per gram liver, the hydroxylation of aniline is as great as in adult liver (Ackermann, 1971), whereas the rate of ethylmorphine demethylation is somewhat lower.

The aromatic hydroxylation of desmethylimipramine (DMI) was also studied in human fetal liver microsomes (unpublished results). This drug belongs to the group of tricyclic antidepressants. Tritiated desmethylimipramine was used, and the 2-hydroxylated metabolite was determined with

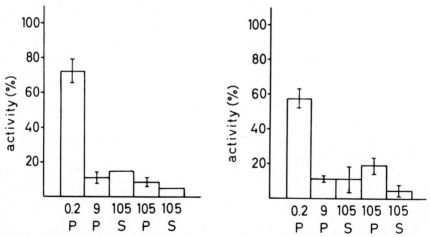

FIG. 4. Para-hydroxylation and aniline (left) and demethylation of ethylmorphine (right) in different fractions of human fetal liver, expressed as percent of total liver activity. $\pm$ SE is indicated. The bars indicate the same fraction as in Fig. 3 (from Rane and Ackermann, 1971b).

TABLE 1. *Hydroxylation of desmethylimipramine in human fetal and adult liver microsomes.*

Liver no.	Gestational age (weeks)	nmoles of hydroxylated metabolites formed from DMI/ml incubate (30 min)[a]	$\dfrac{\text{mg protein}}{\text{ml incubate}}$
Fetal			
1	12	0.026	1.0
2	13	0.087	2.0
3	13	0.203	1.4
4	13	0.000	1.0
5	13	0.000	1.0
6	18	0.147	1.0
7	19	0.168	1.0
8	19	0.184	2.8
9	21	0.073	0.8
Adult			
10	—	0.543	1.0
11	—	0.471	1.0
12	—	0.067	1.0

[a] Note that for the fetal livers the relationship between amount of protein and rate of metabolism has not been checked.

the liquid scintillation technique after differential extraction according to von Bahr and Borga (1971). Table 1 shows the formation of hydroxylated metabolite from DMI in microsomes from adult and fetal livers. The chromatographic mobilities of the recovered metabolites on thin-layer plates are shown in Fig. 5. The main metabolic fraction had a mobility similar to that of the authentic cold reference substance 2-hydroxydesmethylimipramine. This was true both for adult and fetal microsomes.

As mentioned above, the binding of substrates to cytochrome P-450 gives rise to spectral changes, which can be studied by measuring the difference spectra between microsomal suspensions with and without substrate. Table 2 summarizes the spectral changes in human fetal liver microsomes upon addition of different substrates (Rane and Orrenius, *unpublished results*).

Hexobarbital and laurate both caused a type I spectral change in fetal and in adult human liver microsomes. These substrates belong to the group which give a type I spectral change in rat liver microsomes. Aminopyrine and testosterone, which belong to the same group of substrates, caused a different type of spectral change in microsomes derived from human adult liver. This was characterized by a peak of absorption at about 420 nm and a trough in the 390 nm region (modified type II or reversed type I). In fetal

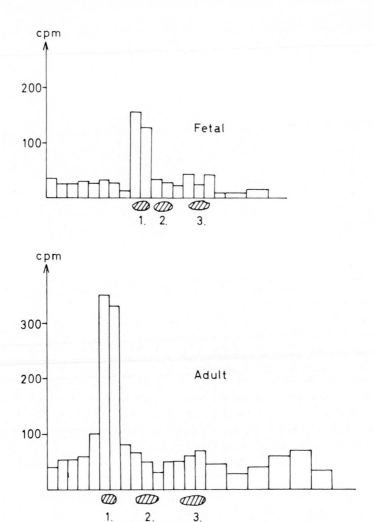

FIG. 5. Thin-layer chromatography of metabolites recovered in chloroform extract obtained by extraction from the incubate. The cold references shown are: (1) 2-hydroxydesmethylimipramine, (2) desmethylimipramine, and (3) didesmethylimipramine.

liver microsomes, aminopyrine caused a modified type II change in the difference spectrum, whereas addition of testosterone was associated with a type I spectral change. Aniline, which usually gives a type II spectral change in rat liver microsomes, produced the same change in human fetal liver microsomes.

TABLE 2. *Substrate-induced spectral changes in human fetal and adult liver microsomes with different substrates*

Substrate	Concentration (mM)	Type of spectral change (in liver microsomes)		
		human fetus	human adult	adult rat
Laurate	0.020– 0.033	I	I	I[a]
Testosterone	0.017– 0.66	I	"II"[b]	I[c]
Hexobarbital	0.5 – 1.5	I	I	I[d]
Aminopyrine	1.0 –10.0	"II"	"II"	I[d]
Ethylmorphine	0.17 – 5.0	"II"	N.I.	I[e]
Aniline	2.16	II	II	II[d]
Nortriptyline	0.003	N.I.	II	I[f]

N.I. means not investigated.
[a] Orrenius and Thor, 1969.
[b] "II" refers to a spectral change characterized by a trough at about 390 nm and a peak at about 420 nm. It is usually called modified type II or reversed type I spectral change.
[c] Schenkman et al., 1967a.
[d] Remmer et al., 1966.
[e] Davies et al., 1969.
[f] von Bahr et al., 1971.

COMMENTS

Research data obtained during the last few years have disclosed the presence of an intact drug-oxidizing enzyme system in the human fetal liver early in gestation. The metabolism of a limited number of drugs has been studied in human fetal liver preparations. Ethylmorphine, aminopyrine, des-methylimipramine, chlorpromazine, and aniline are all oxidized. Many more drugs have to be studied in order to elucidate how compounds with different physico-chemical and structural properties are handled by the fetal liver. Moreover, little is known about the synthetic (conjugation) processes. In the course of this work, specific and sensitive methods for measuring drugs and metabolites should be worked out.

The apparent difference between man and animals in the prenatal development of drug-metabolizing enzymes is not easily understood. The human being is continuously exposed to exogenous compounds such as drugs, food constituents, cigarette smoke, and air pollution. Drugs and polycyclic hydrocarbons are known to induce drug-metabolizing enzymes in the liver of adult animals and man. The human gestational period is much longer than that of the studied animal species, which provides more time for an induction process to take place.

The possibility of such species differences must be considered when evaluating the teratogenicity of new drugs. If drug metabolites are terato-genic, this may remain undetected in animal experiments. This is of particu-lar importance in view of the recent suggestions (Brodie, 1971; Daly, 1971), that certain drug-induced tissue lesions may be related to the formation of highly reactive epoxides, which are metabolic intermediates formed during oxidation of aromatic hydrocarbons. Concern has recently been expressed about the possible teratogenic effects of diphenylhydantoin in man (Mirkin, 1971; see also the chapter by Hill, Horning, and Horning in this volume). This drug contains two benzene rings and is hydroxylated in one of the rings through introduction of either one or two hydroxy groups. The pres-ence of the 3,4-dihydro-dihydroxy-metabolite in the urine from neonates (see chapter by Horning in this volume) offers indirect evidence that epox-ides are formed. This might also be the case during fetal life. The 2-hydrox-ylation of desmethylimipramine is an example of an aromatic hydroxylation taking place in the human fetal liver (see above).

Usually the metabolism of drugs implies a detoxification, but the con-verse possibility also exists (bioactivation). During *in vitro* studies of the metabolism of aniline in human fetal liver, it was shown that methemoglobin was formed from the hemoglobin present in the incubates (Rane and Acker-mann, 1971*b*). It is known that this is caused only by the aniline metabo-lites, predominantly the N-oxidized forms (Wagner, 1969).

In conclusion, the demonstration that the human fetal liver contains the drug-oxidizing cytochrome P-450 system, calls for thorough studies of drug metabolism during fetal development. It is too early to speculate about the true biological role of this enzyme system.

ACKNOWLEDGMENTS

Some of these studies were supported by grants from "Expressen's" Prenatal Research Fund, the National Institutes of Health (GM 13978-06), the Swedish Medical Research Council (B72-14X-1021-07A and B72-13X-2471-05), and the Wallenberg Foundation.

REFERENCES

Ackermann, E. (1970): Die Demethylierung von Aminophenazon und Codein in der Leber des Menschen. *Biochemical Pharmacology*, 19:1955-1973.
Ackermann, E. (1971): Die Michaelis-Menten Konstant und maximalen Reaktionsgesch-

windigkeiten einiger Pharmaka in den Lebermikrosomen des Menschen verglichen mit der Ratte beiderlei Geschlechts. *Biochemical Pharmacology (in press)*.

Ackermann, E., Rane, A., and Ericsson, J. L. E. (1972): The liver microsomal monooxygenase system in the human fetus: Distribution in different subcellular fractions. *Clinical Pharmacology and Therapeutics (in press)*.

Alvares, A. A., Shilling, G., Levin, W., Kuntzman, R., Brand, L., and Mark, L. C. (1969): Cytochromes P-450 and b_5 in human liver microsomes. *Clinical Pharmacology and Therapeutics*, 10:655-659.

von Bahr, C., and Borga, O. (1971): Uptake, metabolism and excretion of desmethylimipramine and its metabolites in the isolated perfused rat liver. *Acta Pharmacologica et Toxicologica*, 29:359-374.

von Bahr, C., Orrenius, S., and Sjöqvist, F. (1971): Interaction of imipramine, desmethylimipramine, nortriptyline and 1-naphthol with microsomal preparations. *Chemico-Biological Interactions*, 3:243-244.

Brodie, B. B. (1971): Possible mechanisms of drug-induced tissue lesions. *Chemico-Biological Interactions*, 3:247.

Brodie, B. B., Gillette, J. R., and La Du, B. N. (1958): Enzymatic metabolism of drugs and other foreign compounds. *Annual Review of Biochemistry*, 27:427-455.

Cooper, D. Y., Narasimhulu, S., Rosenthal, O., and Estabrook, R. W. (1965): Spectral and kinetic studies of microsomal pigments. In: *Oxidases and Related Redox Systems*, edited by T. E. King, H. S. Mason, and M. Morrison. John Wiley & Sons, Inc., New York, London and Sydney, pp. 838-855.

Daly, J. W. (1971): The role of arene oxides in drug metabolism, toxicity and carcinogenicity (personal communication)

Das, M. L., Orrenius, S., and Ernster, L. (1968): On the fatty acid and hydrocarbon hydroxylation in rat liver microsomes. *European Journal of Biochemistry*, 4:519-523.

Davies, D. S., Gigon, P. L., and Gillette, J. R. (1969): Species and sex differences in electron transport systems in liver microsomes and their relationship to ethylmorphine demethylation. *Life Sciences*, 8:85-91.

Done, A. K. (1964): Developmental pharmacology. *Clinical Pharmacology and Therapeutics*, 5:432-479.

Ernster, L., and Orrenius, S. (1965): Substrate-induced synthesis of the hydroxylating enzyme system of liver microsomes. *Federation Proceedings*, 24:1190-1199.

Ernster, L., Siekevitz, P., and Palade, G. E. (1962): Enzyme-structure relationships in the endoplasmic reticulum of rat liver. *Journal of Cell Biology*, 15:541-562.

Estabrook, R. W., Hildebrandt, A., Remmer, H., Schenkman, J. B., Rosenthal, O., and Cooper, D. Y. (1968): The role of cytochrome P-450 in microsomal mixed function oxidation reactions. In: *Biochemie des Sauerstoffs*, edited by B. Hess and Hj. Staudinger. Springer-Verlag, Berlin, Heidelberg, and New York pp. 142-177.

Feuer, G., and Liscio, A. (1970): Effect of drugs on hepatic drug metabolism in the fetus and newborn. *International Journal of Clinical Pharmacology*, 31:30-33.

Fouts, J. R., and Adamson, R. H. (1959): Drug metabolism in the newborn rabbit. *Science*, 129:897-898.

Garfinkel, D. (1958): Studies on pig liver microsomes. I. Enzymic and pigment composition of different microsomal fractions. *Archives of Biochemistry and Biophysics*, 77:493-509.

Gnosspelius, Y., Thor, H., and Orrenius, S. (1969): A comparative study on the effects of phenobarbital and 3,4-benzpyrene on the hydroxylating enzyme system of rat-liver microsomes. *Chemico-Biological Interactions*, 1:125-137.

Gunsalus, I. C. (1968): A soluble methylene hydroxylase system: Structure and role of cytochrome P-450 and iron-sulfur protein components. *Hoppe-Seyler's Zeitschrift für Physiologische Chemie*, 349:1610-1613.

Hayaishi, O. (1962): History and scope. In: *Oxygenases*, edited by O. Hayaishi.

Academic Press, New York and London, pp. 1-29.

Horecker, B. L. (1950): Triphosphopyridine nucleotide-cytochrome *c* reductase in liver. *Journal of Biological Chemistry*, 183:593-605.

Imai, Y., and Sato, R. (1966): Substrate interaction with hydroxylase system in liver microsomes, *Biochemical and Biophysical Research Communications*, 22:620-626.

Jondorf, W. R., Maickel, R. T., and Brodie, B. B. (1958): Inability of newborn mice and guinea pigs to metabolize drugs. *Biochemical Pharmacology*, 1:352-354.

Kamin, H., Masters, B. S. S., Gibson, Q. H., and Williams, C. H. (1965): Microsomal TPNH-cytochrome *c* reductase. *Federation Proceedings*, 24:1164-1171.

Katagiri, M., Ganguli, B. N., and Gunsalus, I. C. (1968): A soluble cytochrome P-450 functional in methylene hydroxylation. *Journal of Biological Chemistry*, 243:3543-3546.

Klingenberg, M. (1958): Pigments of rat liver microsomes. *Archives of Biochemistry and Biophysics*, 75:376-386.

Lang, C. A., and Nason, A. (1959): A triphosphopyridine nucleotide-cytochrome *c* reductase from heart muscle. *Journal of Biological Chemistry*, 234:1874-1877.

Lu, A. Y. H., Junk, K. W., and Coon, M. J. (1969): Resolution of the cytochrome P-450-containing ω-hydroxylation system of liver microsomes into three components. *Journal of Biological Chemistry*, 244:3714-3721.

Mason, H. S. (1957): Mechanisms of oxygen metabolism. *Advances in Enzymology and Related Subjects of Biochemistry*, 19:79-233.

Mirkin, B. L. (1971): Diphenylhydantoin: Placental transport, fetal localization, neonatal metabolism and possible teratogenic effect. *Journal of Pediatrics*, 78:329-337.

Mueller, G. C., and Miller, J. A. (1948): The metabolism of 4-dimethylaminoazobenzene by rat liver homogenates. *Journal of Biological Chemistry*, 176:535-544.

Mueller, G. C., and Miller, J. A. (1953): The metabolism of methylated aminoazo dyes. II. Oxidative demethylation by rat liver homogenates. *Journal of Biological Chemistry*, 202:579-587.

Omura, T., and Sato, R. (1964a): The carbon monoxide-binding pigment of liver microsomes. I. Evidence for its hemoprotein nature. *Journal of Biological Chemistry*, 239:2370-2378.

Omura, T., and Sato, R. (1964b): The carbon monoxide-binding pigment of liver microsomes. II. Solubilization, purification and properties. *Journal of Biological Chemistry*, 239:2379-2385.

Orrenius, S., Berg, A., and Ernster, L. (1969): Effects of trypsin on the electron transport systems of liver microsomes. *European Journal of Biochemistry*, 11:193-200.

Orrenius, S., and Thor, H. (1969): Fatty acid interaction with the hydroxylating enzyme system of rat liver microsomes. *European Journal of Biochemistry*, 9:415-418.

Pelkonen, O., Vorne, M., Arvela, P., Jouppila, P., and Kärki, N. T. (1971a): Drug metabolizing enzymes in human fetal liver and placenta in early pregnancy. *Scandinavian Journal of Clinical and Laboratory Investigations*, 27: suppl. 116, 7.

Pelkonen, O., Vorne, M., Jouppila, P., and Kärki, N. T. (1971b): Metabolism of chlorpromazine and p-nitrobenzoic acid in the liver, intestine and kidney of the human foetus. *Acta Pharmacologica et Toxicologica*, 29:284-294.

Phillips, A. H., and Langdon, R. G. (1962): Hepatic triphosphopyridine nucleotide-cytochrome *c* reductase: Isolation, characterization, and kinetic studies. *Journal of Biological Chemistry*, 237:2652-2660.

Pomp, H., Schnoor, M., and Netter, K. J. (1969): Untersuchungen über die Arzneimitteldemethylierung in der fetalen Leber. *Deutsche Medizinische Wochenschrift*, 94:23, 1232-1240.

Rane, A., and Ackermann, E. (1971a): Evidence for drug metabolism in the human fetal liver. Studies in different cell fractions. Abstract. Joint meeting German and Scandinavian Pharmacological Societies. Copenhagen, July 1971, *Acta Pharmacologica et Toxicologica*, 29: suppl. 4, 84.

Rane, A., and Ackermann, E. (1971b): Metabolism of ethylmorphine and aniline in human fetal liver. *Clinical Pharmacology and Therapeutics* (*in press*).

Remmer, H., Schenkman, J. B., Estabrook, R. W., Sasame, H., Gillette, J. R., Narasimhulu, S., Cooper, C. Y., and Rosenthal, O. (1966): Drug interaction with hepatic microsomal cytochrome. *Molecular Pharmacology*, 2:187-190.

Robbins, K. C. (1961): Enzymatic omega oxidation of fatty acids. *Federation Proceedings*, 20:272.

Sato, R., Omura, T., and Nishibayashi, H. (1965): Carbon-monoxide-binding hemoprotein and NADPH-specific flavoprotein in liver microsomes and their roles in microsomal electron transfer. In: *Oxidases and Related Redox Systems,* edited by T. E. King, H. S. Mason, and M. Morrison. John Wiley & Sons, Inc., New York, London and Sydney, pp. 861-875.

Schenkman, J. B., Frey, I., Remmer, H., and Estabrook, R. W. (1967a): Sex differences in drug metabolism by rat liver microsomes. *Molecular Pharmacology*, 3:516-525.

Schenkman, J. B., Remmer, H., and Estabrook, R. W. (1967b): Spectral studies of drug interaction with hepatic microsomal cytochrome. *Molecular Pharmacology*, 3:113-123.

Short, C. R., and Davies, L. E (1970): Perinatal development of drug-metabolizing activity in swine. *Journal of Pharmacology and Experimental Therapeutics,* 174:185-196.

Strittmatter, P. (1965): Protein and coenzyme interactions in the NADH-cytochrome b_5 reductase system. *Federation Proceedings,* 24:1156-1163.

Uher, J. (1969): Metabolism of the trophoblast in tissue culture under normal and modified conditions. In: *The Foeto-Placental Unit,* edited by A. Pecile and C. Finzi, Excerpta Medica Foundation, Amsterdam.

Wagner, J. (1969): The action of aromatic N-hydroxylated compounds on metabolism of red blood cells. FEBS Symposium, 16:161-181.

Wakabayashi, K., and Shimazono, N. (1961): Studies *in vitro* on the mechanism of ω-oxidation of fatty acids. *Biochimica et Biophysica Acta,* 48:615-617.

Williams, C. H., and Kamin, H. (1962): Microsomal triphosphopyridine nucleotide-cytochrome c reductase of liver. *Journal of Biological Chemistry,* 237:587-595.

Yaffe, S. J., Rane, A., Sjöqvist, F., Boréus, L.-O., and Orrenius, S. (1970): The presence of a monooxygenase system in human fetal liver microsomes. *Life Sciences,* 9:II: 1189-1200.

Zamboni, L. (1965): Electron microscopic studies of blood embryogenesis in humans. I. The ultrastructure of the fetal liver. *Journal of Ultrastructure Research,* 12:509-524.

DISCUSSION

JUCHAU: In the fetal livers obtained from women who smoke, do you observe a shift in the absorption maximum of fetal hepatic cytochrome P-450 from 450 nm to 448 nm?

RANE: We have not observed any changes either in absorption spectrum of the cytochrome or in specific activity of the drug-oxidizing enzymes. Our material is, however, limited.

JOST: The fetal liver is made of a double population of cells—the hematopoietic cells and the hepatocytes. What is the contribution of each category of cells to the microsomal vesicles extracted from the liver? Does the former type of cells participate in drug metabolism?

RANE: The hematopoietic cells contained only sparse endoplasmic reticulum, while this was well developed in the hepatocytes. The proportion of hematopoietic cells may be judged from the $200 \times g$ pellets which we studied with light microscopy. In the $200 \times g$ pellet, we can see hepatocytes which are characterized by their large nuclei; we can also see naked nuclei, erythrocytes, and, finally, small cells which probably are hematopoietic cells. These four components were represented in equal proportions; in other words, the contribution of the hematopoietic cells to the overall activity of microsomal enzymes should not be great. More important in this respect is, perhaps, that the hematopoietic cells are much smaller than the hepatocytes. This has been investigated in fetal rat liver and calculations there have revealed that the volume of the hematopoietic cells is only a few percent of the whole liver volume. Therefore, the contribution of microsomes from the hematopoietic cells to the total should be negligible.

MANN: In his interesting and lucid account, Dr. Orrenius pointed out that when amphetamine interacts with cytochrome P-450, two differential spectral patterns can appear, depending on the concentration of the drug: low concentrations give rise to type I (when amphetamine is metabolized), but high concentrations produce the type II. How differently is the molecule of cytochrome P-450 itself affected by the two concentrations of the same drug? Is there, for instance, any difference in the valency of iron?

ORRENIUS: The two types of spectral change represent different types or sites of interaction between the substance and cytochrome P-450, type I probably interacting with the protein moiety, and type II with the heme iron. There is no difference in the valency of the iron.

RÄIHÄ: I would like to ask Dr. Rane if you have any information concerning the development of the so-called microsomal ethanol-oxidizing system (MEOS), which has been shown by Lieber and Rubin to be fairly active in adult liver.

RANE: We have not looked for the presence of microsomal oxidation of ethanol in the human fetal liver.

KARCZMAR: Dr. Brodie stressed the need of the microsomal metabolism of the foreign substances for the formation of polar, water-soluble metabolites which can be kidney-excreted. He has shown, in fact, that certain water-living animal forms do not possess this system, but develop it if they metamorphose into terrestrial forms. On this basis, it seems that we do not need the microsomal system during our fetal development. Do you have any suggestions for a teleological explanation of the fetal presence of the microsomal system?

RANE: It is known that the drug-metabolizing enzyme system in the rat liver is similar to that metabolizing steroid hormones. The metabolism both of drugs and some steroid hormones has, for instance, been shown to be inhibited by CO. There are also other findings indicating that the two systems are similar, perhaps identical. The situation is probably the same in the human microsomal enzyme system. We know that this system participates in oxidations of steroids. Therefore, one may suggest that the enzyme system has an important natural function in the metabolism of steroids.

Fetal Pharmacology, edited by L. Boréus
Raven Press, New York © 1973

Microsomal Mixed-Function Oxidases in the Fetal and Newborn Rabbit

James R. Fouts

Pharmacology and Toxicology Branch, National Institute of Environmental Health Sciences, National Institutes of Health, Research Triangle Park, North Carolina 27709

HEPATIC DRUG METABOLISM IN THE PERINATAL PERIOD—A REVIEW OF SOME WORK BY THE AUTHOR AND OTHERS

Drug metabolism by hepatic microsomes from fetal and newborn animals

The ability of liver to metabolize drugs can be affected by a variety of factors including the age of the animal. Among some early studies on selected, hepatic, microsomal drug-metabolizing systems in newborn animals were those of Jondorf, Maickel, and Brodie (1959) and Fouts and Adamson (1959). Such early work indicated that most hepatic drug-metabolizing enzymes were either absent or at barely detectable levels in the fetus and newborn of common laboratory animals. The rate of development of these drug metabolic pathways appeared to depend both on the animal species and on the particular drug substrate being used to assay these hepatic enzymes. In most cases, adult levels of hepatic drug-metabolizing enzyme activity were reached only slowly—sometimes several weeks after birth. Exceptions or apparent exceptions can be offered for any generalization and perhaps two of these should be mentioned: certain glucuronidations can be at or above adult levels in the rat liver during the first week of life (Henderson, 1971), and the hepatic hydroxylation of biphenyl at the 2 position is highest soon after birth and disappears before 2 months of age in the rat (Basu, Dickerson, and Parke, 1971). Note that such exceptions are probably species-specific (for rat and not other animals) and substrate-specific (most glucuronidations and most aromatic ring hydroxylations are not detectable or at very low levels in livers from fetus and newborn even in the rat).

Some recent reports deal with hepatic microsomal enzyme components in human fetuses (Yaffe, Rane, Sjöqvist, Boréus, and Orrenius, 1970; Ackermann and Rane, 1971). The results seem to show that drug-metabolizing enzymes may be present in the human before birth, whereas in most animals these systems are undetectable in liver from the fetus. Before such a species "difference" is given too much importance, it must be shown that these pregnant women were not exposed to chemicals which can induce or stimulate these systems in the fetus. This will be discussed below.

Some correlations of enzyme activity with hepatic structure and ultra-structure

Drug-metabolizing enzyme systems are not randomly or evenly distributed throughout the liver. Relatively few studies of these enzyme distributions have been made and the results may not be of general applicability. We do know that Kupfer cells seem to acetylate sulfanilamide and p-aminobenzoic acid, whereas parenchymal cells do this poorly if at all (Govier, 1965). Also, the early studies of Wattenberg and Leong (1962) showed that polycyclic hydrocarbon metabolism was concentrated in parenchymal cells especially in the region of central veins. This latter work has been extended in several other studies on NADPH-requiring systems that (a) can be detected histochemically and (b) probably reflect at least the activity of parts of the hepatic microsomal drug-metabolizing enzyme systems. Nearly all work has been done in adult rats. Most of these studies indicated that enzymes linked with hepatic microsomal drug metabolism were in parenchymal cells and in high quantities in those cells clustered around the central veins. Relatively lower amounts of these enzymes were found midzonally or periportally (Kalina, 1968; Koudstaal and Hardonk, 1969, 1970). Thus, not all liver cells have these systems, and even within a given type of cell (e.g., parenchymal), not all cells are equally active.

Within a given liver parenchymal cell, there may be further localization. Despite some differences of opinion, there is a continually growing body of evidence that these hepatic microsomal enzyme systems may be relatively concentrated in only one kind of endoplasmic reticulum. Thus, oxidative drug metabolisms may have two- to sixfold higher specific activity in hepatic smooth-surfaced endoplasmic reticulum than in rough-surfaced endoplasmic reticulum (Fouts, 1961; Gram, Rogers, and Fouts, 1967a), whereas glucuronide conjugations may be relatively concentrated in rough-surfaced rather than smooth-surfaced endoplasmic reticulum (Gram, Hansen, and Fouts, 1968). Ratios of enzyme activity in rough-surfaced vs. smooth-surfaced hepatic microsomes will depend on the type of metabolism and particular substrate used, as well as the animal species (Gram, Schroeder, Davis, Reagan, and Guarino, 1971), the method of isolation of the microsomes from the liver homogenate (Gram et al., 1967a), which can even include effects by the centrifuge rotor used (Fouts, Rogers, and Gram, 1966; Bergstrand and Dallner, 1969; Fouts, 1971, especially page 310), and—most important—whether the animal has been previously exposed to conditions, chemicals, or drugs which can markedly alter hepatic microsomal drug metabolism. Ratios of enzyme activity in rough- vs. smooth-surfaced microsomes can be shifted dramatically by prior exposure of the animals to microsomal enzyme inducers, especially 3-methylcholanthrene (Gram, Rogers, and Fouts, 1967b; Fouts and Gram, 1969; Glaumann, 1970).

The localization of hepatic drug metabolism in hepatic parenchymal cells, especially those around central veins, and in some cases in only one kind of endoplasmic reticulum, can be most important to understanding drug metabolism by liver in the fetus and newborn. Thus, the inability to detect drug metabolism in the fetus in most species correlates with the small proportion of parenchymal liver cells (relative to reticuloendothelial cells) in the fetal liver and with the absence or very small amounts of smooth-surfaced endoplasmic reticulum in those parenchymal cells that are present in fetal liver. Presence of certain glucuronyl transferase activities at almost adult levels in late fetal or early postnatal life would be compatible with localization of some glucuronyl transferases in rough-surfaced endoplasmic reticulum (rather than smooth-surfaced) and the relative abundance of that rough-surfaced endoplasmic reticulum at these times just before and after birth.

Two recent papers by Leskes, Siekevitz, and Palade (1971a,b) are particularly interesting since these authors studied development of the hepatic endoplasmic reticulum and a microsomal enzyme (glucose-6-phosphatase) in the period just before and after birth. Several points should be mentioned: (1) at and before birth, the only form of endoplasmic reticulum that was identified was rough-surfaced; there was no smooth-surfaced endoplasmic reticulum; (2) not all cells having rough-surfaced endoplasmic reticulum had active glucose-6-phosphatase (histochemical stain)—this was especially true in the fetus; (3) glucose-6-phosphatase appeared simultaneously in all the rough-surfaced endoplasmic reticulum of a given cell, although its appearance was asynchronous in the hepatocyte population as a whole in the fetus; and (4) the smooth-surfaced endoplasmic reticulum developed asynchronously in hepatocytes after birth; various stages of development of smooth-surfaced membranes were found in cells during the first few hours of life. These results seem to indicate (1) that during late fetal life and at the time of birth, there can be cells with highly or at least moderately active endoplasmic reticulum alongside cells which are metabolically silent, and (2) that all parenchymal cells might not acquire drug-metabolizing enzymes at the same time, but that *within* a given cell, all endoplasmic reticulum might become active at the same moment. Such a concept of discontinuity is quite at variance with most "evidence" gathered at gross levels of integration (i.e., age vs. activity of enzyme per gram liver) which appeared to suggest a gradual and generalized assumption of function by all cells. Instead of a gradually increasing "glow" of enzyme activity in all cells, we may have individual cells "turning on" in gradually increasing *numbers*. One caution should be mentioned, however. The enzyme marker used by Leskes et al. (1971a,b) was glucose-6-phosphatase. This has no known structural continuity or functional relationship with microsomal drug-metabolizing enzymes. The study by Leskes et al. (1971a,b) points to a new concept which should now be tested with the hepatic microsomal drug-metabolizing enzyme systems.

Some correlations of enzyme activity with drug toxicity

In many cases, metabolism of a drug by hepatic microsomal enzymes leads to less active and less toxic metabolites. Thus, the hepatic microsomal enzyme systems can be a part of the body's defenses against chemicals and drugs. Other mechanisms for terminating drug action or getting rid of drugs do exist (e.g., storage in body fat, binding to blood and tissue proteins, excretion by lung, kidney, gut), and drug metabolism can produce more, rather than less, active or toxic metabolites. Nevertheless, the relative lack of drug-metabolizing enzyme systems in liver of fetus and newborn has often been cited as one of the major reasons for increased susceptibility of fetus and newborn of animals and humans to drugs and other chemicals to which they may become exposed indirectly via administration to the mother or directly as when treating the sick infant.

Generalized principles of drug usage in premature and newborn infants have been stated often. These can usually be summarized as "give less" and monitor carefully for effects. Quantification of dose for use in such very young infants is often based on some "magic" formula such as mg/kg or mg/square meter of body surface area. Such dose calculations may be extremely desirable, but their use may be most dangerous. Most such calculations are based on an assumption that body mechanisms for eliminating drugs are maturing in proportion to the denominator (e.g., body weight or surface area). This is only an approximation of the facts since these mechanisms involve absorption, distribution, excretion, metabolism, as well as receptor-like sensitivity and response to drugs, and the age dependencies of the functions of these processes are a series of curves that do *not* belong to the same family. Indeed, many of these curves show marked discontinuities, so that a few hours or days can affect function of that system, relative to a given dose of drug or chemical, several-fold. Recognition of the multiple causes and erratic nature of age-related changes in drug action and toxicity cannot be overemphasized, in my opinion.

As hepatic drug-metabolizing enzyme systems mature with age, there is often a marked change in drug action and toxicity in newborn to which metabolizable drugs are given. A recent tabulation of LD_{50} values in newborn and adult animals has been most useful to us in our research and emphasizes this principle (Goldenthal, 1971). In concluding this section I wish to emphasize two points. Drugs or chemicals whose toxicity is largely dependent on metabolism by hepatic microsomal enzymes usually show large shifts in LD_{50} with increasing age (e.g., many barbiturates and tranquilizers). However, drugs eliminated largely by excretion, rather than metabolism, often show quite different patterns of change and even little change in LD_{50} with increasing age (e.g., some antibiotics).

Stimulation or "induction" of hepatic microsomal enzymes in fetus and newborn

One of the first attempts to stimulate hepatic drug-metabolizing enzymes in fetal and newborn animals was made by Inscoe and Axelrod (1960). Many chemicals and drugs exist which, when given to weanling or adult animals, can increase the amount or activity of the hepatic microsomal enzymes metabolizing drugs and steroids. Most of these stimulators or inducers appear to act indirectly. Thus, most of these inducers do not enhance drug metabolism if added directly to the drug-metabolizing enzyme assay systems *in vitro,* but they do act if injected into the whole animal several hours before sacrifice or if they are allowed to perfuse through the intact liver (Juchau, Cram, Plaa, and Fouts, 1965) or be in contact with fetal tissue in culture for several hours (Nebert and Gelboin, 1968) long enough to allow the synthesis of new enzyme by an active enzyme-synthesizing system in liver.

The success of Nebert and Gelboin in inducing active microsomal drug-metabolizing enzymes in cultures of whole hamster embryos is in sharp contrast with the lack of enzyme induction in fetuses from mothers pretreated with enzyme inducers as reported by Inscoe and Axelrod (1960). Our own results also indicated that giving the enzyme inducer phenobarbital to the pregnant rabbit did not cause induction of hepatic microsomal enzymes in the fetus until just before birth (Hart, Adamson, Dixon, and Fouts, 1962). Lack of response of the fetus to enzyme inducers given the mother could be of multiple causation. Since the inducer is given to the mother, it may not reach the fetus in amounts adequate to induce microsomal enzymes in the fetal liver. However, our results showed that, just before birth, the fetus was able to respond to enzyme inducers, and that this response increased (matured) even more with age after birth (Hart et al., 1962). These results would seem to indicate a multiple defect in response to microsomal enzyme induction in the fetus. We postulated that in early fetal life there may be both a defect in enzyme-synthesizing systems as well as a lack of a proper stimulus (inducer) for these hepatic systems. In late fetal life or in the neonatal rabbit, the enzyme-forming systems can respond, but the stimulus is lacking. Providing an *exogenous* stimulus (phenobarbital or benzpyrene) leads to enzyme induction.

A variation on the theme that lack of response of fetus to inducers of drug metabolism is due to a restriction of access of fetus to inducer is indicated in the article by Singer and Litwack (1971). These authors showed that uptake of cortisol by fetal liver is much less than by liver in newborn rats and very much less than in adult rats. Both qualitative and quantitative changes were involved, since the major binder (protein) of cortisol in fetal rat liver cytosol was a minor binder in adult liver cytosol. The ability of cortisol to induce liver tyrosine transaminase could be correlated with these changes in cortisol-binding protein. Extrapolating these findings to the hepatic drug-metabolizing systems, one might postulate that lack of response of the fetal enzymes to inducers like benzpyrene or phenobarbital might be related to inability of these inducers to be bound by the fetal tissue or by the right protein in the fetal tissues. To my knowledge, studies testing such an hypothesis have not been made.

Another explanation for lack of fetal response to inducers of hepatic microsomal drug metabolism might be the presence of a repressor or inhibitor to enzyme synthesis in the fetus and/or newborn. This is an attractive possibility since it would help explain why induction can be seen in tissue culture, but perhaps[1] not in the whole animal. The paper by Klinger, Zwacka, and Ankermann (1968) is therefore most interesting since these workers seem to have found such a repressor in the fetal rat liver. Induction of hepatic drug-metabolizing enzymes in the weanling rat by injections of these rats with phenobarbital could be inhibited by pretreatment of the rat with supernatant fractions prepared from fetal rat liver (but not from other fetal organs or from adult animal liver). Such an inhibitor or repressor might be diluted out in tissue culture, allowing response of such cultured cells to inducers of drug metabolism. Gradually increasing ability to respond to inducers of drug metabolism—seen as the newborn animal matures—would reflect gradually decreasing quantities of the repressor or inhibitor (adult liver did not have the inhibitor of induction according to Klinger et al., 1968). Along these same lines, Netter (1971) reported that in rats the development of glucuronyl transferase in tissue culture is delayed by the presence of fetal serum and enhanced by the presence of adult serum.

I return now to a point mentioned in the first section of this chapter, the apparent presence in the human fetus of detectable levels of hepatic microsomal drug-metabolizing components as reported by Yaffe et al. (1970) and Ackermann and Rane (1971). Because of the ubiquitous nature of chemicals and drugs which can induce or stimulate hepatic microsomal drug metabolism in animals and man, there remains the question of whether the presence of these enzyme systems in the human fetus might not be a result of the pregnant woman's exposure to such enzyme inducers. The widespread use of drugs in pregnancy, and the occurrence of hepatic enzyme-inducing chemicals in so many parts of our environment[2] make a truly "unexposed" human almost impossible to find. It is much easier to isolate experimental

---

[1] The word "perhaps" is used because exactly comparable experiments have not been done. Thus, the same animal species, the same inducer, and the same hepatic microsomal enzyme responses have *not* been studied by all groups. For example, Inscoe and Axelrod (1960) used benzpyrene and methylcholanthrene as inducers, but assayed glucuronide conjugation on rats. Hart et al. (1962) used phenobarbital as the inducer and assayed hexobarbital, aminopyrine, and p-nitrobenzoic acid metabolism in the rabbit. Nebert and Gelboin (1969) have used polycyclic hydrocarbons and related inducers of benzpyrene hydroxylase in cultures of hamster embryos.

[2] Polycyclic hydrocarbons capable of inducing hepatic microsomal enzymes are found in polluted air and in many cooked or smoked meats (charcoal-broiled meats, smoked meat and fish). Insecticides capable of hepatic enzyme effects are found in inhaled dusts and sprays, food, and water. Industrial pollutants capable of causing stimulation of hepatic enzymes are in water, food, and air (e.g., polychlorinated biphenyls).

animals from such effectors than even to minimize exposure to such inducers in the case of humans. In my opinion, the ability of the human fetus to metabolize drugs is likely to be highly variable and to apply to only a few drugs. The *detection* of fetal drug metabolism in humans is probably not an indication of difference from most other animals wherein the fetus seems to lack these systems unless the mother has been exposed to enzyme inducers. Such a prediction (variable, low levels of some drug metabolisms, absence of most in the human fetus) is supported by some recent literature (Netter, 1971; Pelkonen, Vorne, Jouppila, and Karki, 1971).

RECENT WORK BY THE AUTHOR—DRUG METABOLISM IN LIVER AND LUNG OF NEWBORN RABBITS

Liver vs. lung microsomal drug metabolisms in the adult rabbit

It has been known for many years that drugs could be metabolized in tissues other than liver. However, if asked to name the organ where most drugs would be metabolized, or where the quantitatively most important part of one drug's metabolism would occur, most people would probably say the liver. Certainly, the studies that have been made with widely used drugs usually confirm this impression. Although exceptions can be cited, the liver is the site where most drugs and chemicals which enter the body are metabolized most extensively.

Metabolism of drugs and chemicals by nonhepatic tissue may be important in explaining tissue-specific drug-induced pathology or toxicology. We have been most interested in drug metabolism by organs in more-or-less constant contact with the environment. As part of this interest, we have begun a series of studies of chemical and drug metabolisms by the lung.

We have done most of our studies on rabbit lung since we and others (Oppelt, Zange, Ross, and Remmer, 1970; Bend, Hook, and Gram, 1971a; Bend, Hook, Gram, and Fouts, 1971b; Hook, Bend, Fouts, and Gram, 1971; Bend, Hook, Easterling, Gram, and Fouts, 1972; Hook, Bend, Hoel, Fouts, and Gram, 1972) have shown that this species has easily detectable levels of several microsomal drug-metabolizing enzymes and components in lung. We have made a study of methods by which to prepare representative samples of lung drug-metabolizing systems and have described the morphology and some of the biochemistry of the lung microsomal fraction as compared with liver microsomes (Hook et al., 1972). We have also studied optimal conditions for and kinetics of the metabolism *in vitro* of several drugs by lung microsomes, inhibitors of these enzymes, and the drug-microsome difference spectra produced when drugs were added to suspensions of lung microsomes (Bend et al., 1972). Both quantitative and qualitative differences were seen and were numerous. A number of similarities were also seen, and among the most interesting was the level of activity of several drug-metabolizing enzymes. Thus, benzphetamine and ethylmorphine were demethylated and biphenyl was hydroxylated at comparable rates in lung and liver microsomes when activity was expressed per unit of microsomal protein. If enzyme activity was expressed per unit of cytochrome P450, then lung microsomes were *more* active than liver microsomes for many substrates, since lung P450 content was much less than liver P450 content per mg protein (Bend et al., 1972).

Liver and lung microsomal drug metabolisms in the newborn rabbit

Because of my interest in drug metabolism in the fetal and newborn animal, my recent studies have concerned the metabolism of drugs by the lung in the newborn rabbit and a comparison of the rate of development of these systems in lung and liver. Most of these results are being readied for publication and some were presented at the annual meeting of the Society of Toxicology in March 1972.

As with liver, most of the components measured[3] were in very low quantity in the lungs from the just-born animal. We have not yet been able to study enzyme levels in the fetal lung because of the limits in our assay systems.

If one can make generalizations at all, it would seem from our data that the maturation curves of the rabbit liver microsomal systems often showed a discontinuity between 2 and 4 weeks of age—there were large increases in several hepatic microsomal components during this time. With comparable lung systems, we often did not see such marked changes, but instead a more gradual and uniform increase occurred. This is typified by the behavior of cytochrome P450 and benzpyrene hydroxylase (Table 1). Adult tissue levels of the components studied were often reached at or before 1 month of age in the case of liver but not lung. Some of our results are summarized in Tables 1 and 2.

---

[3] Enzymes and components measured in lung microsomes of newborn, 2 weeks, 1-month-old, and adult Dutch-belted rabbits included: (a) cytochrome P450, (b) cytochrome b_5, (c) protein, (d) NADPH-cytochrome c reductase, (f) demethylation of benzphetamine, (g) demethylation of aminopyrine, (h) hydroxylation of benzpyrene, and (i) various difference spectra produced by adding drug substrates to suspensions of microsomes.

TABLE 1. *Microsomal components in rabbit liver and lung at three ages.*

Component	Tissue	Age and % of adult value		
		3-5 days	2 weeks	1 month
Cytochrome P450	liver	22	39	100
	lung	26	35	56
Cytochrome b₅	liver	50	80	100
	lung	50	75	90
TPNH-cytochrome c reductase	liver	75	90	130
	lung	52	61	90
Benzpyrene hydroxylation	liver	25	19	85
	lung	25	50	75
Benzphetamine demethylation	liver	19	24	90
	lung	13	21	62
Aminopyrine demethylation	liver	9	30	100
	lung	10	25	60

Methods for measuring these components in liver and lung microsomes as well as preparation and characterization of liver and lung microsomes are given in the papers by Hook et al. (1972) and Bend et al. (1972). All values are given as % of adult levels of the component.

We have attempted to measure NADPH-cytochrome P450 reductase in rabbit lungs at various ages and have encountered a problem worth discussion. This enzyme may be the rate-limiting step in the metabolism of drugs by the hepatic, microsomal mixed-function oxidase system (Gigon, Gram, and Gillette, 1969; Kupfer and Orrenius, 1970). Its activity is affected by the presence of substrates (Gigon et al., 1969) as well as by ionic strength and cations such as Mg^{++} (Fouts and Pohl, 1971). We have studied this "P450-reductase" in liver microsomes from rats and rabbits of varying ages and in lung microsomes from rabbits of varying ages. A major problem arose when attempts to measure this enzyme were made using microsomes having small amounts of cytochrome P450. The reaction is quantified on the basis of the amount of cytochrome P450 reduced per unit time per unit protein or phospholipid. The reaction rate, especially in the presence of substrates or metal ions, can be very rapid, and zero or even first-order kinetics are obeyed only for short periods of time even with a lot of cytochrome P450 present. Using liver microsomes from adult animals, we have found that a plot of P450 reduced vs. time is usually a curve, although initial time periods can appear to be nearly linear (the first 5 sec of the reaction on the Aminco-Chance spectrophotometer, using the rapid-mixing cell). With the small amounts of cytochrome P450 present in liver, or es-

TABLE 2. *Adult levels of microsomal components of rabbit liver and lung.*

Component	Tissue	N	Adult concentration (mean ± SE)	Units
Cytochrome P450	liver	25	1.81 ± 0.48	nmoles/mg protein
	lung	12	0.39 ± 0.14	nmoles/mg protein
Cytochrome b_5	liver	18	1.10 ± 0.10	nmoles/mg protein
	lung	12	0.19 ± 0.04	nmoles/mg protein
TPNH-cytochrome c reductase	liver	19	89 ± 5	nmoles of cytochrome c reduced per mg protein
(without added KCl)	lung	13	116 ± 11	per min
Benzphetamine demethylation	liver	22	9.8 ± 1.9	nmoles HCHO per
	lung	10	14.7 ± 5.0	mg protein per min
Benzpyrene hydroxylation	liver	11	725 ± 62	fluorescence units per
	lung	10	150 ± 25	mg protein per min
Aminopyrine demethylation	liver	4	9.5 ± 1.0	nmoles HCHO per
	lung	4	3.1 ± 0.6	mg protein per min

Methods of assay: see footnote to Table 1. N refers to number of individual animals used.

pecially lung, microsomes of fetal and newly born rabbits, we have not been able to quantify P450 reductase activity—the reaction runs out of "substrate" (cytochrome P450) too quickly.

Another problem should at least be mentioned. We quantify microsomal drug metabolism in liver in terms of drug metabolized per unit time per milligram of microsomal protein. We can compare adult enzyme activity and fetal or newborn enzyme activity on such a basis or on the basis of total enzyme activity per organ. If we compare on the basis of specific enzyme activity, then we assume that the microsomal fractions of adult and young animals are comparable. If, however, enzymes normally associated with microsomes in the adult are associated with other cell fractions in the fetus, then misleading answers can result. Chatterjee, Price and McKee (1965) have reported that fetal rat liver microsomes sediment at low g forces— much lower than adult or even newborn rats. Thus, the fraction sedimenting between 200 and 8,000 g in fetal liver homogenates contained 95% microsomes with the rest of the pellet having mitochondria and other particles. In the 14-day-old or adult liver, the 8,000 g sediment was almost pure mitochondria (Chatterjee et al., 1965).

We have made studies on some components of the mixed-function oxidase system and on some drug metabolisms that in the adult organ (liver

TABLE 3. *Recovery of benzphetamine-metabolizing enzyme in fractions of liver and lung homogenates of newborn and adult rabbits.*

Animal age and sample	Benzphetamine metabolism per min	
	(nmoles/mg microsomal protein)	(nmoles/g tissue)
Adult liver homogenate	13	207
9,000 *g* supernatant	11	180
microsomes	10	164
Adult lung homogenate	37	183
9,000 *g* supernatant	26	130
microsomes	20	100
6-day-old liver homogenate	2.1	15
9,000 *g* supernatant	1.8	13
microsomes	1.5	11
6-day-old lung homogenate	5.3	24
9,000 *g* supernatant	3.0	15
microsomes	2.3	13

Methods of assay: see footnote to Table 1.

and lung) in the rabbit are concentrated in microsomes. We have compared activity or concentration of these components in homogenate, 9,000 *g* supernatant, or microsomal fractions from these homogenates. A typical experiment is shown in Table 3. We will continue such studies, but some conclusions seem possible and can be summarized:

(1) In the period from birth to 1 month of age in the rabbit, the microsomal fraction from liver homogenates is a representative sample of the hepatic endoplasmic reticulum of these ages. The microsomal fraction contains well over two-thirds of the total mixed-function oxidase activity of the liver homogenate at all ages. This suggests to us that the hepatic microsomal fraction contains most of the microsomes present in the whole homogenate of liver and can be considered a valid measure of liver drug-metabolizing enzyme activity.

(2) Rabbit lung microsomal fractions contain less of the total enzyme activity of the homogenate than do comparable fractions of liver. Nevertheless, the data now in hand indicates that lung microsomes do contain at least 50% of the total component or enzyme activity present in the homogenate. We do not yet have enough data to determine if the fraction of total homogenate activity found in lung microsomes varies significantly with age of the animal. Our data do *not* suggest that such variability, if it occurs, will be huge. The relatively poorer harvest of lung microsomes from the homogenate (in contrast with liver) may be due to less efficient homogena-

tion of lung and/or the fibrous network in which lung microsomes can be enmeshed (Hook et al., 1972).

CONCLUSIONS

Drug-metabolizing enzyme systems normally found in the microsomes of liver and lung in adult animals are absent or in very low quantities in microsomes from these organs of the fetus or newborn. Some stimulation of these "detoxification" systems may be possible in the fetus and newborn of both animals and man. Whether and how much stimulation can be produced may depend on the species of animal, the stimulator used (both amount and route of administration), the time it is given (both in terms of birth as well as duration of treatment with stimulator), and the particular organ and drug metabolism pathway that is being measured. In my opinion, no generalities should be expected because of the many possibilities for modulation of stimulatory response by factors as yet only suspected, e.g., environment, genetics, or unexpected exposures to anti-inducers.

Development of drug-metabolizing enzyme systems in liver and lung (and probably other organs) as the animal matures will affect drug and chemical effects on the animal. Drug and chemical effects may change with age both qualitatively and quantitatively as various activation and inactivation pathways for the chemical (or drug) mature or disappear at different rates. Coupled with changes in drug and chemical metabolism will be changes with age in all other factors governing the body's handling of chemicals, i.e., absorption, distribution, excretion, and interaction of chemicals with active sites for pharmacologic or toxicologic effects. Thus, although chemical or drug metabolism is a major determinant of drug actions, it is but one of the many factors that interact to determine eventually the biological response to the chemical or drug.

REFERENCES

Ackermann, E., and Rane, A. (1971): The monooxygenase system in the human fetal liver: subcellular distribution and studies on *in vitro* metabolism of aniline. *Chemico-Biological Interactions*, 3:233-234.

Basu, T. K., Dickerson, J. W. T., and Parke, D. V. W. (1971): Effect of development on the activity of microsomal drug-metabolizing enzymes in rat liver. *Biochemical Journal*, 124:19-24.

Bend, J. R., Hook, G. E. R., Easterling, R. E., Gram, T. E., and Fouts, J. R. (1972): A comparative study of the hepatic and pulmonary microsomal mixed-function oxidase systems in the rabbit. *Journal of Pharmacology and Experimental Therapeutics* (*in press*).

Bend, J. R., Hook, G. E. R., and Gram, T. E. (1971*a*): Study of the mixed function oxidase system in rabbit lung. *Federation Proceedings*, 30:282.

Bend, J. R., Hook, G. E. R., Gram, T. E., and Fouts, J. R. (1971*b*): Mixed function oxidase (MFO) activity of microsomal fractions from rabbit lung and liver. *Pharmacologist*, 13:245.

Bergstrand, A., and Dallner, G. (1969): Isolation of rough and smooth microsomes from rat liver by means of a commercially available centrifuge. *Analytical Biochemistry*, 29:351-356.

Chatterjee, J. B., Price, Z. H., and McKee, R. W. (1965): Biosynthesis of L-ascorbic acid in different sub-cellular fractions of prenatal and postnatal rat livers. *Nature*, 207:1168-1170.

Fouts, J. R. (1961): The metabolism of drugs by subfractions of hepatic microsomes. *Biochemical and Biophysical Research Communications*, 6:373-378.

Fouts, J. R. (1971): Liver smooth endoplasmic reticulum "microsomal" drug-metabolizing enzyme system. In: *Methods in Parmacology*, Vol. 1, edited by Arnold Schwartz. Appleton-Century-Crofts, New York, pp. 287-325.

Fouts, J. R., and Adamson, R. H. (1959): Drug metabolism in the newborn rabbit. *Science*, 129:897-898.

Fouts, J. R., and Gram, T. E. (1969): The metabolism of drugs by subfractions of hepatic microsomes. The case for microsomal heterogeneity. In: *Microsomes and Drug Oxidations*, edited by J. R. Gillette, A. H. Conney, G. J. Cosmides, R. W. Estabrook, J. R. Fouts, and G. J. Mannering. Academic Press, New York, pp. 81-91.

Fouts, J. R., and Pohl, R. J. (1971): Further studies on the effects of metal ions on rat liver microsomal reduced nicotinamide adenine dinucleotide phosphate-cytochrome P-450 reductase. *Journal of Pharmacology and Experimental Therapeutics*, 179:91-100.

Fouts, J. R., Rogers, L. A., and Gram, T. E. (1966): The metabolism of drugs by hepatic microsomal enzymes. Studies on intramicrosomal distribution of enzymes and relationships between enzyme activity and structure of the hepatic endoplasmic reticulum. *Experimental and Molecular Pathology*, 5:475-490.

Gigon, P. L., Gram, T. E., and Gillette, J. R. (1969): Studies on the rate of reduction of hepatic microsomal cytochrome P450 by reduced nicotinamide adenine dinucleotide phosphate: Effect of drug substrates. *Molecular Pharmacology*, 5:109-122.

Glaumann, H. (1970): Chemical and enzymatic composition of microsomal subfractions from rat liver after treatment with phenobarbital and 3-methyl-cholanthrene. *Chemico-Biological Interactions*, 2:369-380.

Goldenthal, E. I. (1971): A compilation of LD_{50} values in newborn and adult animals. *Toxicology and Applied Pharmacology*, 18:185-207.

Govier, W. C. (1965): Reticuloendothelial cells as the site of sulfanilamide acetylation in the rabbit. *Journal of Pharmacology and Experimental Therapeutics*, 150:305-308.

Gram, T. E., Hansen, A. R., and Fouts, J. R. (1968): The submicrosomal distribution of hepatic UDP-glucuronyl transferases in the rabbit. *Biochemical Journal*, 106:587-591.

Gram, T. E., Rogers, L. A., and Fouts, J. R. (1967*a*): Further studies on the metabolism of drugs by subfractions of hepatic microsomes. *Journal of Pharmacology and Experimental Therapeutics*, 155:479-493.

Gram, T. E., Rogers, L. A., and Fouts, J. R. (1967*b*): Effect of pretreatment of rabbits with phenobarbital or 3-methylcholanthrene on the distribution of drug-metabolizing enzyme activity in subfractions of hepatic microsomes. *Journal of Pharmacology and Experimental Therapeutics*, 157:435-445.

Gram, T. E., Schroeder, D. H., Davis, D. C., Reagan, R. L., and Guarino, A. M. (1971): Enzymic and biochemical composition of smooth and rough microsomal membranes from monkey, guinea pig and mouse liver. *Biochemical Pharmacology,* 20:1371-1381.

Hart, L. G., Adamson, R. H., Dixon, R. L., and Fouts, J. R. (1962): Stimulation of hepatic microsomal drug metabolism in the newborn and fetal rabbit. *Journal of Pharmacology and Experimental Therapeutics,* 137:103-106.

Henderson, P. Th. (1971): Metabolism of drugs in rat liver during the perinatal period. *Biochemical Pharmacology,* 20:1225-1232.

Hook, G. E. R., Bend, J. R., Fouts, J. R., and Gram, T. E. (1971): Comparative distribution of particulate marker enzymes in rabbit liver and lung. *Pharmacologist,* 13:245.

Hook, G. E. R., Bend, J. R., Hoel, D., Fouts, J. R., and Gram, T. E. (1972): Preparation of lung microsomes and a comparison of the distribution of enzymes between subcellular fractions of rabbit lung and liver. *Journal of Pharmacology and Experimental Therapeutics (in press).*

Inscoe, J. K., and Axelrod, J. (1960): Some factors affecting glucuronide formation *in vitro. Journal of Pharmacology and Experimental Therapeutics,* 129:128-131.

Jondorf, W. R., Maickel, R. P., and Brodie, B. B. (1959): Inability of newborn mice and guinea pigs to metabolize drugs. *Biochemical Pharmacology,* 1:353.

Juchau, M. R., Cram, R. L., Plaa, G. L., and Fouts, J. R. (1965): The induction of benzpyrene hydroxylase in the isolated perfused rat liver. *Biochemical Pharmacology,* 14:473-482.

Kalina, M. (1968): Heterogeneity of reduced pyridine nucleotide-tetrazolium reductase system in rat liver. *Laboratory Investigation,* 18:278-282.

Klinger, W., Zwacka, G., and Ankermann, H. (1968): Untersuchungen zum Mechanisms der Enzyminduktion. VIII. Die Übertragung eines zytoplasmatischen Hemmfaktors der Entwicklung Mikrosomaler Leberenzyme aus der Leber von Rattenfoeten auf infantile Ratten. *Acta biologica medizinisch germanica,* 20:137-145.

Koudstaal, J., and Hardonk, M. J. (1969): Histochemical demonstration of enzymes related to NADPH-dependent hydroxylating systems in rat liver after phenobarbital treatment. *Histochemie,* 20:68-77.

Koudstaal, J., and Hardonk, M. J. (1970): Histochemical demonstration of enzymes in rat liver during postnatal development. *Histochemie,* 23:71-81.

Kupfer, D., and Orrenius, S. (1970): Interaction of drugs, steroids, and fatty acids with liver-microsomal cytochrome P450. *European Journal of Biochemistry,* 14:317-322.

Leskes, A., Siekevitz, P., and Palade, G. E. (1971a): Differentiation of endoplasmic reticulum in hepatocytes. I. Glucose-6-phosphatase distribution *in situ. Journal of Cell Biology,* 49:264-287.

Leskes, A., Siekevitz, P., and Palade, G. E. (1971b): Differentiation of endoplasmic reticulum in hepatocytes. II. Glucose-6-phosphatase in rough microsomes. *Journal of Cell Biology,* 49:288-302.

Nebert, D. W., and Gelboin, H. V. (1968): Substrate-inducible microsomal aryl hydroxylase in mammalian cell culture. I. Assay and properties of induced enzyme. *Journal of Biological Chemistry,* 243:6242-6249.

Netter, K. J. (1971): Arzneimittelaufnahme und-abbau während der Fetalperiode. *Archiv für Gynäkologie,* 211:112-133.

Oppelt, W. W., Zange, M., Ross, W. E., and Remmer, H. (1970): Comparison of microsomal drug hydroxylation in lung and liver of various species. *Research Communications in Chemical Pathology and Pharmacology,* 1:43-56.

Pelkonen, O., Vorne, M., Jouppila, P., and Karki, N. T. (1971): Metabolism of chlorpromazine and p-nitrobenzoic acid in the liver, intestine, and kidney of the human fetus. *Acta Pharmacologica et Toxicologica,* 29:284-294.

Singer, S., and Litwack, G. (1971): Effects of age and sex on H³-cortisol uptake, binding and metabolism in liver and on enzyme induction capacity. *Endocrinology,* 88:1448-1455.
Wattenberg, L. W., and Leong, J. L. (1962): Histochemical demonstration of reduced pyridine nucleotide dependent polycyclic hydrocarbon metabolizing systems. *Journal of Histochemistry and Cytochemistry,* 10:412-420.
Yaffe, S. J., Rane, A., Sjöqvist, F., Boréus, L. O., and Orrenius, S. (1970): The presence of a mono-oxygenase system in human fetal liver microsomes. *Life Sciences,* part II, 9:1189-1200.

Fetal Pharmacology, edited by L. Boréus
Raven Press, New York © 1973

Oxidation and Reduction of Foreign Compounds in Tissues of the Human Placenta and Fetus

M. R. Juchau, Q. H. Lee, G. L. Louviaux*, K. G. Symms,
J. Krasner, and S. J. Yaffe

*Departments of Pharmacology and Obstetrics-Gynecology, School of Medicine,
University of Washington, Seattle, Washington 98105, and Department of
Pediatrics, School of Medicine, State University of New York at Buffalo,
Buffalo, New York 14222*

INTRODUCTION

Alterations in the chemical structure of drug molecules very frequently result in profound modifications in the spectrum of pharmacologic and/or toxicologic effects produced by such molecules. This is true whether the alteration occurs as a consequence of chemical manipulation prior to introduction of the molecule into a biological system (e.g., by the medicinal chemist), or as a result of biotransformation following drug administration. Therefore, before the actions of drugs and foreign compounds upon a given biological system can be predicted accurately, an understanding of the chemical modifications which such compounds will undergo during their sojourn within the system must be understood. Realization of these fundamental principles, coupled with an awareness of the enormous dearth of understanding with respect to the effects of drugs on the developing human conceptus, has led us to initiate systematic studies on drug biotransformation in the human feto-

---

* Present address: Los Alamitos Clinic, Los Alamitos, California 90813.

placental unit. Several reviews dealing with drug biotransformation in the human placenta have appeared recently in the literature (Juchau and Yaffe, 1969; Juchau, 1971a,b,c, 1972; Juchau and Dyer, 1972); this chapter is concerned with research results obtained since the submission for publication of the aforementioned reviews.

OXIDATIVE REACTIONS IN THE HUMAN PLACENTA

With respect to the oxidation of drug substrates, biotransformation reactions occur via two principal processes: dehydrogenation (in which hydrogens are removed from the drug substrate and transferred to an endogenous acceptor, such as NAD or NADP), and mixed-function oxidation (in which one atom of molecular oxygen is incorporated into the drug molecule and the second atom reduced to water). Currently, interest is centered about the latter process which proceeds at particularly rapid rates in the presence of enzyme systems concentrated in the endoplasmic reticulum of hepatic cells. Recently, Kuntzman, Lu, West, Jacobson, and Conney (1971) isolated from these subcellular structures two cytochromes (P-450 and P-448), which serve as terminal oxidases for such reactions, and, in reconstituted systems, have demonstrated that each exhibits definitive drug substrate specificity. Drug substrates also have been categorized with respect to the manner in which they bind to the terminal oxidase. Those which bind directly to the heme moiety by virtue of a free primary amino group (i.e., aniline, amphetamine) exhibit type II difference spectra when added to suspensions of rat liver microsomes, with maxima at approximately 430 nm and minima at about 395 nm. Those which bind to hydrophobic sites on the oxidase exhibit type I difference spectra when added to rat liver microsomal suspensions, with maxima at approximately 385 nm and minima at 420 nm. Substrates which produce type I difference spectra, however, may be specific for P-450 (ethylmorphine, aminopyrine, benzphetamine, hexobarbital, etc.) or for P-448 (3,4-benzpyrene, 3-methylcholanthrene, or 3-methyl-4-monomethylaminoazobenzene). Thus, at present, three separate substrate categories may be said to exist with reference to mixed-function oxidations of drugs. These will be referred to as follows: category I, with aminopyrine as prototype; category II, with aniline as prototype; and category III, with 3,4-benzpyrene as prototype. Such a classification is particularly useful in discussions of drug metabolism in the placenta and fetus.

Human placenta and oxidation of substrates in category I

Van Petten, Hirsch, and Cherrington (1968) reported rates of pentobarbital metabolism in 9,000 $\times$ g supernatant fractions of human, term placental homogenates which approached rates observed in corresponding rat liver preparations. Welch, Harrison, Gomni, Poppers, Finster, and Conney, (1969), however, were unable to detect significant pentobarbital-2-^{14}C oxidation. Other investigators (Creaven and Parke, 1965) also have reported negative results with respect to the oxidation of substrates in category I. In our own experience, we have failed repeatedly in attempts to demonstrate significant oxidation of substrates in this category either during early gestation (Juchau, Niswander, and Yaffe, 1968) or at term (Juchau and Yaffe, 1969). Substrates examined included hexobarbital, aminopyrine, chlorpromazine, zoxazolamine, and codeine.

Human placenta and oxidation of substrates in category II

During studies on benzpyrene hydroxylation in human placental homogenate subfractions, we encountered a placenta which exhibited remarkably high levels of benzpyrene hydroxylase activity (Juchau, 1971b). None of the activity could be detected in 104,000 $\times$ g supernatant fractions, but high activity was observed in each of the particulate fractions examined. Specific activity was highest in a post-mitochondrial pellet (microsomes), which also was analyzed for aniline hydroxylase activity. Although no aniline hydroxylation could be detected in the microsomal fraction of human placentas, a detectable reaction was measured in the presence of rat placental 9,000 $\times$ g supernatant fractions. Subsequent studies (Juchau and Symms, 1971) have led to the discovery that purified preparations of hemoglobin would catalyze an easily measurable aniline hydroxylation reaction. Comparisons of characteristics of the hemoglobin catalyzed reaction with those of the reaction occurring in placental homogenates and subfractions have led to the conclusion that most, if not all, of the reaction proceeding in placental homogenates occurs as a result of catalysis by contaminating hemoglobin. In model systems analyses we have demonstrated that cytochrome c also catalyzes aniline hydroxylation, but is much less efficient than hemoglobin, and displayed characteristics which differed from the hemoglobin-catalyzed reaction. For example, the cytochrome c catalyzed reaction was markedly accelerated by supplementation with xanthine oxidase or flavins, whereas the hemoglobin and placental reactions were not profoundly affected by flavins (10^{-5} to 10^{-3} M) and were inhibited by xanthine oxidase. Myoglobin was nearly as effective as hemoglobin at equal monomer heme concentrations. The results obtained from these studies indicated that placental cells possessed little or no capacity for hydroxylation of aniline. They also indicated separate and distinct mechanisms for the hydroxylation of aniline and 3,4-benzpyrene. In addition, the discovery that several purified heme compounds would catalyze aniline hydroxylation may provide useful models for the study of the development of drug oxidative mechanisms in the feto-placental unit.

Van Petten et al. (1968) reported a very rapid catalysis of amphetamine metabolism in $9,000 \times g$ supernatant fractions of homogenates of human placentas at term, but the mechanism for this reaction remains to be elucidated.

Human placenta and oxidation of substrates in category III

Abundant evidence now exists that oxidation of substrates in this category will occur in placental tissues from a variety of species, including humans. The placental reaction appears to be very similar to that catalyzed in the liver, with a few important exceptions. Both are strongly induced by pretreatment with polycyclic aromatic hydrocarbons, as was first demonstrated by Welch et al. (1969), are similarly inhibited by carbon monoxide and steroids (Juchau, 1971a), and exhibit similar K_m values with respect to 3,4-benzpyrene as substrate in the reaction. In addition, recent studies in our laboratory (*unpublished*) with marker enzymes, electron microscopy, and chemical analyses indicate that the placental enzyme is localized in the endoplasmic reticulum of trophoblast cells. However, important differences between the placental and hepatic reactions were observed. In contrast to the hepatic enzyme system, placental benzpyrene hydroxylase does not appear to be induced by phenobarbital pretreatment (Nebert, Winker, and Gelboin, 1969) and has a much lower apparent affinity for the initial electron donor, NADPH (Juchau, 1971a). Studies on placental benzpyrene hydroxylation during early gestation (8 to 16 weeks) indicated that the enzyme first began to appear in placentas of smokers after the first trimester of pregnancy (Juchau, 1971a), a finding which could have important significance relative to the effects of drugs on the fetus during the more critical stages of development. More recent studies in our laboratories (*unpublished*) have demonstrated that, in certain cases (extensive drug abuse frequently is associated), placental benzpyrene hydroxylase at term may approach levels observed in analogous preparations of hepatic tissues.

Mixed-function oxidation of steroids in human placenta

Extremely important steroid biosynthetic reactions are catalyzed by mixed-function oxidative enzymes present in human placental tissues. The rate-limiting step in the placental conversion of cholesterol to progesterone appears to be the oxidation of the cholesterol side-chain which results in the formation of the intermediate pregnenolone. Rate-limiting for production of placental estrogens is the oxidation of carbon 19 catalyzed by a poorly defined mixed-function oxidative system referred to as aromatase. This system catalyzes the conversion of androgens (testosterone and androstenedione) to estrogens (β-estradiol and estrone). Since studies from several independent laboratories showed that cigarette smoking could profoundly increase placental benzpyrene hydroxylase activity, it was of interest to determine whether smoking could affect other placental monooxygenases. Results of these studies are presented in Table 1. It appears evident from the data that no correlations exist between smoking habits and aromatase or cholesterol side-chain oxidase. Nor were any correlations found between placental benzpyrene hydroxylase and the two latter parameters. Recently, in a preliminary study, Conney et al. (1971) obtained results which indicated no correlations between placental aromatase and benzpyrene hydroxylase, although placentas from only four smokers and three non-smokers were analyzed. Studies by Meigs and Ryan (1968) and Juchau (1971a) with various inhibitors also strongly indicated that these two systems differed in many important respects. Whether or not other placental steroid hydroxylation reactions may be catalyzed by the same system which catalyzes benzpyrene hydroxylation, however, remains to be determined.

REDUCTION REACTIONS IN THE HUMAN PLACENTA

As a general rule, reduction reactions are somewhat less complex than oxidative reactions, and frequently allow a more direct approach to the study of electron-transport systems in tissues. Catalysis of the transfer of electrons to one, two, four, and six electron-acceptor xenobiotic molecules has been demonstrated in human placental homogenates (Juchau and Yaffe, 1969), but only two of these reactions have been studied in any detail: reduction of the azo-linkage of neoprontosil (Juchau, Krasner, and Yaffe, 1968), and the aromatic nitro group of p-nitrobenzoic acid (PNBA) (Juchau, 1969; Juchau, Krasmer, and Yaffe, 1970; Symms and Juchau, 1971).

Reduction of azo-linkages in human placenta

A fairly rapid rate of azo-linkage reduction was observed in the presence of placental homogenates and homogenate subfractions. Characteristics of the placental reaction were strikingly different from those observed in liver homogenates. In the placenta, flavins inhibited the reaction, carbon monoxide did not affect it, activity was highest in the soluble portion of placental homogenates, and azo-reduction was not affected by inducing agents such as phenobarbital or 3-methylcholanthrene. Subsequent investigations revealed that the

TABLE 1. *Influence of cigarette smoking on placental mixed-function oxidases.*

Exp.	Product Formation[a]	Smokers[b]	Non-Smokers
1	Estrone	354 ± 82	180 ± 69
2	β-Estradiol	943 ± 97	1,140 ± 103
3	Total estrogens	1,297 ± 143	1,272 ± 154
4	Testosterone	1,863 ± 126	2,734 ± 182
5	Pregnenolone	31 ± 12	31 ± 10
6	Progesterone	23 ± 13	47 ± 16
7	17α-hydroxyprogesterone	2.2 ± 1.7	3.0 ± 1.9
8	Total side-chain oxidase products	57 ± 19	80 ± 26
9	Hydroxylated benzpyrene	628 ± 213	9 ± 6

[a] In experiments 1 through 4, androstenedione 4-[14]C (0.2 μC) was utilized as substrate and was incubated together with 2.5 ml placental 9,750 × g supernatant fraction, 5 μmoles NADPH, 65 μmoles glucose-6-phosphate, 0.7 μmoles unlabeled androstenedione, and 0.6 ml buffer containing 0.25 M sucrose, 0.04 M nicotinamide, and 0.05 M potassium phosphate at a final pH of 7.05 in a total volume of 3.7 ml. Incubations were carried for 60 min at 37.5°C under an atmosphere of 100% oxygen. Methods for quantitation of metabolites formed (estrone, β-estradiol, and testosterone) are described by Juchau and Lee (*manuscript submitted*). In experiments 5 through 8, cholesterol-4-[14]C (0.5 μC) was utilized as substrate and was incubated together with 3 ml solubilized acetone powder enzyme preparation (in sucrose-nicotinamide-phosphate buffer, pH 7.2), 10 μmoles NADPH, 130 μmoles glucose-6-phosphate, and 15 units glucose-6-phosphate dehydrogenase (Sigma) in a total volume of 3.65 ml. Incubations were carried out for 60 min at 37.5°C under an atmosphere of air. Methods employed to quantitate the amounts of oxidized products formed are described by Juchau and Lee (*manuscript in preparation*). Numbers in the Table indicate nmoles product formed per g protein per hr with standard deviations.

[b] Smokers averaged slightly less than one pack per day.

Six placentas were analyzed for smokers and seven for non-smokers.

enzymic generation of reducing equivalents (NADPH) through a very active placental hexose-monophosphate shunt pathway was the single most important factor in the explanation of enhanced rates of the reduction of the azo-linkage of neoprontosil in human placental tissues. Comparatively large amounts of glucose-6-phosphate and 6-phosphogluconate were found in the soluble fraction. Removal of these substances by dialysis reduced the rate of the placental reaction to that of the spontaneous reaction, strongly suggesting that the only observable enzymic components involved were placental glucose-6-phosphate dehydrogenase and 6-phosphogluconate dehydrogenase. The mechanisms by which placental particulate fractions enhance rates of azo-linkage reduction, however, have not yet been determined.

Since it has been discovered that a variety of heme-containing compounds, including hemoglobin, hematin, and myoglobin, will catalyze aromatic nitro group reduction (next section), it was of interest to determine if such compounds would catalyze azo-linkage reduction in model system (tissue-free) reactions. Utilizing optimal conditions for hemoglobin catalysis of nitro group reduction, however, it was found that this heme compound would not increase the rate of the reaction. Whether other heme compounds catalyze the reaction has yet to be determined.

Reduction of aromatic nitro groups in human placenta

Recent studies with tissue-free (model) systems have indicated that in addition to compounds containing free sulfhydryl groups (reduced glutathione, mercaptoethanol, etc.), several heme-containing compounds, including hematin, are much more effective catalysts in the conversion of PNBA to the corresponding amine, p-aminobenzoic acid (PABA) (Symms and Juchau, 1972). Hemoglobin, methemoglobin, metmyoglobin, myoglobin, cytochrome c, hematin, peroxidase, and catalase were all effective catalysts for the reduction reaction when incubated with FMN or FAD. In addition, purified milk xanthine oxidase catalyzed the six-electron transfer in the absence of added flavins but, unlike heme catalysts, exhibited heat lability. Cyanocobalamin, chlorophyllin, copper phthalocyanine, and ferrous salts (with or without EDTA) were not measurably active, indicating that the structure of the porphyrin compound is critical in the catalytic mechanism (Symms and Juchau, 1971). Studies tend to indicate that reduced flavins or flavoproteins will reduce the aromatic nitro group to the nitroso and hydroxylamino intermediates, but that the heme moiety is essential for catalysis of conversion of the hydroxylamine to the primary amine. On the basis of separation techniques and comparisons with reactions in tissue-free model systems, the principal non-dialyzable, heat-stable, carbon monoxide-sensitive catalyst for aromatic nitro group reduction (Juchau, 1971a,b,c) present in soluble fractions of human placental homogenates tentatively has been identified as hemoglobin. More importantly, however, the studies which led to this conclusion have provided important models for the investigation of mechanisms of aromatic nitro group reduction in particulate fractions of placental tissue homogenates, as well as in other tissues of the feto-placental unit.

OXIDATION REACTIONS IN HUMAN FETAL TISSUES

Classical concepts of drug metabolic processes have implied that capacity for mixed-function oxidations of drug substrates is essentially nonexistent in fetal tissues, particularly during the earlier stages of gestation. Such concepts have arisen largely as a result of research with experimental animals (Jondorf, Maickel, and Brodie, 1959; Fouts and Hart, 1965; Short and Davis, 1970). However, very recent studies originating from the Karolinska Institute (Yaffe, Rane, Sjöqvist, Boréus, and Orrenius, 1970; Rane, Sjöqvist, and Orrenius, 1971; Ackermann and Rane, 1971) tend to imply that the human fetus may differ from fetuses of other animal species with regard to drug metabolizing capabilities. Studies in our own laboratories tend to confirm these concepts.

Human fetus and oxidation of substrates in category I

Yaffe et al (1970) reported variable levels of aminopyrine N-demethylase activity in microsomes derived from human fetal livers at 14 to 25 weeks of gestation. These investigators reported that each of the electron-transport components essential for mixed-function oxidation of drug substrates was present in human fetal liver microsomes during this early period of gestation. In a more recent report, Rane et al. (1971) reported oxidation of desmethylimipramine, testosterone, and laurate in similar microsomal preparations. Pelkonen, Vorne, Jouppila, and Kärki (1971) also recently have reported significant oxidation of chlorpromazine in 12,000 $\times$ g supernatant fractions of fetal livers between the 8th and 26th weeks of gestation. We have been unable to detect significant levels of aminopyrine N-demethylase or hexobarbital oxidase activities in 9,000 $\times$ g supernatant fractions of human fetal livers between the 10th and 16th weeks of gestation.

Human fetus and oxidation of substrates in category II

Ackermann and Rane (1971) have recently reported the detection of aniline hydroxylase activity in 200 $\times$ g pellet fractions of human fetal livers. In our laboratories, we have detected readily measurable *p*-aminophenol formation following incubation of several fetal tissue homogenates (*unpublished results*). These include 9,000 $\times$ g supernatant and pellet fractions of human fetal liver, adrenal, lung, kidney, and brain. In the first four tissues, specific activities were higher in the supernatant fraction and followed this order: adrenal > liver > kidney > lung. In brain tissues, on the other hand, activity was localized in the 9,000 $\times$ g pellet fraction. In view of the results indicating that any of a number of heme compounds would catalyze aniline hydroxylation *in vitro* (as mentioned earlier), considerably more effort will be required to determine the mechanism by which this xenobiotic is hydroxylated in human fetal tissues. Of particular interest, however, is the high specify activity exhibited in the human fetal adrenal gland. This high specific activity observed in fetal adrenal gland homogenates corresponds with observations (reported later) on benzpyrene hydroxylase, nitro-reductase, and azo-reductase activities, each of which exhibited highest specific activities in the adrenal gland between the 12th and 16th weeks of gestation. The adrenal may play a very important role in the metabolism of drugs in the human fetus.

Human fetus and oxidation of substrates in category III

Utilizing 9,000 $\times$ g supernatant fractions of human fetal liver homogenates, we were unable to detect significant benzpyrene hydroxylase activity between the 8th and 16th weeks of gestation, regardless of the smoking habits of the mother (Juchau, 1971a). Other investigators have also failed to detect activity of this enzyme system in human fetal liver microsomes (Yaffe et al., 1970; Rane et al., 1971). Recently, however, we have been able to observe comparatively high levels of activity in whole homogenates of human fetal adrenal, kidney, and liver tissues at 16 weeks gestation (*unpublished results*). Very low levels were also detected in placental homogenates, but significant activity could not be observed in brain or lung tissues. One mother had a history of considerable drug-taking but had smoked cigarettes only during the first month of pregnancy (two packs per week). Another had been on chronic diphenylhydantoin therapy. Specific activity in the adrenal gland approached that observed in rat liver 9,000 $\times$ g supernatant fractions, whereas that in the liver was significantly lower. Since tissue-free model systems which catalyzed aniline hydroxylation and nitrobenzoic acid reduction would not carry the benzpyrene hydroxylase reaction, we feel that these findings are particularly interesting and significant.

REDUCTION REACTIONS IN HUMAN FETAL TISSUES

Reduction of aromatic nitro groups

Several investigators have reported that human fetal liver tissues contain catalysts for the reduction of aromatic nitro groups (Stambaugh and Manthei, 1970; Pelkonen et al., 1971; Juchau, 1971c). In our laboratories, human fetal liver, adrenal gland, kidney, brain, and lung were investigated during early gestation (7 to 18 weeks), with respect to capacity for aromatic nitro group reduction. Of the tissues studied, the adrenal glands displayed the highest specific activities, particularly near mid-term gestation. Catalytic activity was readily demonstrable in whole homogenates of fetal liver, even at 7 weeks gestation. The catalytic activity in liver, adrenal, kidney, and lung was shown to be due to factors other than hemoglobin or methemoglobin, since heat denaturation (boiling) of dialyzed fractions markedly reduced nitro-reductase activity (*unpublished results*), whereas denaturation of hemoglobin or methemoglobin by heating or a variety of other procedures does not affect its catalytic activity with respect to aromatic nitro group reduction (Symms and Juchau, 1972). In the absence of added flavins, however, significant activity was observed only in adrenal and liver preparations. Again, most adrenal preparations exhibited considerably higher specific activities than corresponding liver preparations.

Reduction of azo-linkages

Comparatively high specific activities with respect to the reduction of the azo-linkage of neoprontosil were observed in whole homogenates of human fetal tissues (*unpublished results*). Unlike the reaction which proceeds in the presence of preparations of placental tissues at term, however, addition of flavins (FMN or FAD at 5×10^{-4} M final concentration) accelerated rather than inhibited the reaction catalyzed by components of fetal tissues. Again the fetal adrenal gland and liver displayed the highest specific activities, emphasizing the potential of these organs to modify the effects of drugs in the developing human conceptus.

ACKNOWLEDGMENTS

The authors gratefully acknowledge the technical assistance of Mrs. Carolyn Tocha, Miss Patricia Loftis, and Mr. Mark Pedersen in these studies. We also wish to acknowledge the excellent cooperation of the Department of Obstetrics and Gynecology and Pathology of the Children's Hospital, Buffalo, New York, and of the Central Embryology Laboratory in the University Hospital, Seattle, Washington. Special thanks are extended to Dr. Kenneth Niswander and Dr. Thomas Shepard, who were particularly helpful in securing the necessary human tissues for these studies, as well as supplying competent advice and information. Original research reported was supported by NICHD Grant HD-04839 and a grant from the National Foundation (March of Dimes).

REFERENCES

Ackermann, E., and Rane, A. (1971): The monooxygenase system in human fetal liver: Subcellular distribution and studies on *in vitro* metabolism of aniline. *Chemico-Biological Interactions,* 3:233-234.

Conney, A. H., Welch, R., Kuntzman, R., Chang, R., Jacobson, M., Munroe-Faure, A. D., Peck, A. W., Bge, A., Poland, A., Poppers, P. J., Finster, M., and Wolff, J. A. (1971): Effects of environmental chemicals on the metabolism of drugs, carcinogens and normal body constituents in man. *Annals of the New York Academy of Sciences,* 179:155-172.

Creaven, P. J., and Parke, D. V. (1965): The effect of pregnancy on the microsomal metabolism of foreign compounds. *Federation of the European Biochemical Society,* 128:88A.

Fouts, J. R., and Hart, L. G. (1965): Hepatic drug metabolism in the perinatal period. *Annals of the New York Academy of Sciences,* 123:245-251.

Jondorf, W. R., Maickel, R. P., and Brodie, B. B. (1958): Inability of newborn mice and guinea pigs to metabolize drugs. *Biochemical Pharmacology,* 1:352-354.

Juchau, M. R. (1969): Studies on the reduction of aromatic nitro groups in human and rodent placental homogenates. *Journal of Pharmacology and Experimental Therapeutics,* 165:1-8.

Juchau, M. R. (1971a): Human placental hydroxylation of 3,4-benzpyrene during early gestation and at term. *Toxicology and Applied Pharmacology,* 18:665-675.

Juchau, M. R. (1971b): Mechanisms of drug biotransformation reactions in the placenta *Federation Proceedings,* 31:48-53.

Juchau, M. R. (1971c): Drug biotransformation in the human fetus: Nitro group reduction. *Archives Internationales de Pharmacodynamie et de Thérapie,* 194:204-216.

Juchau, M. R. (1972): Drug biotransformation reactions in the placenta. In: *Perinatal Pharmacology,* edited by B. Mirkin. Academic Press, New York.

Juchau, M. R., and Dyer, D. C. (1972): Pharmacology of the placenta. *Pediatric Clinics of North America,* 19:65-79.

Juchau, M. R., Krasner, J., and Yaffe, S. J. (1968): Studies on reduction of azo-linkages in human placental homogenates. *Biochemical Pharmacology* 17:1969-1979.

Juchau, M. R., Krasner, J., and Yaffe, S. J. (1970): Model systems for aromatic nitro group reduction—relationships to tissue catalyzed reactions. *Biochemical Pharmacology,* 19:443-455.

Juchau, M. R., Niswander, K. R., and Yaffe, S. J. (1968): Drug metabolizing systems in homogenates of human immature placentas. *American Journal of Obstetrics and Gynecology,* 100:348-357.

Juchau, M. R., and Symms, K. G. (1971): Mechanism of catalysis of aniline hydroxylation in placental homogenates. *The Pharmacologist,* 13:465A.

Juchau, M. R., and Yaffe, S. J. (1969): Biotransformations of drug substrates in placental homogenates. In: *The Foeto-Placental Unit,* edited by A. Pecile and C. Finzi. Excerpta Medica Foundation, Amsterdam.

Kuntzman, R., Lu, A. Y. H., West, S., Jacobson, M., and Conney, A. H. (1971): The importance of cytochrome P-450 and P-448 in determining the specificity of the reconstituted liver microsomal hydroxylation system. *Chemico-Biological Interactions,* 3:287-289.

Meigs, R. A., and Ryan, K. J. (1968): Cytochrome P-450 and steroid biosynthesis in the human placenta. *Biochimica et Biophysica Acta,* 165:476-487.

Nebert, D. W., Winker, J., and Gelboin, H. V. (1969): Aryl hydrocarbon hydroxylase activity in human placenta from cigarette smoking and non-smoking women. *Cancer Research,* 29:1763-1768.

Pelkonen, O., Vorne, M., Jouppila, P., and Kärki, N. T. (1971): Metabolism of chlorpromazine and *p*-nitrobenzoic acid in the liver, intestine and kidney of the human fetus. *Acta Pharmacologica et Toxicologica,* 29:284-294.

Rane, A., Sjöqvist, F., and Orrenius, S. (1971): Cytochrome P-450 in human fetal liver microsomes. *Chemico-Biological Interactions,* 3:305-307.

Short, C. R., and Davis, L. E. (1970): Perinatal development of drug-metabolizing enzyme activity in swine. *Journal of Pharmacology and Experimental Therapeutics,* 174:185-192.

Stambaugh, J. E., and Manthei, R. W. (1970): The development of drug metabolizing enzymes in human fetal liver. *Federation Proceedings,* 29:348A.

Symms, K. G., and Juchau, M. R. (1971): Heme catalysis of aromatic nitro group reduction in model systems. *The Pharmacologist,* 13:223A.

Symms, K. G., and Juchau, M. R. (1972): The mechanism of aromatic nitro group reduction in the soluble fraction of human placenta. *Biochemical Pharmacology,* 21:2417-2426.

Van Petten, G. R., Hirsch, G. H., and Cherrington, A. D. (1968): Drug metabolizing activity of the human placenta. *Canadian Journal of Biochemistry,* 46:1057-1064.

Welch, R. M., Harrison, Y. E., Gomni, B. W., Poppers, P. J., Finster, M., and Conney, A. H. (1969): Stimulatory effect of cigarette smoking on the hydroxylation of 3,4-benzpyrene and the N-demethylation of 3-methyl-4-monomethyl aminoazobenzene by enzymes in human placenta. *Clinical Pharmacology and Therapeutics,* 10:100-109.

Yaffe, S. J., Rane, A., Sjöqvist, F., Boréus, L. O., and Orrenius, R. (1970): The presence of a monooxygenase system in human fetal liver microsomes. *Life Sciences,* 9:1189-1200.

DISCUSSION

RÄIHÄ: You showed that benzpyrene hydroxylase was not inducible in the placenta by smoking early in gestation, whereas it could be induced later. At what stage of gestation did this inducibility appear, and could you also show this lack of inducibility in early rat placentas?

JUCHAU: We were unable to demonstrate significant induction in human placentas by cigarette smoking at very early periods of gestation, and it appears to us that the capacity of the placental system to be induced increased with gestational age. The inducibility did not suddenly appear at a certain stage of gestation but appeared to increase as a continuum. We have shown marked induction of rat-placental enzyme hydroxylase by pretreatment with 3-methylcholanthrene as early as 13 days in gestation, but inducibility appears to be maximal at approximately 17 days gestation.

NEUBERT: Microsomal drug oxidizing systems certainly are rather unspecific with respect to drugs. But, on the other hand, evidence has accumulated on the existence of multiple systems. Almost 10 years ago, we found in hepatomas the absence of most N-demethylating systems but presence of the capacity to oxidize cocaine. Therefore, many drugs have to be included in such studies with fetal tissues, and it is hard to extrapolate on the metabolism of drugs from data that have been obtained on other foreign substances.

JUCHAU: I agree. We have chosen to study drug substrates that have been intensively investigated in the rat liver, a common model in studies of drug metabolic processes. By choosing model substrates for each of the various reaction types and studying these reactions in detail, we hope to gain insights into aspects of drug biotransformation in tissues of the fetus and placenta.

MIRKIN: Have you investigated any species which demonstrate the stage in phylogeny at which the sub-human liver begins to resemble the human in its drug metabolizing capacity?

JUCHAU: We have investigated tissues of the monkey (*Macaca nemestrina*) fetus in which the pattern of drug biotransformation appears to be similar, although only very preliminary studies have been completed in this respect. The pattern of development of drug metabolizing enzymes in human hepatic systems, however, appears to differ markedly from that observed in common laboratory animals such as rabbits, rats, mice, etc.

McBRIDE: From your study, have you any definite views on the advisability of women smoking during pregnancy?

JUCHAU: Studies in cell cultures have shown that those cells which metabolize 3,4-benzpyrene are more susceptible to the toxicity (cell death) of 3,4-benzpyrene than are cells which do not metabolize this compound. The epoxide intermediate is very reactive and is suspected to be a primary factor in cellular toxicity of polycyclic hydrocarbons and are presumed also to be proximate carcinogens. On the other hand, induction of benzpyrene hydroxylase has been shown to protect against the carcinogenicity of such compounds. Recent studies have suggested that separate enzymes catalyze conversion to the epoxide and to the subsequent hydroxylated product. It may be that the relative activity of such enzymes could be a principal determinant of the cellular effects produced by polycyclic aromatic hydrocarbons. The fact that human placental and fetal tissues can hydroxylate benzpyrene quite actively does not indicate that cigarette smoking is advisable during pregnancy.

Fetal Pharmacology, edited by L. Boréus
Raven Press, New York © 1973

Possible Influence of Drugs on Fetal Steroid Metabolism

Gyula Telegdy

Department of Physiology, University Medical School, Pecs, Hungary

Over the last 10 years, increased attention has been centered on the steroidogenesis in the human fetus. It became evident that the human fetus develops in a special hormonal environment which is formed from maternal, placental, and fetal sources. The placenta and fetus, forming the feto-placental unit, play a special and probably the most important role in establishing this hormonal environment. The function of the feto-placental unit in steroid metabolism has been repeatedly reviewed (Diczfalusy, 1967, 1968, 1970*a*; Mitchell, 1967; Solomon, Bird, Lind, Iwamiya, and Young, 1967). At midgestation, the fetus and placenta complement each other in such a way that the unit is able to elaborate all biologically important steroids that the fetus and placenta are unable to produce alone in significant quantities (Diczfalusy, 1970*b*). Steroids produced in one compartment will reach the other compartment via the umbilical circulation and then be further metabolized. When the steroids return to the original compartment, the metabolism may proceed further. In this way, the feto-placental unit is able to synthesize all biologically active steroids.

STEROIDOGENESIS IN THE HUMAN FETO–PLACENTAL UNIT

In this section the most important steroidogenetic steps taking place in the human feto-placental unit at midgestation are summarized. For further details the following reviews are recommended: (Diczfalusy, 1967, 1968, 1970a,b); Mitchell (1967); and Solomon et al. (1967).

The results presented here are based mainly on perfusion experiments carried out by E. Diczfalusy and co-workers at the Swedish Medical Research Council, Reproductive Endocrinology Research Unit, Karolinska Hospital, Stockholm. The period of gestation was between the 14th and 20th weeks.

The midterm fetus is able to utilize acetate for sterol (squalene, lanosterol, and cholesterol) synthesis (Telegdy, Weeks, Lerner, Stakeman, and Diczfalusy, 1970b; Mathur, Archer, Wiqvist, and Diczfalusy, 1970; Van Leusden, Siemerink, Telegdy, and Diczfalusy, 1971), while the placenta is unable to carry out these reactions (Telegdy et al., 1970b; Telegdy, Weeks, Wiqvist, and Diczfalusy, 1970c; Van Leusden, Siemerink, Telegdy, and Diczfalusy, 1971). In the fetus, the *de novo* synthesized cholesterol is metabolized to pregnenolone and dehydroepiandrosterone (DHA) mainly via a conjugated pathway (Telegdy, Weeks, Archer, Wiqvist, and Diczfalusy, 1970a; Archer, Mathur, Wiqvist, and Diczfalusy, 1971), circulating cholesterol mainly via an unconjugated pathway (Telegdy et al., 1970a) (Fig. 1).

The placenta utilizes circulating cholesterol for the synthesis of pregnenolone and progesterone (Solomon, Lenz, Vande Wiele, and Lieberman, 1954; Solomon, 1960; Jaffe, Eriksson, and Diczfalusy, 1965; Jaffe and Peterson, 1966; Telegdy et al., 1970c). Progesterone is the major precursor of corticosteroids in the fetus where it can also be reduced and hydroxylated (Bird, Solomon, Wiqvist, and Diczfalusy, 1965; Bird, Wiqvist, Diczfalusy, and Solomon, 1966) (Fig. 2). Pregnenolone reaching the fetus from the placenta is mainly sulfurylated in the fetus, and the free pregnenolone is converted to DHA and conjugated to dehydroepiandrosterone sulfate (DHA-S) and then to 16α-DHA and 16α-DHA-S. (Pion, Jaffe, Wiqvist, and Diczfalusy, 1967; Solomon et al., 1967).

The conjugated steroids are hydrolyzed in the placenta. Androstenedione

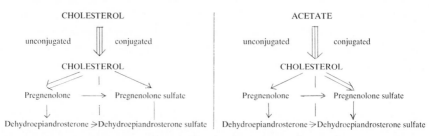

FIG. 1. Acetate and cholesterol metabolism in the human midterm fetus.

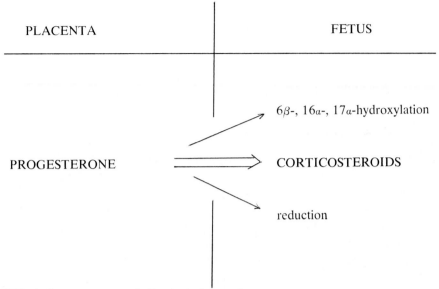

PLACENTA | FETUS

6β-, 16α-, 17α-hydroxylation

PROGESTERONE ⟹ CORTICOSTEROIDS

reduction

FIG. 2. Progesterone metabolism in the human fetus.

and testosterone are formed from DHA. From androstenedione estrone is synthesized, and from testosterone estradiol-17β (Bolte, Mancuso, Eriksson, Wiqvist, and Diczfalusy, 1964; Dell'Acqua, Mancuso, Eriksson, Ruse, Solomon, and Diczfalusy, 1967; Lamb, Mancuso, Dell'Acqua, Wiqvist, and Diczfalusy, 1967; Reynolds, Mancuso, Wiqvist, and Diczfalusy, 1968; Schwers, Vancrombreucq, Govaerts, and Diczfalusy, 1971). In the fetus, estriol is formed from estrone via 16-hydroxylation and subsequent reduction of the 17-oxo group, and via 16-hydroxylation from estradiol-17β (Schwers, Eriksson, and Diczfalusy, 1965; Benagiano, Kincl, Zielske, Wiqvist, and Diczfalusy, 1967). This is the "phenolic" pathway leading to estriol synthesis. Physiologically this pathway is probably the less important pathway leading to estriol synthesis (Fig. 3). 16α-DHA and 16α-DHA-S formed in the fetus reaching the placenta will be hydrolyzed and then converted to 16α-androstenedione and to estriol. This is the most important "neutral" pathway of estriol synthesis in the feto-placental unit (Dell'Acqua et al., 1967) (Fig. 4).

The estrogens in the fetal organism are extensively conjugated into sulfates (Diczfalusy, 1953; Diczfalusy, Cassmer, Alonso, and De Micquel, 1961a,b; Diczfalusy, Cassmer, Alonso, De Micquel, and Westin, 1961c),

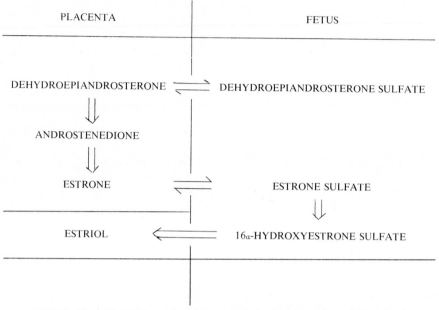

FIG. 3. Phenolic pathway of estriol synthesis in the human feto-placental unit.

glucosiduronates, or sulfate-glucosiduronate double conjugates (Mikhail, Wiqvist, and Diczfalusy, 1963).

The fetus is unable to convert significant amounts of Δ^5-compounds to the corresponding Δ^4-steroids because of insufficient activity of the Δ^4-Δ^5 isomerase-3β-hydroxysteroid dehydrogenase enzyme (Bolte, Wiqvist, and Diczfalusy, 1966; Solomon et al., 1967). However, some Δ^4-androgens formed in the placenta can also be aromatized in the fetal liver (Mancuso, Dell'Acqua, Eriksson, Wiqvist, and Diczfalusy, 1965; Mancuso, Benagiano, Dell'Acqua, Shapiro, Wiqvist, and Diczfalusy, 1968).

The major steroidogenetic pathways described above are operating in the human feto-placental unit at midterm. Whether the conditions are the same at very early or late pregnancy has yet to be determined.

The biological role of free steroids, steroid conjugates, and reductive and oxidative metabolites are poorly understood. Any extrapolation as to the function of these compounds must rely on the uncertain supposition that these steroids are acting in a similar way in animal and human adults. Also, little is known about the regulation of steroid formation in prenatal life. The fetus alone is capable of synthesizing mainly the Δ^5-type of steroids

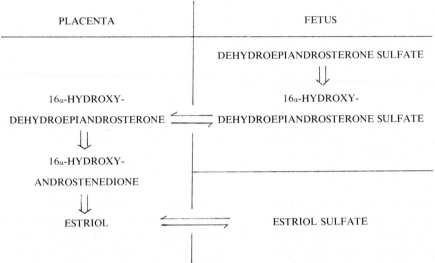

FIG. 4. Neutral pathway of estriol synthesis in the human feto-placental unit.

from small molecules. A large number of steroids, however, are formed from placental precursors. Because of the distribution of steroidogenetic enzymes between the fetus and placenta, certain drugs may effect the fetal steroidogenetic reactions primarily in the fetus or secondarily in the placenta by altering its steroid production.

The amount of information available about drug action on human fetal steroidogenesis is very limited. Even data from animal experiments are scarce. At present one must operate on the assumption that certain drugs can influence steroidogenesis in the fetal and feto-placental unit in the same way as in animals and in human adults.

FACTORS INFLUENCING STEROIDOGENESIS

Hormones

ACTH. It is still open for discussion if ACTH, under physiological conditions, can cross the placental barrier. It has been shown that in the decapitated rat fetus the decreased fetal liver glycogen cannot be restored by adrenalectomy of the mother (e.g., Jost, 1969). However, significant adrenal enlargement can be induced (Knobil and Briggs, 1955). This finding would indicate that some of the ACTH from the maternal side may enter into the fetal circulation. In the human, metopirone induces an endogenous increase of ACTH in the fetus which will increase the androgen production in the fetus and a concomitant increase in estrogen production in the feto-placental unit (Oakey and Heys, 1970). The same effect can be achieved by intravenous administration of ACTH (Dässler, 1966). This would indicate that in the human fetus ACTH may be one of the factors controlling the adrenal androgen production.

HCG. The role of human chorionic gonadotrophin (HCG) in steroidogenesis is still not clear. It has been shown that HCG given intraamniotically at midpregnancy induces ultrastructural changes in the fetal adrenal cortex, indicating increased secretory activity (Johannisson, 1968). HCG given to the newborn results in a significant increase in urinary DHA excretion (Lauritzen, 1966). On the basis of placental perfusion experiments carried out on midterm and term placentas, it has been suggested that HCG may control the conversion of androgens to estrogens in the placenta (Cedar, Alsat, Urtasun, and Varangot, 1968). These data would indicate that HCG may influence both fetal and placental steroidogenesis.

Corticoids given to the fetus in animal experiments produce atrophy of the fetal adrenals (e.g., Jost, 1969). In the human, corticoids suppress the androgen production in the fetal adrenal, decrease the androgen level in cord blood (Simmer, Dignam, Easterling, Frankland, and Naftolin, 1966), and reduce estriol production (Warren and Cheatum, 1967; Oakley and Heys, 1970). It has also been shown that cortisone and cortisol treatment is teratogenic, causing cleft palate in the mouse and cardiac abnormalities in the rabbit (e.g., Tuchmann-Duplessis, 1969). In the human no definite conclusion can be drawn. However, the data of Popert (1962) would indicate that there is a possible teratogenic hazard of corticoid treatment given to pregnant women. It remains to be established if there is any correlation between changes in steroidogenesis induced by exogenous corticoid treatment and malformation of the fetus.

Drugs influencing steroidogenesis

In this section the drugs effecting sterol synthesis and metabolism are not included: readers may consult the review of Dorfman (1963). Some of these drugs have been used for therapeutical purposes in certain endocrine disorders (for review see Temple, 1970).

Clofibrate (chlorophenoxyisobutyrate) is used clinically to reduce the serum level of lipids including cholesterol (e.g., Best and Duncan, 1965). In rats, after clofibrate treatment, the corticosterone secretion is decreased *in vivo* (Huffman and Azarnoff, 1967), and the effect of ACTH on corticoid production is blocked (Saffran, Saffran, and Salhanick, 1970). It has been shown that in bovine adrenal mitochondrial preparations the activity of 11β-hydroxylase is inhibited (McIntosh, Uzgiris, and Salhanick, 1970). In human adults, clofibrate does not seem to influence the unstimulated adrenal function (Berry, Smith, Moxham, Kellie, and Nabarro, 1963). How this drug would influence the fetal adrenal function is not known.

AY-9944 [*trans*-1,4-*bis*(2-chlorobenzylaminomethyl)cyclohexane dihydrochloride] inhibits cholesterol synthesis by inhibiting the reduction of the Δ^7 double bound in the steroid nucleus (Dvornik, Kraml, Dubuc, Givner, and Gaudry, 1963; Kraml, Bagli, and Dvornik, 1964). In rats, AY-9944 decreases the adrenal corticoid production *in vivo* and *in vitro* (Givner, Rochefort, and Dvornik, 1967) and blocks the steroidogenic response to stress (Rochefort, Givner, and Dvornik, 1968).

Aminoglutethimide (Elipten®, Ciba; α-ethyl-*p*-aminophenyl-glutarimide) was used as an anticonvulsant drug until it was established that its prolonged use led to side effects such as hypoadrenocorticism, sexual precocity, and virilization (e.g., Hughes and Burley, 1970).

In animal experiments, aminoglutethimide has been shown to block the conversion of cholesterol to Δ^5-pregnenolone (Camacho, Cash, Brough, and Wilroy, 1967; Cash, Brough, Cohen, Satoh, 1967; Cohen, 1968). Studies carried out on beef adrenal slices and monolayer cultures of functional adrenal tumor cells suggest that this drug inhibits the 20α-hydroxylation of cholesterol (Kahnt and Neher, 1966; Kowal, 1967). In higher concentrations it is a competitive inhibitor of 11β-hydroxylation (Kowal, 1967, 1969).

In the human, aminoglutethimide blocks the synthesis of adrenal cortisol, aldosterone, and androgens (Camacho et al., 1967; Cash et al., 1967; Fishman, Liddle, Island, Fleisher, and Kuchel, 1967). The catabolism of cortisol is also altered possibly by inhibition of 11β-dehydrogenase and by stimulation of Δ^4-3-ketoreductase enzyme (Hagen and Buttler, 1969).

It has been reported that aminoglutethimide induces congenital female pseudohermaphroditism when taken by the mother during pregnancy (Iffy, Ansell, Bryant, and Herrmann, 1965). However, in adult women after several weeks treatment, no significant alterations in estrogen or pregnanediol excretion were observed (Philbert, Laudat, Laudat, and Bricaire, 1966). Long treatment (6 yr) may cause ovarian dysfunction and virilization in young women (Cash, Petrini, and Brough, 1969).

Glutethimide is a compound closely related to aminoglutethimide and is used as a non-barbiturate hypnotic in the human. In rats high doses *in vivo* and *in vitro* are able to block 11-hydroxylation and also 21-hydroxylation (Johnston, Krisle, and Troop, 1968). In human adults, a normal dose (up to 1 g/day) has no significant effect on steroidogenesis (MacMahon and Foley, 1967; Cohen, 1968).

Paraaminoglutethimide and orthoaminoglutethimide can block the 20α-hydroxylation of cholesterol while other closely related drugs such as phenylglutethimide and glutethimide have no effect (Kahnt and Neher, 1966).

Metopirone [Metyrapone®; SU-4885; 2 methyl-1,2,*bis*-(3-pyridyl-1-propanone)] and *SKF 12185* [2-(*p*-aminophenyl)-2-phenyl-ethylamine]. Both compounds are potent inhibitors of 11β-hydroxylase (Jenkins, Meakin, Nelson, and Thorn, 1958; Gabrilov, Nicolis, and Gallagher, 1967 a,b). It has been shown that in higher concentration metopirone is capable of inhibiting 18-hydroxylation (Stachenko and Giroud, 1964; Kraulis and Birmingham, 1965; Erikson, Ertel, and Ungar, 1966; Kahnt and Neher, 1966) and 19-hydroxylation (Griffith, 1963; Giles and Griffith, 1964; Kahnt and Neher, 1966).

In the previable fetus perfused with progesterone and metopirone, the 11β-hydroxylation, 16α- and 17α-hydroxylation of progesterone is blocked. It has been claimed that there was a partial block of 17α-hydroxylation whereas the conjugation with sulfuric acid was unimpaired (Shimao, Wiqvist, Diczfalusy, and Solomon, 1968).

SU-8000 [3-(6-chloro-3-methyl-idenyl)-pyridine], *SU-9055* [3-(1,2,3,4-tetrahydro-1-oxo-2-naphtyl)-pyridine], and *SU-10603* [2-methyl-1,2-*bis*-(3-pyridyl)-1-propanone] are potent inhibitors of 17α-hydroxylation (Chart, Sheppard, Allen, Bencze, and Gaunt, 1958; Givner, Kraml, Dvornik, and Gaudry, 1964). In the rabbit testis, SU-8000 inhibits the biosynthesis of testosterone (Hall, Eik-Nes, and Samuels, 1963) and in rat testicular microsomes the 17-20 lyase activity (Shikita, Ogiso, and Tamaoki, 1965). In pregnant rats treated with SU-8000, a partial inhibition of 17-20 lyase, 17β- and 20α-hydroxysteroid dehydrogenase activity in the fetal testicles could be demonstrated (Bloch, Lew, and Klein, 1971). In adrenal preparations, SU-8000 is also able to block 11β-hydroxylase activity (Sharma, Forchielly, and Dorfman, 1963). The dehydrogenation process of 18-hydroxycorticosterone leading to aldosterone formation is impaired by SU-8000; the 18-hydroxylation of corticosterone can be blocked by SU-9055 (Raman, Sharma, and Dorfman, 1966). The 16α-hydroxylation in the human testis can also be inhibited by SU-9055 (Colla, Liberti, and Ungar, 1966).

Cyanoketone (WIN, 2α-cyano-4,4,17α-trimethyl-17β-hydroxyandrost-5-en-3-one) inhibits the 3β-hydroxysteroid dehydrogenase-Δ^4-Δ^5-isomerase system (Goldman, Yakovac, and Bongiovanni, 1965) thus blocking the conversion of pregnenolone to progesterone (Goldman, 1967). Cyanoketone given to pregnant rats causes retarded development of external genitalia in male fetuses and inhibits the 3β-hydroxysteroid dehydrogenase activity (Goldman, Yakovac, Bongiovanni, 1966). Testicles of cyanoketone-exposed fetuses convert less pregnenolone to DHA, testosterone, and androstenedione (Bloch et al., 1971). In the human fetus, cyanoketone may also interfere with testicular androgen production which may lead to impaired development of sexual organs and altered placental progesterone and androgen production.

F 6060 [*bis*-(*p*-hydroxyphenyl) cyclohexylidene methane; Ferrosan®] and its derivatives *F 6066* and *F 6103* have been shown to alter the progesterone synthesis from pregnenolone in *in vitro* studies of ovaries and adrenals (Larsson and Stensson, 1967). This finding has been supported by histochemical observations (Appelgren, 1969). In mice and rats, F 6060 is an effective abortifacient (Einer-Jensen, 1968), but in the human it has no effect either on implantation or early gestation (Bacic, Engström, Johannisson, Leideman, and Diczfalusy, 1970). How this drug would affect the steroidogenesis in other stages of pregnancy is unknown.

Heparin and heparinoid. It has been repeatedly reported that heparin is able to block aldosterone production via inhibition of 18-hydroxylation of corticosterone (Fachet, Stark, Vallent, and Palkovits, 1962; Gláz and Sugár, 1964; Abbot, Gornall, Sutherland, Stiefel, and Laidlaw, 1966). In rat adrenal tissue, the 11β-hydroxylation of androgens is impaired in the presence of heparin (Lakatos, Koref, Stechek, Holló, and Furr, 1970), and adrenal corticosterone production is also decreased (Fachet et al., 1962; Casperie, Benraad, Kloppenborg, and Majoor, 1967).

Ubiquinone inhibits the production of 18-hydroxycorticosterone and aldosterone in the rat adrenal. It acts most probably as an 18-hydroxylase inhibitor (Kumagai, Nishino, Kimm, Shimomura, Nananhoshi, and Yamamura, 1970). It has been used successfully in the treatment of Conn's syndrome (Kumagai, 1967).

17α-methyltestosterone (17α-methylandrost-4-en-17β-ol-3-one) has been used as an anabolic agent in man. In the rat adrenal, it suppresses the 11β-hydroxylation and possibly 18-hydroxylation *in vitro*. It appears to act as a competitive substrate for hydroxylating enzymes (Rembiesa, Young, and Saffran, 1968). *In vivo* 17α-methyltestosterone may arise from the metabolism of 17α-methylandrost-5-ene-3β-17β-diol (Rembiesa, Holzbauer, Young, Birmingham, and Saffran, 1967).

Danazol [17α-pregn-4-4n-20-yno-(2,3-d) isoxazol-17-ol] inhibits the androgen formation in the Leydig cells and blocks gonadotrophin release in human and in hypophysectomized male rat (Sherins, Gandy, Thorslund, and Paulsen, 1971). The site of action is unknown.

Ethanol increases the reduction of 17-ketosteroids to 17β-hydroxysteroids in superfused guinea pig liver (Admirand, Cronholm, and Sjövall, 1970). In the human, ethanol enhances the concentration of plasma 17-hydroxysteroid sulfates (Cronholm and Sjövall, 1968; Cronholm, Sjövall, and Sjövall, 1969).

Phenobarbital, diphenylhydantoin, and phenylbutazone increase the metabolism of cortisol via the hydroxylation pathway, thus increasing the excretion of 6β-hydroxycortisol in man (Werk, MacGee, and Sholiton, 1964; Burstein and Klaiber, 1965; Kuntzman, Jacobson, and Conney, 1966).

N-Phenylbarbital (phetarbital) increases the polar metabolites of testosterone and excretion of 6β-hydroxycortisol in the human (Southren, Gordon, Tochimoto, Krikun, Kriger, Jacobson, and Kuntzman, 1969).

Thalidomide (N-phthalyl-glutamic acidimide) is a sedative and hypnotic and teratogen in the human. In animal experiments, with high doses of thalidomide a transient stimulation of adrenal corticoid secretion can be achieved. However, long treatment causes a decrease in corticoid production possibly by blocking the neural system (Brode, 1968).

TABLE 1. *Steroidogenic enzymes in the midterm human fetus and placenta and drugs possibly influencing their activities.*

Enzyme	Fetus	Placenta	Drugs[a]
1. Squalene cyclohydroxylase	+	+	
2. C-20-C-22 Lyase	+	+	aminoglutethimide (I)
3. C-17-C-20 Lyase	+	?	SU-8000 (I)
Hydroxysteroid dehydrogenase			
4. 3α-	+	—	
5. 3β-	?	+	cyanoketone (I), F 6060 (I)
6. 6β-	+	+	
7. 11β-	+	+	aminoglutethimide (I)
8. 17α-	+	—	
9. 17β-	+	+	SU-8000 (I), ethanol (S)
10. 18-	+	—	SU-8000 (I), ubiquinone (I)
11. 20α-	+	+	SU-8000 (I)
12. 20β-	+	+	
13. Δ⁴-Δ⁵-isomerase	?	+	cyanoketone, F 6060 (I)
14. Δ⁴-5α-reductase	+	—	aminoglutethimide (S)
15. Δ⁴-5β-reductase	+	—	
16. Aromatizing enzyme system	+	+	HCG (S)

TABLE 1 (continued).

Enzyme	Fetus	Placenta	Drugs[a]
Steroid hydroxylase			
17. 2-	+	+	
18. 6α-	+	+	
19. 6β-	+	+	phenobarbital, diphenylhydantoin, phenylbutazone, phetarbital (S)
20. 7α-	+	—	
21. 7β-	+	—	
22. 11β-	+	—	clofibrate (I), aminoglutethimide (I), glutethimide (I), metyrapone (I), SU-8000 (I), heparin (I), 17α-methyltestosterone (I)
23. 15α-	+	—	
24. 16α-	+	—	metyrapone (I), SU-9055 (I)
25. 16β-	+	—	
26. 17α-	+	?	metyrapone (I), SU-8000 (I), SU-9055 (I), SU-10603 (I)
27. 18-	+	—	metyrapone (I), SU-9055 (I), ubiquinone (I), 17α-methyltestosterone (I)
28. 19-	+	+	aminoglutethimide (I), para-aminoglutethimide (I), ortho-aminoglutethimide (I)
29. 20α-	+	?	aminoglutethimide (I), para-aminoglutethimide (I), ortho-aminoglutethimide (I)
30. 21-	—	+	glutethimide (I)
31. O-Methyltransferase	+	?	
32. Arylsulfotransferase	+	?	
Hydroxysteroid sulfotransferase			
33. 3β-	+	—	
34. 21-	+	—	
35. UDP-Glucuronyltransferase	+	—	
36. β-Glucuronidase	+	—	
37. Arylsulfatase	—	+	
38. Sterolsulfatase	—	+	

? = quantitative significance is questionable or not known.
[a] (I) = inhibition; (S) = stimulation.

Ampicillin [D(-)-α-aminobenzylpenicillin] decreases the maternal plasma and urinary estrogen level in pregnant women (Willman and Pulkkinen, 1971). The mechanism of action is unknown.

The enzymes detected in the fetus and placenta are summarized in Table 1. Some of these enzyme reactions can be influenced by drugs, but for most of these reactions no specific inhibitors or stimulants are known. The distribution of the enzymes shows that certain enzymes are absent in one of the compartments but are present in the other compartment. In this way, the drug may selectively influence the steroidogenesis in one compartment. However, the feto-placental unit is an interdependent system, and a change in steroidogenesis in one compartment will also affect the metabolism in the other compartment. Since the site of action of some of these drugs listed in this review is not known, they are not included in Table 1.

CONCLUDING REMARKS

Although considerable information is available about steroidogenesis in the human fetus, the function of the different steroids formed during pregnancy and the factors regulating this delicate hormonal balance are poorly understood. Further research should be devoted to clarify this problem. Since drugs can influence certain steroidogenetic reactions, this interaction can be used to investigate the physiological significance of these pathways. Furthermore, some of these drugs are also known to interfere with the development of the fetus. Teratogenic nature of specific drugs can be resolved by an investigation of these drugs with relation to steroid synthesis, metabolism, and cellular site of steroid action.

REFERENCES

Abbott, E. C., Gornall, A. G., Sutherland, D. J. A., Stifel, M., and Laidlow, C. (1966): The influence of heparin-like compounds on hypertension, electrolyte and aldosterone in man. *Canadian Medical Association Journal*, 94:1155-1164.

Admirand, W. H., Cronholm, T., and Sjövall, J. (1970): Reduction of dehydroepiandrosterone sulfate in the liver during ethanol metabolism. *Biochimica et Biophysica Acta*, 202:343-348.

Appelgren, L. (1969): Histochemical demonstration of drug interference with progesterone synthesis. *Journal of Reproduction and Fertility*, 19:185-186.

Archer, D. F., Mathur, R. S., Wiqvist, N., and Diczfalusy, E. (1971): Quantitative assessment of the *de novo* sterol and steroid synthesis in the human foeto-placental unit. 2. Synthesis and secretion of steroids and steroid sulphates by the midgestation foetus. *Acta Endocrinologica*, 66:666-678.

Bacic, M., Engström, L., Johannisson, E., Leideman, T., and Diczfalusy, E. (1970): Effect of F-6103 on implantation and early gestation in women. *Acta Endocrinologica*, 64:705-717.

Benagiano, G., Kincl, F. A., Zielske, F., Wiqvist, N., and Diczfalusy, E. (1967): Studies on the metabolism of C-19 steroids in the human foeto-placental unit. *Acta Endocrinologica*, 56:203-220.

Berry, C., Smith, E., Moxham, A., Kellie, A. E., and Nabarro, J. D. N. (1963): The effects of Astromid on the metabolism of adrenal steroids and on plasma lipid fractions. *Journal of Atherosclerosis Research*, 3:380-395.

Best, M. M., and Duncan, C. H. (1965): Reduction of serum triglycerides and cholesterol by ethyl p-chlorophenoxy-isobutyrate (CPIB). *American Journal of Cardiology,* 26:230-233.

Bird, C. E., Solomon, S., Wiqvist, N., and Diczfalusy, E. (1965): Formation of C-21 steroid sulphates and glucosiduronates by previable human foetuses perfused with 4-^{14}C-progesterone. *Biochimica et Biophysica Acta,* 104:623-626.

Bird, C. E., Wiqvist, N., Diczfalusy, E., and Solomon, S. (1966): Metabolism of progesterone by the perfused previable human fetus. *Journal of Clinical Endocrinology and Metabolism,* 26:1144-1159.

Bloch, E., Lew, M., and Klein, M. (1971): Studies on the inhibition of fetal androgen formation: Inhibition of testosterone synthesis in rat and rabbit fetal testes with observation on reproductive tract development. *Endocrinology,* 89:16-31.

Bolté, E., Mancuso, S., Eriksson, G., Wiqvist, N., and Diczfalusy, E. (1964): Studies on the aromatization of neutral steroids in pregnant women. 1. Aromatization of C-19 steroids by placentas perfused *in situ. Acta Endocrinologica,* 45:535-559.

Bolté, E., Wiqvist, N., and Diczfalusy, E. (1966): Metabolism of dehydroepiandrosterone sulphate by the human foetus at midpregnancy. *Acta Endocrinologica,* 52:583-597.

Brode, E. (1968): Experimentelle Untersuchungen mit cyclishen Imiden. *Arzneimittelforschung,* 18:661-665.

Burstein, S., and Klaiber, E. L. (1965): Phenobarbital-induced increase in 6β-hydroxycortisol excretion: Clue to its significance in human urine. *Journal of Clinical Endocrinology and Metabolism,* 25:293-296.

Camacho, A. M., Cash, R., Brough, A. J., Wilroy, R. S. (1967): Inhibition of adrenal steroidogenesis by amino-glutethimide and mechanism of action. *Journal of the American Medical Association,* 202:20-26.

Cash, R., Brough, A. J., Cohen, M. N. P., Satoh, P. S. (1967): Aminoglutethimide (Elipten®, Ciba) as an inhibitor of adrenal steroidogenesis: Mechanism of action and therapeutic trial. *Journal of Clinical Endocrinology and Metabolism,* 27:1239-1248.

Cash, R., Petrini, M. A., and Brough, A. J. (1969): Ovarian dysfunction associated with an anticonvulsant drug. *Journal of the American Medical Association,* 208:1149-1152.

Casperie, A. F., Benraad, T. J., Kloppenborg, P. W. C., and Majoor, C. L. H. (1967): Effect of heparin on the corticosterone secretion rate with description of the double isotope method used. *Acta Endocrinologica,* Suppl. 119:140.

Cédard, L., Alsat, E., Urtasun, M. J., and Varangot, J. (1968): Kinetic study of the action of gonadotropins on estrogenic biosynthesis and glicidic metabolism by human placenta perfused *in vitro.* In: Abstracts of the *International Symposium on the Foeto-placental Unit,* Milan, edited by A. Pecile and G. B. Carruthers. Excerpta Medica, Amsterdam.

Chart, J. J., Sheppard, H., Allen, M. J., Bencze, W. L., and Gaunt, R. (1958): New amphenone analogs as adrenocortical inhibitors. *Experientia,* 14:151-152.

Cohen, M. P. (1968): Aminoglutethimide inhibition of adrenal desmolase activity. *Proceedings of the Society for Experimental Biology and Medicine,* 127:1086-1089.

Colla, J. C., Liberti, J. P., and Ungar, F. (1966): Inhibition of 16α-hydroxylation in human testis by SU-9055. *Steroids,* 8:25-32.

Cronholm, T., and Sjövall, J. (1968): Effect of ethanol on the concentration of solvolyzable plasma steroids. *Biochimica et Biophysica Acta,* 152:233-236.

Cronholm, T., Sjövall, J., and Sjövall, K. (1969): Ethanol induced increase of the ratio between hydroxy- and ketosteroids in human pregnancy. *Steroids,* 13:671-678.

Dässler, C.-G. (1966): Der Einfluss von Corticotropin auf die Östrogen-Ausscheidung in der Schwangerschaft und bei intrauterinem Fruchttod. *Acta Endocrinologica,* 53:401-406.

Dell'Acqua, S., Mancuso, S. S., Eriksson, G., Ruse, J. L., Solomon, S., and Diczfalusy, E. (1967): Studies on the aromatization of neutral steroids in pregnant women. 6.

Aromatization of 16α-hydroxylated C-19 steroids by midterm placentas perfused *in situ. Acta Endocrinologica*, 55:401-414.

Diczfalusy, E. (1953): Chorionic gonadotropin and oestrogen in the human placenta. *Acta Endocrinologica*, Suppl. 12:1-175.

Diczfalusy, E. (1967): Oestrogen and progesterone metabolism in the human foetoplacental unit. *Memoires de l'Academie Royale de Medicine de Belgique*. II, Ser. 6:111-140.

Diczfalusy, E. (1968): *The Foeto-Placental Unit*. Excerpta Medica International Congress Series No. 183, pp. 65-109.

Diczfalusy, E. (1970a): Role of the foetus, placenta and mother in steroidogenesis at midgestation. In: *Advances in the Biosciences*, Vol. 6, edited by G. Raspé. Pergamon Press, Vieweg.

Diczfalusy, E. (1970b): A modified theory of steroid synthesis in the human foetoplacental unit. *Transactions of the 17th Meeting of the German Endocrine Socity*. Springer-Verlag, Berlin, pp. 32-46.

Diczfalusy, E., Cassmer, O., Alonso, C., and De Micquel, M. (1961a): Estrogen metabolism in the human fetus and newborn. *Recent Progress in Hormone Research*, 17:147-206.

Diczfalusy, E., Cassmer, O., Alonso, C., and De Miquel, M. (1961b): Oestrogen metabolism in the human foetus. I. Tissue levels following the administration of 17β-oestradiol and oestriol. *Acta Endocrinologica*, 37:353-375.

Diczfalusy, E., Cassmer, O., Alonso, C., De Miquel, M., and Westin, B. (1961c): Oestrogen metabolism in the human foetus. II. Oestrogen conjugation by foetal organs *in vitro* and *in vivo. Acta Endocrinologica*, 37:516-528.

Dorfman, R. I. (1963): Inhibitors of steroid actions and cholesterol and steroid biosynthesis. In: *Metabolic Inhibitors*, Vol. 1, edited by R. M. Hochster and J. H. Ouastel. Academic Press, New York, pp. 567-585.

Dvornik, D., Kraml, M., Dubuc, J., Givner, M., and Gaudry, R. (1963): A novel mode of inhibition of cholesterol synthesis. *Journal of the American Chemical Society*, 85:3309.

Einer-Jensen, N. (1968): Antifertility properties of two diphenylethenes. *Acta Pharmacologica*, 26, Suppl. 1:1-97.

Erikson, R. E., Ertel, R. J., and Ungar, F. (1966): Effect of SU-4885 on steroid 18-hydroxylation in the mouse adrenal *in vitro. Endocrinology*, 78:343-349.

Fachet, J., Stark, E., Vallent, K., and Palkovits, M. (1962): Some observations on the functional interrelationship between the thymus and the adrenal cortex. *Acta Medica Hungarica*, 18:461-466.

Fishman, L. M., Liddle, G. W., Island, D. P., Fleisher, N., and Kuchel, O. (1967): Effect of aminoglutethimide on adrenal function in man. *Journal of Clinical Endocrinology and Metabolism*, 27:481-490.

Gabrilov, J., Nicolis, G. L., and Gallagher, T. F. (1967a): Effect of SK&F-12185 [DL-2(p-aminophenyl)-2-phenylethylamine] on adrenocortical function in primary aldosteronism. *Journal of Clinical Endocrinology and Metabolism*, 27:1337-1340.

Gabrilov, J. L., Nicolis, G. L., and Gallagher, T. F. (1967b): Effect of DL-2(p-aminophenyl)-2-phenylethylamine on adrenocortical function in Cushing's syndrome due to nontumorous adrenocortical hyperfunction. *Journal of Clinical Endocrinology and Metabolism*, 27:1550-1557.

Giles, C., and Griffith, K. (1964): Inhibition of the aromatization activity of human placenta by SU 4885. *Journal of Endocrinology*, 28:343-344.

Givner, M. L., Kraml, M., Dvornik, D., and Gaudry, R. (1964): An inhibitor of adrenal steroid 11 beta-hydroxylase. *Nature*, 203:317.

Givner, M. L., Rochefort, J. G., and Dvornik, D. (1967): Effect of AY-9944 on rat adrenal function. *Endocrinology*, 81:976-980.

Gláz, E., and Sugár, K. (1964): Effect of heparin and heparinoids on the synthesis of aldosterone and corticosterone by the rat adrenal gland. *Endocrinology,* 74:159-164.

Goldman, A. S. (1967): Experimental congenital adrenocortical hyperplasia: Persistent postnatal deficiency in activity of 3β-hydroxysteroid dehydrogenase produced. *Journal of Clinical Endocrinology and Metabolism,* 27:1041-1049.

Goldman, A. S., Yakovac, W. C., and Bongiovanni, A. M. (1965): Persistent effects of a synthetic androstene derivative on activities of 3β-hydroxysteroid dehydrogenase and glucose-6-phosphate dehydrogenase in rats. *Endocrinology,* 77:1105-1118.

Goldman, A. S., Yakovac, W. C., and Bongiovanni, A. M. (1966): Production of congenital adrenal cortical hyperplasia, hypospadiasis and clitoral hypertrophy (adrenogenital syndrome) in rats by inactivation of 3-beta-hydroxysteroid dehydrogenase. *Proceedings of the Society for Experimental Biology and Medicine,* 121:757-766.

Griffith, K. (1963): Inhibition of 19-hydroxylase activity in the golden hamster adrenal by SU 4884. *Journal of Endocrinology,* 26:445-446.

Hagen, A. A., and Buttler, F. M. (1969): The influence of aminoglutethimide on the catabolism of cortisol-4-C^{14} in the human. *Federation Proceedings,* 28:579.

Hall, P. F., Eik-Nes, K. B., and Samuels, L. T. (1963): Influence of an inhibitor of 17α-hydroxylation on the biosynthesis of testosterone by testicular tissue. *Endocrinology,* 73:547-553.

Huffman, D. H., and Azarnoff, D. L. (1967): The effect of hypocholesterolemic drugs on adrenal corticosteroid secretion. *Steroids,* 9:41-51.

Hughes, S. W. M., and Burley, D. M. (1970): Aminoglutethimide: A side effect turned to therapeutic advantage. *Postgraduate Medical Journal,* 46:409-416.

Iffy, L., Ansell, J. S., Bryant, J. S., and Herrmann, W. L. (1965): Nonadrenal female pseudohermaphroditism: An unusual case of fetal masculinization. *Journal of Obstetrics and Gynecology,* 26:59-65.

Jaffe, R. B., Eriksson, G., and Diczfalusy, E. (1965): *In situ* perfusion of the midterm human placenta with cholesterol. In: Abstracts VI Pan American Congress of Endocrinolgy, Mexico City, edited by A. Stuart Mason and A. Moragas Redecilla. *Excerpta Medica International Congress Series 99.*

Jaffe, R. B., and Peterson, E. P. (1966): *In vivo* steroid biogenesis and metabolism in the human term placenta. 2. *In situ* placental perfusion with cholesterol-7α-^{3}H. *Steroids,* 8:695-710.

Jenkins, J. S., Meakin, J. W., Nelson, D. H., and Thorn, G. W. (1958): Inhibition of adrenal steroids 11-oxygenation in the dog. *Science,* 128:478-480.

Johannisson, E. (1968): The foetal adrenal cortex in the human. Its ultrastructure at different stages of development and in different functional stages. *Acta Endocrinologica,* Suppl. 130:1-107.

Johnston, G. G., Krisle, J. R., Troop, R. C. (1968): Inhibition of adrenal steroidogenesis by glutethimide. *Proceedings of the Society for Experimental Biology and Medicine,* 129:20-23.

Jost, A. (1969): The extent of foetal endocrine autonomy. In: *Foetal Autonomy,* edited by G. E. W. Wolstenholme and M. O'Connor. A. Churchill Ltd., London.

Kahnt, F. W., and Neher, R. (1966): On the adrenal biosynthesis of steroids *in vitro.* Part III. Selective inhibition of adrenocortical function. *Helvetica Chimica Acta,* 49:725-732.

Knobil, E., and Briggs, N. F. (1955): Fetal-maternal interrelations: The hypophyseal-adrenal system. *Endocrinology,* 57:147-152.

Kowal, J. (1967): A possible system for studying ACTH action during complete blockade. *Clinical Research,* 15:455.

Kowal, J. (1969): Adrenal cells in tissue culture. IV. Use of an inhibitor of steroid synthesis for the study of ACTH action. *Endocrinology,* 85:270-279.

Kraml, M., Bagli, J., and Dvornik, D. (1964): Inhibition of the conversion of 7-dehydro-cholesterol to cholesterol by AY-9944. *Biochemical and Biophysical Research Communications,* 15:455-457.

Kraulis, I., and Birmingham, M. K. (1965): Inhibition of the biosynthesis of 18-hy-droxyl-11-desoxycorticosterone by SU-4885. *Canadian Journal of Biochemistry,* 43: 1471-1476.

Kumagai, A. (1967): Cited in: A. Kumagai, K. Nishino, T. Kimm, A. Shimomura, M. Nananhosi, and Y. Yamamura (1970): Inhibitory effect of ubiquinone on biosynthesis of aldosterone in rat adrenal *in vitro. Endocrinologica Japonica,* 17:143-148.

Kumagai, A., Nishino, K., Kimm, T., Shimomura, A., Nananhoshi, M., and Yamamura, Y. (1970): Inhibitory effect of ubiquinone on biosynthesis of aldosterone in rat adrenal *in vitro. Endocrinologica Japonica,* 17:143-148.

Kuntzman, R., Jacobson, M., and Conney, A. H. (1966): Effect of phenylbutazone on cortisol metabolism in man. *The Pharmacologist,* 8:195.

Lakatos, K., Koref, O., Steczek, K., Holló, I., and Furr, L. (1970): The effect of heparin on androgen metabolism of incubated rat adrenal slices. *Acta Endocrinologica,* 65:731-736.

Lamb, E., Mancuso, S., Dell'Acqua, S., Wiqvist, N., and Diczfalusy, E. (1967): Studies on the metabolism of C-19 steroids in the human foeto-placental unit. 1. Neutral metabolites formed from dehydroepiandrosterone and dehydroepiandrosterone sulphate by the placenta at midpregnancy. *Acta Endocrinologica,* 55:263-277.

Larsson, H., and Stensson, M. (1967): Effect of *bis*(*p*-hydroxyphenyl)-cyclohexylidene-methane (F 6060) on the conversion of pregnenolone to Δ^4-3-ketosteroids *in vitro. Acta Endocrinologica,* 55:673-684.

Lauritzen, C. (1966): Action of HCG and steroids on physiological processes in the neonatal period. In: *Research on Steroids,* Vol. 2, edited by C. Cassano. Il Pensiero Scientifico, Rome, p. 109.

MacMahon, F. G., and Foley, J. (1967): Lack of glutethimide effect on adrenal. *Journal of Clinical Endocrinology and Metabolism,* 27:1495-1496.

Mancuso, S., Benagiano, G., Dell'Acqua, S., Shapiro, M., Wiqvist, N., and Diczfalusy, E. (1968): Studies on the metabolism of C-19 steroids in the human foeto-placental unit. 4. Aromatization and hydroxylation products formed by previable foetuses perfused with androstenedione and testosterone. *Acta Endocrinologica,* 57:208-227.

Mancuso, S., Dell'Acqua, S., Eriksson, G., Wiqvist, N., and Diczfalusy, E. (1965): Aromatization of androstenedione and testosterone by the human fetus. *Steroids,* 5:183-197.

Mathur, R. S., Archer, D. F., Wiqvist, N., and Diczfalusy, E. (1970): Quantitative assessment of the de novo sterol and steroid synthesis in the human foeto placental unit I. Synthesis and secretion of cholesterol and cholesterol sulphate. *Acta Endocrinologica,* 65:663-674.

McIntosh, E. N., Uzgiris, V. I., and Salhanick, H. A. (1970): Clofibrate inhibition of 11β-hydroxylation in bovine adrenal cortex mitochondria. *Endocrinology,* 86:656-657.

Mikhail, G., Wiqvist, N., and Diczfalusy, E. (1963): Oestriol metabolism in the previable human foetus. *Acta Endocrinologica,* 42:519-532.

Mitchell, F. L. (1967): Steroid metabolism in the foeto-placental unit and in early childhood. *Vitamins and Hormones,* 25:191-269.

Oakey, R. E., and Heys, R. F. (1970): Regulation of the production of oestrogen precursors in the foetus. *Acta Endocrinologica,* 65:502-508.

Philbert, M., Laudat, M. H., Laudat, Ph., and Bricaire, A. (1966): Étude clinque et biologique d'un inhibiteur de l'hormonosynthese corticosurrenale: L'aminoglutethi-mide. *Annales d'Endocrinologie,* 29:189-210.

Pion, R. J., Jaffe, R. B., Wiqvist, N., and Diczfalusy, E. (1967): Formation of dehydroepiandrosterone sulphate by previable human foetuses. *Biochimica et Biophysica Acta,* 137:584-587.

Popert, A. J. (1962): Pregnancy and adrenocortical hormones. Some aspects of their interaction in rheumatic disease. *British Medical Journal,* 5283:967-972.

Raman, P. B., Sharma, D. C., and Dorfman, R. I. (1966): Studies on aldosterone biosynthesis *in vitro. Biochemistry,* 5:1795-1804.

Rembiesa, R., Holzbauer, M., Young, P. C. M., Birmingham, M. K., and Saffran, M. (1967): Metabolism of 17α-methylandrostenediol and 17α-methyltestosterone by rat adrenal gland *in vitro. Endocrinology,* 81:1278-1284.

Rembiesa, R., Young, P. C. M., and Saffran, M. (1968): Effect of 17α-methyltestosterone on steroid formation by rat adrenal tissue. *Canadian Journal of Biochemistry,* 46:433-440.

Reynolds, J. W., Mancuso, S., Wiqvist, N., and Diczfalusy, E. (1968): Studies on the aromatization of neutral steroids in pregnant women. 7. Aromatization of 3β, 17β-dihydroxy-androst-5-en-16-one by placentas perfused *in situ* at midpregnancy. *Acta Endocrinologica,* 58:377-395.

Rochefort, J. G., Givner, M. L., and Dvornik, D. (1968): Alteration of adrenocortical steroidogenesis in the rat by inhibition of cholesterol biosynthesis. *Endocrinology,* 83:555-564.

Saffran, J., Saffran, M., and Salhanick (1970): Clofibrate inhibits lipid synthesis and ACTH-stimulated steroidogenesis by rat adrenal tissue. *Endocrinology,* 86:652-655.

Schwers, J, Eriksson, G., and Diczfalusy, E. (1965): Metabolism of oestrone and oestradiol in the human foeto-placental unit at midpregnancy. *Acta Endocrinologica,* 49:65-82.

Schwers, J., Vancrombreuq, T., Govaerts, M., Eriksson, G., and Diczfalusy, E. (1971): Metabolism of dehydroepiandrosterone sulphate following *in situ* placental perfusion at midpregnancy. *Acta Endocrinologica,* 66:637-647.

Sharma, D. C., Forchielli, E., and Dorfman, R. I. (1963): Inhibition of enzymatic steroid 11β-hydroxylation by androgens. *Journal of Biological Chemistry,* 238:572-575.

Sherins, R. J., Gandy, H. M., Thorslund, T. W., and Paulsen, C. A. (1971): Pituitary and testicular function studies. I. Experience with a new gonadal inhibitor, 17α-pregn-4-en-20yno-(2,3-*d*)isooxazol-17-ol (Danazol). *Journal of Clinical Endocrinology and Metabolism,* 32:522-531.

Shikita, M., Ogiso, T., and Tamaoki, B. (1965): Effect of inhibitors on testicular microsomal steroid 17-alpha-hydroxylase and 17-alpha-hydroxypregnene C_{17}-C_{20} lyase. *Biochimica et Biophysica Acta,* 105:516-522.

Shimao, S., Wiqvist, N., Diczfalusy, E., and Solomon, S. (1968): The effect of metopirone (SU-4885) on the metabolism of progesterone by the perfused previable human fetus. *Canadian Journal of Biochemistry,* 46:663-669.

Simmer, H. H., Dignam, W. J., Easterling, W. E., Frankland, M. V., and Naftolin, F. (1966): Neutral C^{19}-steroids and steroid sulfates in human pregnancy. III. Dehydroepiandrosterone sulfate. 16α-hydroxydehydroepiandrosterone and 16α-hydroxydehydroepiandrosterone sulfate in cord blood and blood of pregnant women with and without treatment with corticoids. *Steroids,* 8:179-193.

Solomon, S. (1960): Synthesis of steroids by the placenta. In: *The Placenta and Fetal Membranes,* edited by C. A. Villee. Williams and Wilkins, Baltimore.

Solomon, S., Bird, C. E., Lind, W., Iwamiya, M., and Young, P. C. P. (1967): Formation and metabolism of steroids in the fetus and placenta. *Recent Progress in Hormone Research,* 23:297-347.

Solomon, S., Lenz, A. L., Vande Wiele, R., and Lieberman, S. (1954): Pregnenolone an intermediate in the biosynthesis of progesterone and the adrenal cortical hormones. *Abstracts of the 126th Meeting of the American Chemical Society,* New York, p. 29C.

Southren, L., Gordon, G. G., Tochimoto, S., Krikun, E., Kriger, D., Jacobson, M., and Kuntzman, R. (1969): Effect of N-phenylbarbital (Phetarbital) on the metabolism of testosterone and cortisol in man. *Journal of Clinical Endocrinology and Metabolism,* 29:251-256.

Stachenko, J., and Giroud, C. J. P. (1964): Further observations on the functional zonation of the adrenal cortex. *Canadian Journal of Biochemistry,* 42:1777-1786.

Telegdy, G., Weeks, J. W., Archer, D. F., Wiqvist, N., and Diczfalusy, E. (1970a): Acetate and cholesterol metabolism in the human foeto-placental unit at midgestation. 3. Steroids synthesized and secreted by the foetus. *Acta Endocrinologica,* 63:119-133.

Telegdy, G., Weeks, J. W., Lerner, U., Stakeman, G., and Diczfalusy, E. (1970b): Acetate and cholesterol metabolism in the human foeto-placental unit at midgestation. 1. Synthesis of cholesterol. *Acta Endocrinologica,* 63:91-104.

Telegdy, G., Weeks, J. W., Wiqvist, N., and Diczfalusy, E. (1970c): Acetate and cholesterol metabolism in the human foeto-placental unit at midgestation. 2. Steroid synthesized and secreted by the placenta. *Acta Endocrinologica,* 63:105-118.

Temple, T. E., and Liddle, G. W. (1970): Inhibitors of adrenal steroid biosynthesis. *Annual Review of Pharmacology,* 10:199-218.

Tuchmann-Duplessis, H. (1969): Reactions of the foetus to drugs taken by the mother. In: *Foetal Autonomy,* edited by G. E. W. Wolstenholme and M. O'Connor. J. & A. Churchill Ltd., London, pp. 245-270.

Van Leusden, H. A., Siemerink, M., Telegdy, G., and Diczfalusy, E. (1971): Squalene and lanosterol synthesis in the foeto-placental unit at midgestation. *Acta Endocrinologica,* 66:711-719.

Warren, J. C., and Cheatum, S. G. (1967): Maternal urinary estrogen excretion: Effect of adrenal suppression. *Journal of Clinical Endocrinology and Metabolism,* 27:433-436.

Werk, E. E., Macgee, J., Jr., and Sholiton, L. J. (1964): Effect of diphenylhydantoin on cortisol metabolism in man. *Journal of Clinical Investigation,* 43:1824-1835.

Willman, K., and Pulkkinen, M. O. (1971): Reduced maternal plasma and urinary estriol during ampicillin treatment. *American Journal of Obstetrics and Gynecology,* 109:893-896.

DISCUSSION

PAOLETTI: Have you any experience or information on the inhibition of 11β-hydroxylase in man by clofibrate? After prolonged clinical treatment with clofibrate, the human steroid pattern is often reported to be normal, suggesting a different effect on animal and human 11β-hydroxylase systems.

TELEGDY: The 11β-hydroxylase inhibition with clofibrate refers to rat experiments. It is true that in man the corticoid secretion is normal after clofibrate treatment.

JUCHAU: In studies of drug hydroxylation reactions, it is frequently observed that inhibitors can also act as inducers. Has this also been observed with respect to the inhibitors which you have mentioned—could they act as inducers of steroid hydroxylations?

TELEGDY: Diphenylhydantoin and phenylbutazone are acting as stimulators, possibly as inducers, of 6β-hydroxylase enzyme. I don't know of any other data concerning inhibitors acting as inducers of other enzymes.

MIRKIN: What evidence exists to demonstrate that the enzymes which hydroxylate steroids are the same as those hydroxylating drugs?

TELEGDY: There is no such direct evidence. However, studies on other enzyme systems such as sulfatase in the placenta show that certain sulfates such as DHA-sulfate or pregnenolone sulfate can be hydrolyzed, but that corticoid sulfates or testosterone sulfate cannot. This would indicate substrate specific sulfatase reactions. Whether the same is true also for hydroxylation remains to be seen.

ORRENIUS: Clear evidence that the same enzymes catalyze aromatic drug hydroxylation and steroid hydroxylation in the liver has to await demonstration that both reactions are catalyzed by the same solubilized and purified enzyme system. There is presently, however, some indirect evidence that common enzyme components are involved in both reactions, such as enhanced activity following phenobarbital pretreatment, carbon monoxide inhibition of the reaction, mutual competitive inhibition of the metabolism, and so on.

Fetal Pharmacology, edited by L. Boréus
Raven Press, New York © 1973

Placental Transfer of Drugs

M. G. Horning, C. Stratton, J. Nowlin, A. Wilson, E. C. Horning, and R. M. Hill

Institute for Lipid Research and Department of Pediatrics, Baylor College of Medicine, Houston, Texas 77025

INTRODUCTION

Although studies of placental transfer (Villee, 1965; Moya and Thorndike, 1963) indicated that most drugs will cross the placenta and enter the fetal circulation, the impression has remained that a placental barrier, similar to the blood-brain barrier, protects the fetus from pharmacologically active agents administered to the mother. In fact, however, equilibration between the maternal and fetal circulation is extremely rapid, and blood concentrations of drugs and metabolites in the fetal circulation are comparable to the maternal blood concentrations (Flowers, 1959; Ploman and Persson, 1957; Root, Eichner, and Sunshine, 1961). As a result, the fetus receives the maternal or adult dose of most drugs.

The term "placental transfer" does not fully describe what happens when drugs are administered to pregnant females; more than simple transfer to the fetal circulation is involved. The drugs and metabolites are stored in fetal tissues, particularly liver, brain, and the adrenals. The disposal of stored drugs must be carried out by the fetus *in utero* and by the neonate at birth.

We have been concerned with placental transfer of the drugs administered to mothers just prior to (4 to 5 days) and during delivery and the subsequent disposition of the stored drugs by the newborn infant; the metabolism of drugs by the fetus was not investigated. The initial studies have been concerned with secobarbital, phenobarbital, pentobarbital, aspirin, caffeine, theophylline, and theobromine, the drugs ingested most frequently during this period. The anticonvulsant drugs diphenylhydantoin, primidone, mephobarbital, and ethylmethylsuccinimide have also been investigated since several epileptic mothers have participated in the study.

Placental transfer was difficult to investigate with earlier analytical procedures based on spectrophotometric analyses. The biological samples were small and difficult to obtain, and the results were sometimes questionable since spectrophotometric measurements do not define chemical structures. The development of gas-phase analytical systems (gas chromatograph-mass spectrometer-computer) has made it possible to study the placental transfer of drugs at the microgram and submicrogram level and to identify unequivocally drugs and drug metabolites in biological samples.

Procedures have been developed for the isolation of drugs and drug metabolites from blood and urine based on ion-exchange (DEAE-Sephadex) chromatography (Horning and Horning, 1970) or potassium carbonate-isopropanol extraction (Horning, Boucher, Stafford, and Horning, 1972). Both procedures provide a fraction that can be converted directly to derivatives for analysis by gas chromatography and gas chromatography-mass spectrometry. The potassium carbonate-isopropanol procedure is rapid (30 min), but the extracts contain compounds in addition to drugs and drug metabolites which may interfere with quantification and identification of some drugs. The DEAE-Sephadex procedure yields a fraction that contains only neutral and basic compounds (including drugs and drug metabolites) but requires several hours to carry out. Both isolation procedures are being used for urine analysis. All blood samples, however, are analyzed by the potassium carbonate-isopropanol method.

Analyses have been carried out on urine and plasma obtained from both the mother and infant. Twenty-four-hour urine samples are collected from both male and female newborn infants using a pediatric urine col-

TABLE 1. *Drugs administered during labor and delivery to 100 gravid females.*

Drug	% Ps
Narcotic	97
Belladonna alkaloid	74
Oxytocin	56
Sedative	46
Ataraxic	45
Tranquilizer	34

lector, usually on day two. A urine sample is obtained from the mother as close to delivery as possible. Plasma samples are obtained from the mother at delivery, and, whenever possible, arterial and venous blood (plasma) are obtained from the placenta. A blood sample is obtained from the infant during the period of urine collection. Multiple urine collections are obtained from the infant when feasible.

DRUG METABOLISM STUDIES

The administration of drugs to mothers during labor and delivery is probably more extensive in the United States than in many European countries. Table 1 lists the drugs given to 100 gravid females during labor and delivery in the private hospital where this study was carried out. Diazepam

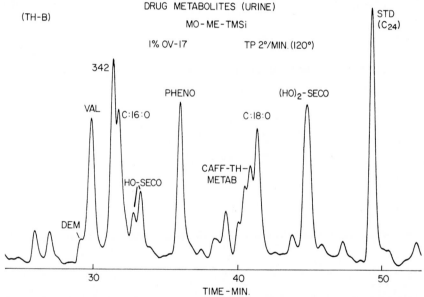

FIG. 1. Gas chromatographic separation of the MO-ME-TMSi derivatives of a urinary fraction containing neutral and basic metabolites. An internal standard, n-tetracosane [24], was added to the sample. The drugs and drug metabolites identified are meperidine (Demerol®; DEM), a metabolite of diazepam (VAL), hydroxysecobarbital (HO-SECO), dihydroxysecobarbital [(HO)$_2$-SECO], phenobarbital (PHENO), and caffeine metabolites (CAFF-TH). The urine was a 24-hr collection made on day 1. The compounds were separated on a 1% OV-17 column by temperature programming at 2°/min from 120°C. All drugs and metabolites reached the infant by placental transfer except phenobarbital which was given to the infant.

(Valium®), which has come into wide use in obstetrics since this summary was prepared, should be added to the list. As anticipated, the infants delivered in this hospital excreted several drugs and drug metabolites immediately after birth. Typical urinary drug profiles are shown in Figs. 1 and 2. Although there is considerable variation among the infants, these may be considered as average neonatal drug profiles.

In Fig. 1 the infant was excreting meperidine, a metabolite of diazepam, two metabolites of secobarbital, phenobarbital, hydroxyphenobarbital, caffeine, and caffeine metabolites. The mother had received meperidine, diazepam, and secobarbital during labor and delivery. Caffeine was self-administered, and phenobarbital had been administered to the neonate. The infant in Fig. 2 was excreting two secobarbital metabolites, phenobarbital, and hydroxyphenobarbital. These two examples, of the many obtained in our laboratory over the past 3 years, demonstrate that drugs readily cross the placenta and reach the fetus.

The origin of the metabolites in neonatal urine is of considerable

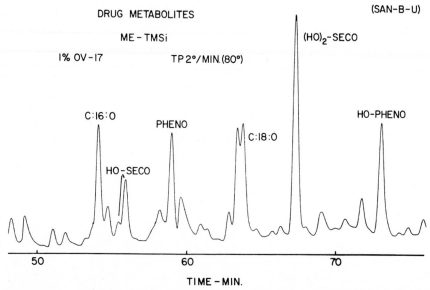

FIG. 2. Gas chromatographic separation of the ME-TMSi derivatives of a urinary fraction containing neutral and basic metabolites. The metabolites identified were phenobarbital (PHENO), hydroxyphenobarbital (HO-PHENO), hydroxysecobarbital (HO-SECO), and dihydroxysecobarbital [(HO)$_2$-SECO]. A 24-hr urine was collected on day 2 from an infant who had received the drugs by placental transfer. The separation was carried out on a 1% OV-17 column by temperature programming at 2°/min from 80°C.

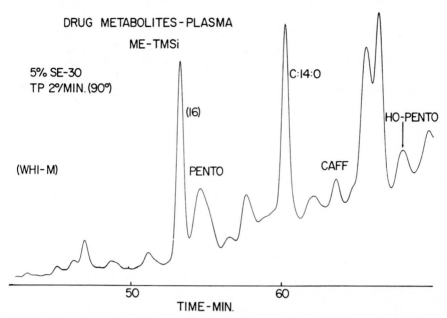

FIG. 3. Gas chromatographic separation of drugs and metabolites extracted from maternal plasma. An internal standard, *n*-hexadecane [16], was added to the sample. The compounds identified were pentobarbital (PENTO), hydroxypentobarbital (HO-PENTO), caffeine (CAFF), and myristic acid [C:14:0]. The separation was carried out on a 5% SE-30 column by temperature programming at 2°/min from 90°C.

interest since it has been reported that newborn mammals (mice, guinea pigs, and rabbits) do not have active enzyme systems for metabolizing drugs (Fouts and Adamson, 1959; Jondorf, Maickel, and Brodie, 1959). If this were true for the human as well, all of the metabolites excreted by the neonate would have been formed in maternal tissues and transferred to the fetus for subsequent excretion after birth.

It is possible to demonstrate that the same metabolites are present in the maternal and neonatal circulation. Figure 3 shows the metabolites in plasma obtained from a mother addicted to pentobarbital; both pentobarbital and hydroxypentobarbital were still present in blood drawn from the mother 32.5 hr after delivery. Blood was obtained from the infant 11.5 hr after birth; Figure 4 shows the presence of pentobarbital and hydroxypentobarbital in the neonatal plasma. In this instance, there is little doubt that both the metabolite and the parent drug were transferred to the fetus and stored in the fetal tissues.

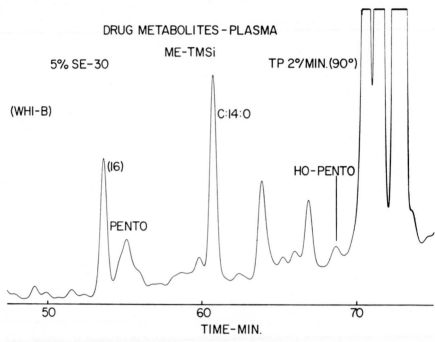

FIG. 4. Gas chromatographic tracing of the ME-TMSi derivatives of drugs and metabolites extracted from neonatal plasma. An internal reference compound, *n*-hexadecane [16], was added to the sample. The compounds identified were pentobarbital (PENTO), hydroxypentobarbital (HO-PENTO), and myristic acid [C:14:0]. The separation conditions were the same as those listed in Fig. 3.

Urine was collected from this infant 30 to 54 hr after birth and a urinary drug profile was obtained (Fig. 5). Pentobarbital, hydroxypentobarbital [5-ethyl-5-(3-hydroxy-1-methylbutyl)-barbituric acid], and dihydroxypentobarbital (a mixture of diols) were identified in the urine. Hydroxypentobarbital was the major metabolite; 3.4 mg was excreted in 24 hr. The total excretion of pentobarbital and metabolites other than hydroxypentobarbital was 0.9 mg/24 hr. The amounts of hydroxypentobarbital (1.7 μg/ml) and pentobarbital (2.8 μg/ml) transferred from the maternal circulation to the fetus were comparable.

It has been possible to demonstrate that the human infant is capable of metabolizing some drugs from birth and that the enzyme systems necessary for carrying out various types of hydroxylation are operative. It is sometimes necessary to administer drugs (barbiturates, anticonvulsants) to

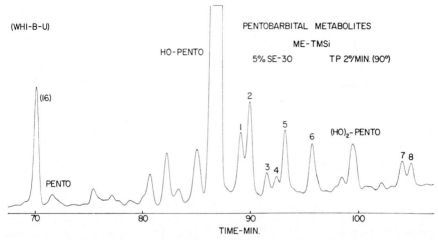

FIG. 5. Gas chromatographic separation of the ME-TMSi derivatives of a urinary fraction containing neutral and basic compounds. An internal reference compound, *n*-hexadecane [16], was added to the sample. The compounds identified were pentobarbital (PENTO), hydroxypentobarbital (HO-PENTO), and dihydroxypentobarbital [(HO)₂-PENTO]. The compounds numbered 1–8 were isomeric hydroxypentobarbital metabolites. The urine was a 24-hr collection from a newborn infant on day 2 who received pentobarbital and hydroxypentobarbital by placental transfer (Figs. 3 and 4). The separation conditions were the same as those for Fig. 3.

newborn infants for medical reasons. Several infants receiving secobarbital, diphenylhydantoin, and phenobarbital during the first few days after birth have been studied; none of the drugs administered to the infants had been given to the mothers. The usual metabolites were present in the neonatal urines.

SECOBARBITAL

Secobarbital was administered to two infants on days 1 and 1 to 3 after birth. A total of 70 mg was given to Baby GAR both intramuscularly and intravenously on days 1 to 3, and a 24-hr urine was collected on day 5. A second infant (Baby MID) received a total of 31 mg intravenously from the 5th to the 28th hr; a 24-hr urine was collected from the 26th to the 50th hr. Hydroxysecobarbital [5-allyl-5-(3-hydroxy-1-methylbutyl)-barbituric acid] and dihydroxysecobarbital [5-(2,3-dihydroxypropyl)-5-(1-methylbutyl)-barbituric acid] were identified as the major metabolites in both urines;

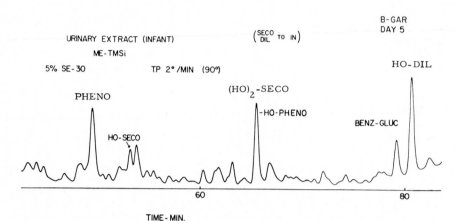

FIG. 6. Gas chromatographic separation of the ME-TMSi derivatives of drugs and metabolites present in a solvent extract of urine. The compounds identified were phenobarbital (PHENO), hydroxyphenobarbital (HO-PHENO), hydroxysecobarbital (HO-SECO), dihydroxysecobarbital [(HO)₂-SECO], hydroxydiphenylhydantoin (HO-DIL), and benzoyl glucosiduronic acid (BENZ-GLUC). Secobarbital and diphenylhydantoin had been given directly to the infant, while phenobarbital had been given to the mother. A 24-hr urine collection was made on day 5. The separation conditions were the same as those for Fig. 3.

secobarbital was not found. The urinary drug profile of Baby GAR is shown in Fig. 6.

Aliphatic hydroxylation of secobarbital to form hydroxysecobarbital is presumably carried out by the same enzyme system that hydroxylates pentobarbital. Secobarbital is marketed as a *dl*-mixture, and hydroxysecobarbital is excreted as a mixture of diastereoisomers. These are partially resolved by gas chromatography when OV-17 is used as the liquid phase (Figs. 1 and 2). The mass spectra of the diastereoisomers are almost identical.

The other major metabolite, dihydroxysecobarbital, was first identified by Waddell (1965) and called secodiol. The oxidation of the allylic side chain to the diol probably involves a different enzyme system from the one involved in the oxidation of the 1-methylbutyl side chain, and the reaction may take place by way of the 2,3-epoxide. Hydrolysis of the epoxide would result in formation of dihydroxysecobarbital.

Since both metabolites were present in urines collected on day 2 (Baby MID) and day 5 (Baby GAR), the infants evidently had active enzyme systems for carrying out both aliphatic and allylic (epoxidation) hydroxylations on days 2 and 5, and probably from the time of delivery.

Hydroxysecobarbital and dihydroxysecobarbital have been identified in the urines of all infants (25) receiving secobarbital by placental transfer. The amounts excreted in urine have varied from 0.02 to 0.57 mg/24 hr for dihydroxysecobarbital and from 0.07 to 0.14 mg/24 hr for hydroxysecobarbital.

PHENOBARBITAL

Phenobarbital was administered to an infant; the urinary analysis is shown in Fig. 7. A total of 50 mg was given intramuscularly from the 6th to the 31st hr after birth. Phenobarbital and hydroxyphenobarbital [5-ethyl-5-(4-hydroxyphenyl)-barbituric acid] were identified in the urine collected from the 5th to the 28th hr. In contrast to secobarbital, unchanged drug (0.15 mg/24 hr) was excreted in the urine.

Enzymatic hydroxylation of the phenyl ring occurs through an oxygenated intermediate which may be an arene oxide (epoxide) (Jerina, Daly,

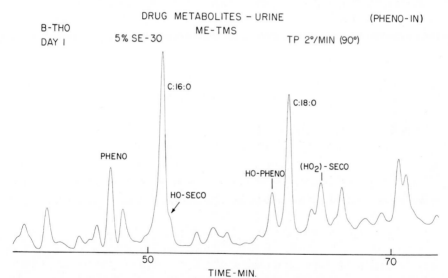

FIG. 7. Gas chromatographic separation of the ME-TMSi derivatives of a urinary fraction containing neutral and basic metabolites. The compounds identified were phenobarbital (PHENO), hydroxyphenobarbital (HO-PHENO), hydroxysecobarbital (HO-SECO), and dihydroxysecobarbital [(HO)$_2$-SECO]. The urine was a 24-hr collection made on day 1 from an infant who had been given phenobarbital and who had received secobarbital and/or its metabolites by placental transfer.

Witkop, Zaltzman-Nirenberg, and Udenfriend, 1968). The possible products arising from this metabolic pathway are *p*- and *m*-hydroxyphenobarbital, the phenolic diol [5-ethyl-5-(3,4-dihydroxyphenyl)-barbituric acid], and the di-hydroxycyclohexadiene derivative [5-ethyl-5-(3,4-dihydroxy-1,5-cyclohexa-dien-1-yl)-barbituric acid].

The phenolic diol has not yet been identified in neonatal urines after direct administration or placental transfer. It is present in the urines of rats receiving a single dose (100 mg/kg) of phenobarbital. The amount is small, however, compared to *p*-hydroxyphenobarbital; conversion of the inter-mediate arene oxide (epoxide) to *p*-hydroxyphenobarbital is preferred in the rat. Small amounts of an isomeric hydroxyphenobarbital, probably *m*-hy-droxyphenobarbital, have also been detected in rat urines following pheno-barbital ingestion (Horning and Horning, 1971).

The dihydroxycyclohexadien-1-yl metabolite has not yet been found in human or rat urine, although it might be an intermediate in the formation of the dihydroxyphenyl metabolite.

Both phenobarbital and hydroxyphenobarbital were found in the urines of eight newborn infants receiving the drug and/or the metabolite by pla-cental transfer. The amount of phenobarbital excreted varied from 0.15 to 0.62 mg/24 hr; the infant excreting 0.62 mg/24 hr of phenobarbital ex-creted 0.39 mg/24 hr of hydroxyphenobarbital.

DIPHENYLHYDANTOIN

Diphenylhydantoin was administered to two infants, and 24-hr urine samples were obtained. A total of 100 mg was given intramuscularly to Baby GAR (Fig. 6) on days 1 to 6; a 24-hr urine was collected on the 5th day. Diphenylhydantoin (84 mg) was administered intramuscularly and orally to a second infant (Baby CAN) daily from the 5th to the 11th day. A 24-hr urine was obtained on day 8.

p-Hydroxydiphenylhydantoin [5-ethyl-5-(*p*-hydroxyphenyl)-hydantoin] was identified in the urine of both infants. Small quantities of unchanged diphenylhydantoin were identified in the urine of Baby CAN. In addition, the new metabolite [5-phenyl-5-(3,4-dihydroxy-1,5-cyclohexadien-1-yl)-hydantoin] (Chang, Savory, and Glazko, 1970) was identified in the urine of Baby CAN (Horning, Stratton, Wilson, Horning, and Hill, 1971). The phenolic diol [5-phenyl-5-(3,4-dihydroxyphenyl)-hydantoin] was not found.

Presumably *p*-hydroxydiphenylhydantoin and the dihydroxycyclohexadien-1-yl metabolite were formed by the same enzyme system that metabolizes phenobarbital; the oxygenated intermediate may be an epoxide of diphenylhydantoin. Although the same enzyme system is probably involved in the metabolism of phenobarbital and diphenylhydantoin, the products identified in urine are quite different. The major metabolite of phenobarbital in neonatal urine is p-hydroxyphenobarbital, and comparable amounts of unchanged phenobarbital are also usually excreted (Fig. 7). The dihydroxycyclohexadien-1-yl metabolite has not been found, and, if present in neonatal urine, is excreted in trace amounts. In contrast, the major metabolites of diphenylhydantoin in neonatal urine are 5-phenyl-5-(4-hydroxyphenyl)-hydantoin and 5-phenyl-5-(3,4-dihydroxy-1,5-cyclohexadien-1-yl)-hydantoin; only small amounts of unchanged diphenylhydantoin are present in urine. The mass spectrum of the dihydroxycyclohexadien-1-yl metabolite identified in the urine of Baby CAN is shown in Fig. 8.

The two infants treated with diphenylhydantoin were also able to carry out an additional reaction necessary for the disposal of drugs and drug metabolites: conjugation with glucuronic acid. When the acidic fraction isolated from urine was analyzed, the glucuronide of 5-phenyl-5-(4-hydroxyphenyl)-hydantoin was identified by both gas chromatography and gas chromatography-mass spectrometry as the methyl ester-trimethylsilyl ether derivative of the intact glucuronide. Thus the two infants had an active UDP-glucuronyl transferase system for the conjugation of p-hydroxydiphenylhydantoin on days 5 and 8 after 5 and 4 days, respectively, on diphenylhydantoin therapy. The glucuronide of p-hydroxyphenobarbital was not present in the urine collected on day 2 from the infant receiving phenobarbital (Baby TH). It is possible that this enzyme system does not become activated until an infant is 4 or 5 days old or that it takes more than 1 day for phenobarbital to induce the glucuronyl transferase. Phenobarbital has been given, however, to jaundiced infants to induce glucuronyl transferase for bilirubin conjugation.

CAFFEINE

Caffeine has, of course, not been given to newborn infants, and the excretion of caffeine and caffeine metabolites has been followed only in infants receiving the drug and/or metabolites by placental transfer. However, differences were observed in the excretion patterns of the neonates and their mothers. If the urinary extract of drugs and metabolites was methylated,

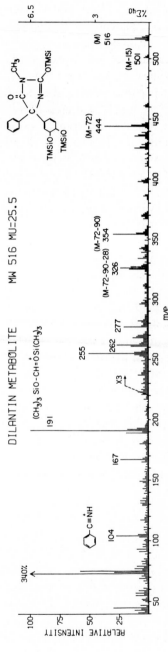

FIG. 8. Mass spectrum of the ME-TMSi derivative of the metabolite (HO)₂-DIL; a combined GC-MS instrument was used. The ion at 255 amu corresponds to the cyclohexadien-1-yl substituent with two TMSi groups, and the ion at 262 amu corresponds to the remainder of the molecule with the addition of a proton. An electron-impact cleavage of this kind also occurs for other ME-TMSi derivatives of hydantoins in this series.

only caffeine was identified in the urine since methylation with diazomethane converted the monomethyl- and dimethylxanthine metabolites to caffeine (1,3,7-trimethylxanthine). However, when the extracts were ethylated with diazoethane, monomethylxanthines were converted to methyldiethylxanthines, dimethylxanthines were converted to dimethylethylxanthines, and caffeine remained unchanged. The three types of xanthines were separated by gas chromatography. The ethyldimethylxanthines were not resolved but chromatographed as a single but somewhat wider peak than caffeine; the methyldiethylxanthines also separated as a single but somewhat wider peak than caffeine (Fig. 9).

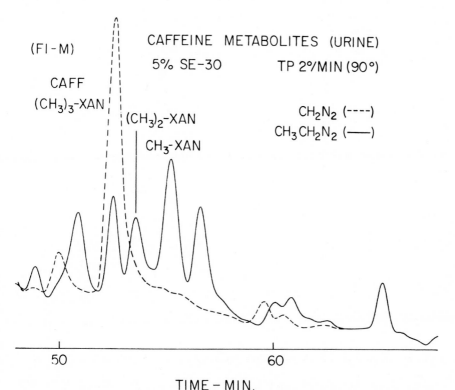

FIG. 9. Gas chromatographic separation of the ME and ET derivatives from a urinary fraction containing neutral and basic metabolites. After methylation, all metabolites were converted to caffeine. After ethylation, the trimethyl (CAFF), dimethyl [(CH₃)₂-XAN], and the methyldiethylxanthines (CH₃-XAN) separated into three groups. The major metabolites in the urine sample collected from the mother (FI-M) at delivery were methyldiethylxanthines. The separation conditions were the same as those for Fig. 3.

The major metabolites in the maternal urine (obtained at delivery) were monomethylxanthines (46% of the total xanthine excretion). Caffeine and dimethylxanthines were excreted in equal amount (26% of the total xanthine excretion) (Fig. 9).

The xanthine profile of an infant (Baby FI on day 1) was quite different (Fig. 10). The major urinary xanthine was unchanged caffeine (75% of the total xanthine excretion); dimethylxanthines accounted for 16% and monomethylxanthines for 9% of the total xanthine excretion.

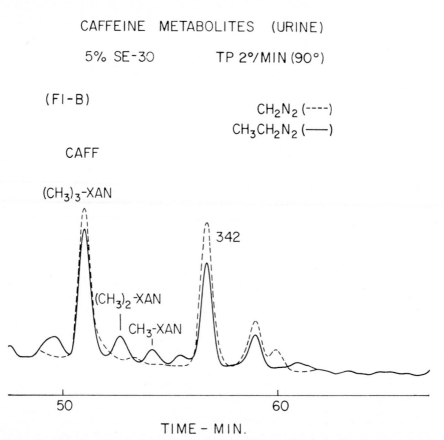

FIG. 10. Gas chromatographic separation of the ME and ET derivatives from a urinary fraction containing neutral and basic metabolites. The urine was a 24-hr collection on day 1 from the infant of the mother in Fig. 9. The major metabolite in the neonatal urine was caffeine. Only small amounts of methyldiethyl- and dimethylethylxanthines were found in the neonatal urine. The separation conditions were the same as those for Fig. 3.

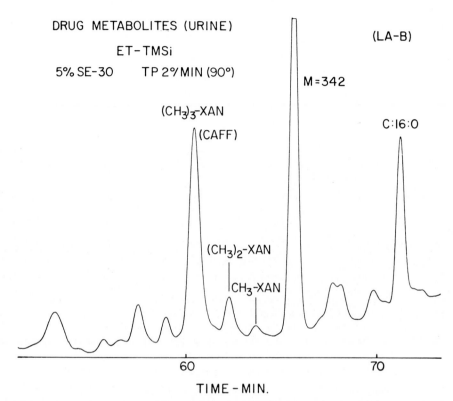

FIG. 11. Gas chromatographic separation of ET-TMSi derivatives from a urinary fraction containing neutral and basic compounds. The major metabolite is caffeine; only small amounts of the methyldiethyl and dimethylethylxanthines were present in the 24-hr urine collected on day 2 from Baby LA. The separation conditions were the same as those for Fig. 3.

In another infant (Baby LA, Fig. 11), a similar profile was obtained for urine collected on day 2 (24 to 48 hr). Caffeine was again the major urinary xanthine (83%); the excretion of dimethylxanthines was 15%, and of monomethylxanthines, 4% of the total xanthine excretion.

Plasma was obtained from the umbilical vein after delivery of the infant, and the drug metabolites were isolated using the potassium carbonate-isopropanol procedure (Horning et al., 1972). After ethylation, the only xanthine derivative identified in the umbilical vein plasma was caffeine (Fig. 12). The neonate evidently received caffeine by placental transfer, and the major compound excreted in urine was caffeine. Thus it seems that the neo-

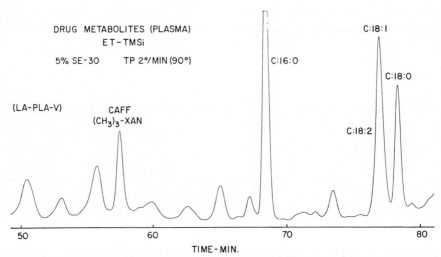

FIG. 12. Gas chromatographic separation of the ET-TMSi derivatives of an extract of placental vein plasma obtained from mother LA. Only caffeine (CAFF) was identified in the blood going to the infant. Other compounds identified in this sample were palmitic acid [C:16:0], linoleic acid [C:18:2], oleic acid [C:18:1], and stearic acid [C:18:0]. The separation conditions were the same as those for Fig. 3.

natal enzyme(s) for demethylation of caffeine is not very active during the first few days after delivery and that caffeine largely remains in neonatal tissues as caffeine.

Caffeine, theophylline, and theobromine, and their metabolites have been found in 90% of the urines that have been studied. This is not surprising when one considers the extensive consumption of coffee, cola drinks, and various proprietary preparations that contain caffeine.

CONCLUSION

All drugs investigated thus far have been transferred from maternal to fetal circulation when administered to mothers; the newborn infant is faced with the necessity of disposing of pharmacologically active agents administered before birth. Unlike some newborn mammals (mice, guinea pigs, rabbits), the human is able at birth to carry out some of the important enzymatic transformations by which drugs are metabolized. Oxidation reactions involving alkyl hydroxylation and epoxidation followed by diol formation occur from birth. It is possible that the ability of the neonate to metabolize drugs is due to induction of the necessary microsomal enzymes, since all mothers in this study received four to five drugs during labor and delivery.

An exception to this generalization is the demethylation of caffeine. This substance is almost always present in the newborn, apparently as a consequence of the ingestion of coffee and other caffeine-containing beverages, and some proprietary products which contain caffeine. The ability of the neonate to demethylate caffeine is far less than that of mothers. The demethylation of other drugs has not yet been studied, but this may also be slower for neonates than for mothers. It is known that some adult methylation reactions do not occur in the newborn, and this may be an important difference between neonates and older infants and adults.

ACKNOWLEDGMENT

This work was supported by U.S. Public Health Service Grant GM-16216 from the National Institute of Medical Sciences.

REFERENCES

Chang, T., Savory, A., and Glazko, A. J. (1970): A new metabolite of 5, 5-diphenylhydantoin (Dilantin). *Biochemical and Biophysical Research Communications,* 38:444-449.

Flowers, C. E. (1959): The placental transmission of barbiturates and thiobarbiturates and their pharmacological action on the mother and the infant. *American Journal of Obstetrics and Gynecology,* 78:730-742.

Fouts, J. R., and Adamson, R. H. (1959): Drug metabolism in the newborn rabbit. *Science,* 129:897-898.

Horning, E. C., and Horning, M. G. (1970): Metabolic profiles: Chromatographic methods for isolation and characterization of a variety of metabolites in man. In: *Methods of Medical Research,* Vol. 12, edited by R. E. Olson. Yearbook Medical Publishers, Chicago, pp. 369-411.

Horning, E. C., and Horning, M. G. (1971): Metabolic profiles: Gas phase methods for analyses of metabolites. *Clinical Chemistry,* 17:802-809.

Horning, M. G., Boucher, E. A., Stafford, M., and Horning, E. C. (1972): A rapid procedure for the isolation of drugs and drug metabolites from plasma. *Clinica Chimica Acta,* 37:381-386.

Horning, M. G., Stratton, C., Wilson, A., Horning, E. C., and Hill, R. M. (1971): Detection of 5-(3,4-dihydroxy-1,5-cyclohexadien-1-yl)-5-phenylhydantoin as a major metabolite of 5,5diphenylhydantoin (Dilantin) in the newborn human. *Analytical Letters,* 4:537-545.

Jerina, D. M., Daly, J. W., Witkop, B., Zaltzman-Nirenberg, P., and Udenfriend, S.

(1968): The role of arene-oxide oxepin systems in the metabolism of aromatic substrates. III. Formation of 1,2-naphthalene oxide from naphthalene by liver microsomes. *Journal of the American Chemical Society,* 90:6525-6527.

Jondorf, W. R., Maickel, R. P., and Brodie, B. B. (1959): Inability of newborn mice and guinea pigs to metabolize drugs. *Biochemical Pharmacology,* 1:352-354.

Moya, F., and Thorndike, V. (1963): Passage of drugs across the placenta. *American Journal of Obstetrics and Gynecology,* 84:1778-1798.

Ploman, L., and Persson, B. H. (1957): On the transfer of barbiturates to the human foetus and their accumulation in some of its vital organs. *Journal of Obstetrics and Gynaecology of the British Commonwealth,* 64:706-711.

Root, B., Eichner, E., and Sunshine, I. (1961): Blood secobarbital levels and their clinical correlation in mothers and newborn infants. *American Journal of Obstetrics and Gynecology,* 81:948-957.

Villee, C. A. (1965): Placental transfer of drugs. *Annals of the New York Academy of Science,* 123:237-244.

Waddell, W. J. (1965): The metabolic fate of 5-allyl-5-(1-methylbutyl)-barbituric acid (secobarbital). *Journal of Pharmacology and Experimental Therapeutics,* 149:23-28.

DISCUSSION

SJÖQVIST: The finding of drug metabolism in the newborn is in excellent agreement with our previous demonstration of cytochrome P-450 in early human fetal life. I would like to make a plea for kinetic studies in order to differentiate between metabolites originating from the maternal circulation and from the newborn. If one can show a parallelism between the urinary excretion of the main metabolites of a drug and its plasma disappearance curve in the newborn, then this is good evidence that the metabolites are formed in the baby. We have recently shown such a parallelism for nortriptyline in a newborn (the mother took an overdose just before delivery) indicating that this drug is effectively hydroxylated immediately after birth (*J. Pediatrics,* in press). We are presently studying the kinetics of the urinary excretion of diphenylhydantoin metabolites (*p*-OH-diphenylhydantoin and its glucuronide) in newborns of mothers treated therapeutically.

HOLMSTEDT: How do you explain the lack of conjugation of phenobarbital when Dilantin is conjugated by the infant?

HORNING: Most infants can conjugate hydroxyphenobarbital with glucuronic acid. This particular infant did not excrete the glucuronide of hydroxyphenobarbital on day 2 after receiving phenobarbital on day 1, suggesting that the necessary enzyme system(s) was (were) not operative in this infant.

BORÉUS: What is the proportion of unchanged versus hydroxylated phenobarbital in the urine of the newborn baby during the first days of life? Do you have a time table? Since the plasma half-life of phenobarbital, according to our findings, is 4 to 5 days, a single injection would be enough to measure the changes with time of the percentage urinary output of the metabolites consecutively in the same patient.

HORNING: We have no data on the changes in the ratio of phenobarbital and its metabolites with time in the neonate. In the rat, equal amounts of phenobarbital, hydroxyphenobarbital, and the glucuronide of hydroxyphenobarbital are excreted during the first 24 hours; the glucuronide becomes the major metabolite on day 2.

DAWES: What was the postnatal course of the infant born to the mother who had been taking large quantities of pentobarbital during pregnancy?

HORNING: In the immediate newborn period, the suck reflex was poor to absent. On the 4th day of life, the suck reflex improved and the infant fed well. We were unable to follow the infant after the first month of life.

KARCZMAR: Some of your very beautiful data seem to indicate the general capacity of the "brand new" infant to conjugate a number of different compounds. Is this a nonspecific capacity? If so, do you have any ideas about why the infant has such a problem with conjugating chloramphenicol, resulting in the "grey baby" syndrome?

HORNING: The newborn infant can form the glucuronides of hydroxyphenobarbital, hydroxypentobarbital, and hydroxydiphenylhydantoin, indicating that the glucuronyl transferase system is active. Chloramphenicol toxicity in the newborn infant, especially in the premature, is caused by two factors: (1) an immature or depressed liver conjugating mechanism, and (2) immature or depressed mechanisms for excretion of chloramphenicol by the kidneys.

LEVY: In collaboration with Dr. Lorne Garrettson, we are studying the kinetics of elimination of salicylate in newborn infants of mothers who took aspirin some hours before delivery. The cumulative excretion of total salicylates by a neonate was measured. Most of the salicylate appeared in the first urine, but its content of nonmetabolized drug is negligible. This indicates appreciable transfer of salicylate metabolites from mother to fetus. Therefore, the initial urine sample(s) does (do) not necessarily reflect the newborn's biotransformation capability. The salicylate metabolite composition in the subsequent urine samples suggests that the human newborn can form salicyluric acid and salicyl glucuronide(s) on the first days of life.

Fetal Pharmacology, edited by L. Boréus
Raven Press, New York © 1973

Antiepileptic Drugs and Fetal Well-Being

R. M. Hill, M. G. Horning, and E. C. Horning

*Department of Pediatrics and Institute for Lipid Research,
Baylor College of Medicine, Houston, Texas 77025*

A characteristic clustering of congenital malformations has been observed in infants born to mothers receiving anticonvulsant medications during their gestation. On January 28, 1969, a 24-year-old multipara was delivered of an infant with multiple malformations. The mother required phenobarbital, diphenylhydantoin, and primidone during her pregnancy for control of seizures. The malformations observed in the infant were a large anterior and posterior fontanelle, low hairline, separation of the metopic suture, broad nasal bridge, wide-set eyes, cleft lip and palate involving the premaxilla, gingival hypertrophy, wide-set nipples, bilateral inguinal hernias, hypoplasia of the distal phalanx of the hands and feet, hypoplasia of the nails, digital thumbs, and pilonidal sinus. Chromosome analysis on the infant revealed a normal karyotype. The cleft lip and palate and hypoplasia of the nails and distal phalanx observed in this infant are shown in Figs. 1 and 2. When this child was delivered, the mother had a child 2 years of age and has subsequently been delivered of a third infant. All three infants have identical malformations with the exception of the cleft lip and palate and inguinal hernia. There was no history of cleft lip or palate in the family, and neither parent had shortening of the distal phalanx, hypoplastic nails, or digitalization of the thumbs. The nails of the three children have grown since birth which suggests some temporary effect on nail formation *in utero* and not agenesis. The nails of the third sibling were less involved, but digitalization of the thumbs was more obvious.

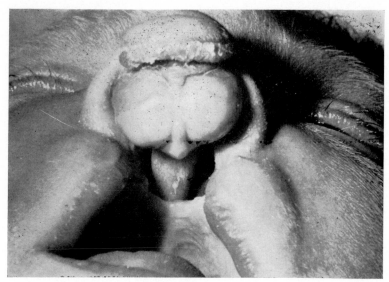

FIG. 1. Cleft lip and palate involving the premaxilla in an infant born to a mother receiving diphenylhydantoin, phenobarbital, and primidone during pregnacy.

Melchior et al. (1967) first called attention to the occurrence of congenital malformations in infants born to mothers receiving anticonvulsant medication during their pregnancy. Earlier, Massey (1966) had reported diphenylhydantoin as a teratogen in mice and this was confirmed by Harbison and Becker (1969). Meadow (1968) reported six children with similar anomalies. In his report the mothers received primidone, phenytoin, trimethadione, and phenobarbital during pregnancy.

Table 1 demonstrates the anomalies observed in 17 additional infants born to mothers receiving anticonvulsant therapy compared to 124 infants who were not exposed to these agents during intrauterine development. Anticonvulsant drugs ingested by the mothers were diphenylhydantoin, primidone, mephobarbital, diazepam, and ethosuximide. Two mothers experienced seizures after oral contraceptive medications were prescribed. Only one mother had a previous history of seizures as a child.

Major congenital anomalies consisted of congenital heart disease (Tetrology of Fallot), cleft lip and palate, hypospadius, dislocation of the hip, epidermal cyst connected to dura, inguinal hernia, and pyloric stenosis. Both infants delivered of a twin pregnancy manifested digital thumbs, hypoplastic nails, hypoplastic distal phalanx, inguinal hernia, low wide-set nipples, pilonidal sinus, and large anterior and posterior fontanelle; only one twin had congenital heart disease and urinary tract anomalies. One twin is represented in Table 1.

Fourteen infants have been followed from 3 months to 2½ years of age. Two infants were hospitalized at 3 and at 6 months of age for diagnostic studies because of failure to thrive. The growth and development of seven infants has been followed for 1 year or longer. Somatic growth in three infants is in the 3rd percentile or less for chronological age, but all seven infants are small since the parents of these children are of average physical stature. Two infants are significantly delayed in mental development at 1 year and 18 months of age.

Folate determinations have been completed in 11 mothers and their infants. Only the mother whose infant had a cleft lip and palate was reported to have a low (2.3 ng/ml) folate level. During the mother's subsequent pregnancy, folic acid supplementation was prescribed and normal folate levels were maintained. She received diphenylhydantoin, amitriptyline, phenobarbital, and diazepam during this pregnancy. Three mothers had a borderline folate level (4 ng/ml).

By the method of gas chromatography-mass spectrometry, metabolites of the various anticonvulsant drugs have been identified in biological samples obtained from these infants. Hydroxyphenylhydantoin, dihydroxyphenylhy-

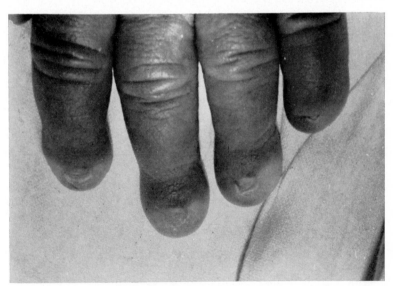

FIG. 2. Hypoplastic fingernails and hypoplastic distal phalanyx observed in an infant born to a mother receiving diphenylhydantoin, phenobarbital, and primidone during pregnancy.

TABLE 1. *Physical findings observed in infants delivered of mothers requiring anticonvulsant therapy[a] during pregnancy.*

Physical Finding	Anticonvulsant Group		Control Group	
Sydney line	9/20	45%	14/124	11%
Inguinal hernia	3/20	15%	7/124	6%
Pilonidal sinus	7/20	35%	4/124	3%
Large anterior and posterior fontanelle	5/20	25%	4/124	3%
Hypoplastic distal phalanx	5/20	25%	1/124	1%
Hypoplastic nails	5/20	25%	0/124	0%
Broad alveolar ridge	6/20	30%	8/124	7%
Metopic ridging	4/20	20%	3/124	2%
Short neck	3/20	15%	2/124	1.6%
Failure to thrive	2/20	10%	0/124	0%
Major anomalies[b]	7/20	35%	7/124[c]	6%
Slow mental development (pts. followed)	2/14	14%	7/124	6%
Digital thumb	4/20	20%	0/124	0%
Low hairline	4/20	20%	0/124	0%

[a] Mephobarbital, primidone, diphenylhydantoin, ethosuximide, phenobarbital, diazepam.
[b] Two infants had two major anomalies.
[c] One infant had two major anomalies.

dantoin, and hydroxydiphenylhydantoin glucuronide have been identified in 24-hr urine collections. The new metabolite identified by Chang et al. (1970) in rat and monkey urine was identified by Horning et al. (1971) in the 24-hr urine samples obtained in an infant between 11 and 34 hr of age. Baughman and Randinitis (1970) reported the half-life for diphenylhydantoin in the neonate as 19 hr. Mirkin (1971) subsequently reported that plasma concentrations of diphenylhydantoin in mother and infant are similar, and the plasma half-life in the infant is 55 to 69 hr. Excretion of diphenylhydantoin was complete in 5 days. Anomalies observed in his series were cleft lip in two infants and microcephaly in one. Only a small quantity of diphenylhydantoin was identified in breast milk.

Mephobarbital was prescribed for control of seizure in one gravid patient. The infant manifested severe tremors and hyperirritability within the first hours of life. These symptoms were interpreted as withdrawal symptoms from placental transfer of mephobarbital and were observed to continue for the first 4 months of life. Irritability was severe enough to require treatment with phenobarbital. Phenobarbital and hydroxyphenobarbital were identified in the urine collected on this infant in the first 26 hr of life before treatment was started. The colic-like symptoms observed in this infant were similar to the withdrawal and/or toxic manifestation seen by Desmond et al. (1969) in infants born to mothers who ingested tranquilizers during pregnancy. Desmond et al. (1972) recently described withdrawal symptoms in infants whose mothers ingested barbiturates in the last trimester of pregnancy and compared their symptomatology to those of infants experiencing narcotic withdrawal. Five additional infants manifested a colic-like syndrome, but the most constant drug ingested by the mother was diphenylhydantoin. In only two cases was phenobarbital consumed by the mother in combination with diphenylhydantoin. Transplacentally acquired phenobarbital has been identified in the urine of a neonate as long as 7 days post-delivery.

Mountain et al. (1970), Davies (1970), and Evans et al. (1970) have reported a coagulation defect similar to vitamin K deficiency in infants born to mothers on diphenylhydantoin and phenobarbital. No evidence of bleeding tendency was observed in 17 patients examined in the immediate newborn period.

The most consistent anomaly reported in infants born to patients on anticonvulsant therapy is a cleft lip and palate. Of interest is the report by Dronamraju (1970) on the incidence of epilepsy in first- and second-degree relatives of patients who have cleft lip and palate. The role which genetic predisposition plays in the occurrence of this anomaly as evidence of intrauterine fetal insult is unclear. Individuality in metabolism of anticonvulsant drugs may be the most important factor in teratogenesis. Westmoreland (1971) reported that the gravid rat is more susceptible to diphenylhydantoin toxicity than the rat in the non-gravid state. A correlation between human maternal plasma levels of anticonvulsant drugs and outcome of their progeny may clarify the sporadic occurrence of anomalies in these infants.

REFERENCES

Baughman, F. A., Jr., and Randinitis, E. J. (1970): Passage of diphenylhyantoin across the placenta. *Journal of the American Medical Association,* 213:466.

Chang, T., Savory, A., and Glazko, A. J. (1970): A new metabolite of 5, 5-diphenylhydantoin (Dilantin). *Biochemical and Biophysical Research Communications,* 38:444.

Davies, P. P. (1970): Coagulation defect due to anticonvulsant drug treatment in pregnancy. *Lancet,* 1:413.

Desmond, M. M., Rudolph, A. J., Hill, R. M., Claghorn, J. L., Dressen, P. R., and Burgdorff, I. (1969): Behavioral alterations in infants born to mothers on psychoactive medication during pregnancy. In: *Proceedings of the Symposium on Congenital Mental Retardation,* edited by Gordon Farrell. University of Texas Press, Austin.

Desmond, M. M., Schwanecke, R. P., Wilson, G. E., Yasunaga, S., and Burgdorff, I. (1972): Maternal barbiturate utilization and neonatal withdrawal symptomatology. *Journal of Pediatrics,* 80:190-197.

Dronamraju, K. R. (1970): Epilepsy and cleft lip and palate. *Lancet,* 2:876-877.

Evans, A. R., Forrester, R. M., and Discombe, C., (1970): Neonatal hemorrhage following maternal anticonvulsant therapy. *Lancet,* 1:517-518.

Harbison, R. D., and Becker, B. A. (1969): Relation of dosage and time of administration of diphenylhydantoin to its teratogenic effect in mice. *Teratology,* 2:305-311.

Horning, M. G., Stratton, C., Wilson, A., Horning, E. C., and Hill, R. M. (1971): Detection of 5-(3,4-dihydroxy-1.5-cyclohexadien-1-yl)-5-phenylhydantoin as a major metabolite of 5,5-diphenylhydantoin (Dilantin) in the newborn human. *Analytical Letters,* 4:537-545.

Massey, K. M. (1966): Teratogenic effects of diphenylhydantoin sodium. *Journal of Oral Therapeutics and Pharmacology,* 2:380-385.

Meadow, S. R. (1968): Anticonvulsant drugs and congenital abnormalities. *Lancet,* 2:1296.

Melchior, J. C., Svensmark, O., and Trolle, D. (1967): Placental transfer of phenobarbitone in epileptic women, and elimination in newborns. *Lancet,* 2:860-861.

Mirkin, B. (1971): Diphenylhydantoin: Placental transport, fetal localization, neonatal metabolism, and possible teratogenic effects. *Journal of Pediatrics,* 78:329-337.

Mountain, K. R., Hirsh, J., and Gallus, A. S. (1970): Neonatal coagulation defect due to anticonvulsant drug treatment in pregnancy. *Lancet,* 1:265-266.

Stevenson, M. M., and Gilbert, E. F. (1970): Anticonvulsants and hemorrhagic disease of newborn infant. *Journal of Pediatrics,* 77:516.

Westmoreland, B., and Bass, N. (1971): Diphenylhydantoin intoxication during pregnancy. *Archives of Neurology,* 24:158-164.

DISCUSSION

MCBRIDE: Could you give the time period over which these abnormalities were collected? How many epileptic women were included in the study?

HILL: We started our study in January 1969, and these cases were collected from this time through 1971. They do not represent all the epileptic women delivering in the city of Houston but only those willing to go on the study. All the patients were selected before delivery. There were only 20 epileptic gravid females in the study.

MCBRIDE: How many of the babies had cleft palate? What was the dose of diphenylhydantoin to the pregnant women?

HILL: Only one infant had a cleft lip and palate, and one infant had a congenital heart malformation. The dose of diphenylhydantoin was 300 to 350 mg/day but diphenylhydantoin was not the only drug consumed. Barbiturates were taken by at least three-quarters of the patients.

LARSSON: What was the frequency of cleft lip and of cleft lip and palate, respectively, in the group of children whose mothers were treated with diphenylhydantoin? It is generally accepted that the cleft lip and palate is more often caused by genetic factors than the isolated cleft palate.

HILL: There was only one infant with a cleft lip and palate. The palate was very unusual in that it only involved the premaxilla. There was no history of cleft lip or palate in the family.

Fetal Pharmacology, edited by L. Boréus
Raven Press, New York © 1973

A Theoretical Analysis of Fetal
Drug Equilibration

G. S. Dawes

*Nuffield Institute of Medical Research, University of Oxford,
Oxford OX3 9DS, England*

An analysis by Goldstein, Aronow, and Kalman (1968) suggested that the kinetics of drug equilibration in the fetus might repay further study. This analysis was carried out in numerical form. A general solution, also based on a simplified diagram of the fetal circulation, is now presented. It will be assumed throughout that no drug is removed by metabolism.

The fetal circulation is composed of a series of parallel circuits through the placenta and through the fetal tissues (Fig. 1). It is convenient to sim-

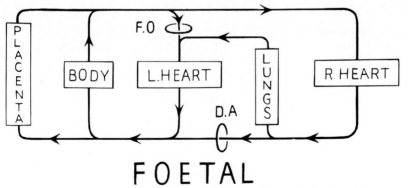

FOETAL

FIG. 1. Diagram of the fetal circulation simplified to illustrate the fact that the combined output of both ventricles supplies the placenta and fetal tissues in parallel.

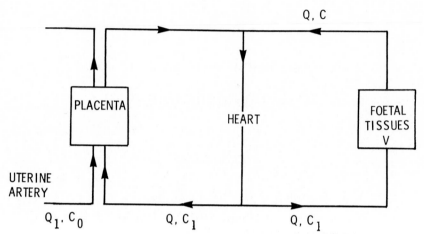

FIG. 2. Diagram of the fetal circulation simplified yet further for analysis.

plify this even further, as shown diagrammatically in Fig. 2. Umbilical blood flow is assumed to be half the output of both ventricles. Blood returning from the placenta is thoroughly mixed in the heart with that returning from the fetal tissues; blood entering the tissues is mixed instantaneously in a fluid volume V. It is also assumed that maternal and fetal bloods pass through the placenta in cross-current streams such that the volumes of bloods and of placental tissue within which equilibration occurs are negligibly small in relation to flow rates, and the equilibration is complete so that drug concentration in maternal and fetal placental effluents are identical. This concentration is:

$$\frac{Q_1 \cdot C_0 + Q \cdot C_1}{Q_1 + Q}$$

Since the quantity of drug leaving and entering the heart is identical, we have

$$2Q \cdot C_1 = \frac{Q(Q_1 \cdot C_0 + Q \cdot C_1)}{Q_1 + Q} + Q \cdot C$$

or

$$2C_1 = \frac{Q_1 \cdot C_0 + Q \cdot C_1}{Q_1 + Q} + C$$

Let
$$Q_1 = \sigma Q$$

Then
$$2\,C_1 = \frac{\sigma \cdot C_0 + C_1}{\sigma + 1} + C$$

and
$$C_1 = \frac{\sigma C_0 + C\,(\sigma + 1)}{2\sigma + 1}$$

The rate of change of drug concentration in the fetal tissue is

$$V \cdot \frac{dc}{dt} = Q \cdot C_1 - Q \cdot C$$

$$= \frac{\sigma}{2\sigma + 1} \cdot Q\,(C_0 - C)$$

whence
$$C = C_0\,(1 - e^{-t/\tau})$$

with a time constant
$$\tau = \left[\frac{2\sigma + 1}{\sigma}\right] \cdot \frac{V}{Q} \tag{1}$$

When $\sigma = 1$ (i.e., when maternal placental and umbilical flows are identical), $\tau = 3V/Q$. This is an interesting result. It shows that the time constant for drug equilibration is three times that which would obtain if the fetal tissues were supplied directly by maternal blood. It is a direct consequence of the geometry of the fetal circulation. When maternal flow is greater than umbilical flow (i.e., $\sigma > 1$), this increase is less, and vice versa (Table 1).

Changes in placental homogeneity (leading to variations in maternal: fetal perfusion ratio) or the introduction of shunts on either side of the

TABLE 1. *Effects of changing fetal tissue volume and maternal placental blood flow.*

Maternal Placental Flow (Q^1) (ml/min/kg)	Fetal Tissue Volume (V) (ml/kg)	σ (Q_1/Q)	Time constant (τ) (min)
200	100	1	1.5
200	900	1	13.5
400	900	2	11.25
100	900	0.5	18
50	900	0.25	27

Conditions as given by Fig. 2 and Eq. (1), with umbilical and fetal tissue blood flows (Q) 200 ml/min/kg (fetal weight).

placenta will have an effect which also can be estimated as variations in σ; so also will variations in the affinity of a drug as between maternal and fetal bloods (e.g., different binding to plasma protein or, with oxygen, variations in Hb O_2 affinity and in O_2-carrying capacity).

Table 1 also shows that if the fetal tissue volume is reduced to 100 ml/kg (e.g., as with a substance whose volume of distribution is confined to the vascular compartment), the time constant for equilibration is correspondingly less.

Incomplete cardiac mixing

Let us suppose that mixing in the heart and great vessels is incomplete. This may be defined by a factor x (where $x \leq 1$) such that the blood entering the fetal tissues has a drug concentration of:

$$C_2 - x \left(\frac{C_2 - C}{2} \right)$$

where C_2 is the concentration in blood returning from the placenta and C that returning from fetal tissues. Otherwise, the vascular arrangement assumed is as in Fig. 2 with maternal placental and umbilical blood flows equal. Then the time constant for drug equilibration is:

$$\tau = \frac{4 - x}{2 - x} \cdot \frac{V}{Q}$$

When $x = 1$, cardiac mixing is complete and $\tau = 3V/Q$ as before. When mixing is only half complete, $x = 0.5$ and $\tau = 2.33V/Q$. When x becomes very small, the fetal circulation tends to become figure-of-eight and $\tau \to 2V/Q$.

Changes in maternal blood concentration

With complete cardiac mixing, we shall consider the situation where the maternal blood concentration falls exponentially with time constant τ_1, such that

$$C_0 = C_m e^{-t/\tau_1}$$

where C_m is the initial maternal arterial drug concentration. Then it can be shown that:

$$C_2 = \frac{C_m \cdot \tau_1}{\tau_1 - \tau} \cdot (e^{-t/\tau_1} - e^{-t/\tau})$$

where τ, as before, is the time constant for fetal drug equilibration. And, when $\tau = \tau_1$,

$$C_2 = \frac{C_m t}{\tau} \cdot e^{-t/\tau}$$

Figure 3 illustrates this result when $\tau = \tau_1 = 10$ min. The maternal arterial drug concentration falls exponentially and crosses to become lower than fetal tissue drug concentration at 10 min. Umbilical vein and artery concentrations are intermediate. In this model, carotid arterial concentration is identical with that in the umbilical artery.

Figure 4 illustrates the result when τ (the fetal time constant) is constant at 10 min, while τ_1 (the maternal time constant) is varied from 5 min to infinity. When τ_1 is infinite, fetal tissue concentration (Fig. 4, uppermost solid line) rises exponentially as rapidly as possible. When τ_1 is finite, fetal tissue concentration rises to a maximum at the point of crossover, i.e.,

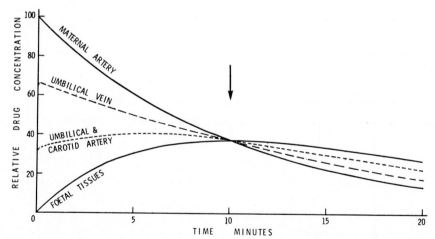

FIG. 3. Changes in fetal blood and tissue concentrations of a drug whose maternal arterial concentration falls exponentially with a time constant, 10 min, identical to that of the fetal circulation (as in Fig. 2).

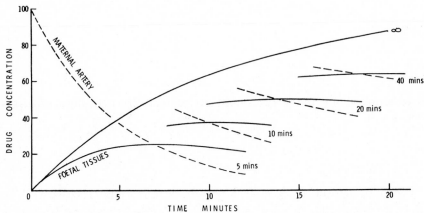

FIG. 4. As in Fig. 3. Changes in maternal arterial blood (- - -) and fetal tissue (—) drug concentrations when the time constant for exponential fall in maternal arterial concentration is varied, that for the fetal circulation being constant (10 min).

where maternal arterial and fetal tissue concentrations coincide. Thereafter, fetal tissue concentration rises to a maximum at the point of crossover, i.e., noted that this model takes no account of drug destruction.) The maximum fetal tissue concentration is 25% of the peak maternal arterial concentration when τ_1 is 5 min, and 50% when τ_1 is 20 min.

The effect of placental volume

We may also consider the situation where the placenta has volume V, and the drug is soluble in placental tissue. We compare the effect of supply

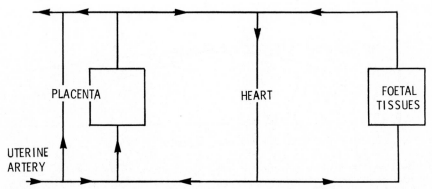

FIG. 5. The fetal circulation, with the uterine artery supplying the placental tissues and exchange area in parallel.

in parallel or *in series* with the area of drug transfer (or gas exchange). If in parallel (Fig. 5), effective maternal blood flow is correspondingly reduced by a shunted flow. At term in sheep, the weight of the placenta (about 350 g) is one-tenth that of the fetus (3.5 kg). If blood flow is correspondingly adjusted, one might suppose that about one-tenth of maternal flow to the placenta would not reach the exchange area, [σ would be 0.9 in Eq. (1)], resulting in a small increase in τ (e.g., Table 1, from 13.5 to 14.0 min).

If the placental tissues are supplied in series with the area of drug transfer, there are two possible arrangements, shown in Figs. 6 and 7. In Fig. 7, equilibration is effected between maternal and umbilical bloodstreams and with placental tissue; the placenta is assumed to be homogeneous.

The general solution for Fig. 6 is given by

$$C_2 = C_0 \left[1 - \frac{\tau_1 \cdot e^{-t/\tau_1}}{\tau_1 - \tau_2} - \frac{\tau_2 \cdot e^{-t/\tau_2}}{\tau_2 - \tau_1} \right] \tag{2}$$

Where $\tau_1 = V_1/Q_1$ (for the placenta)

and $\tau_2 = V \cdot \dfrac{Q_1 Q_2 + Q_2 Q_3 + Q_3 Q_1}{Q_1 Q_2 Q_3}$ (for the fetal tissue)

When $Q_1 = Q_2 = Q_3 = Q$, $\tau_2 = 3V/Q$ as before. The general solution for Fig. 7 is identical with Eq. (2), but τ_1 and τ_2 have different values. Whereas in the circumstances shown in Fig. 6, the time constants τ_1 and τ_2

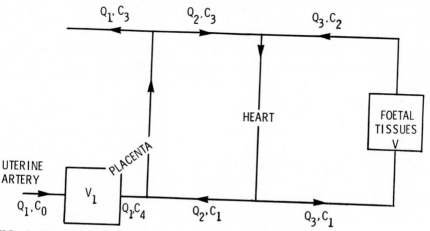

FIG. 6. The fetal circulation, with the uterine artery supplying the placental tissue and exchange area in series.

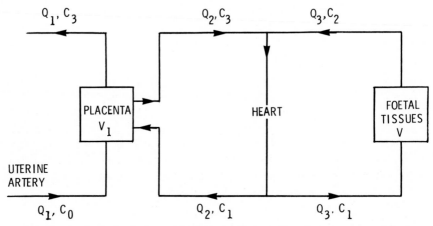

FIG. 7. The fetal circulation, with placental tissue and exchange area combined.

apply to the placenta and fetal tissues (V_1 and V) respectively and independently, in Fig. 7 there is interaction between the two systems. In this condition, τ_1 and τ_2 are each dependent on both V and V_1 (see Appendix).

For Fig. 7, when V/V_1 is large,

$$\tau_1 = \frac{3V}{Q} \quad \text{and} \quad \tau_2 = \frac{2V_1}{3Q}$$

Of the three conditions examined (Figs. 5-7), that depicted in Fig. 7 most closely approximates reality, as it combines simultaneous equilibration between maternal and fetal blood and placental tissue. During gestation, the relative size of placenta and fetus changes considerably. The effect of change in placental volume from 0.1 to 1.8 liter/kg fetal weight has been examined with fetal tissue volume (900 ml/kg) constant and with maternal placental and fetal blood flows (200 ml/kg/min) equal and constant. The effective time constant [i.e., τ_1 when $C_2/C_0 = (e - 1)/e = 0.63$] was calculated from Eq. (2). When $Q_1 = Q$ (i.e., when maternal placental flow is equal to umbilical blood flow), the effect of an increase in placental volume is to cause a small increase in the effective time constant for drug equilibration, as in the lowest curve of Fig. 8. With reduction in maternal placental flow ($Q_1 = Q/2$ or $Q/4$), the increase in time constant is greater, especially as placental volume is increased. We may note first that the increase in placental volume must be large to cause much change in the effective time constant for fetal drug equilibration, and secondly that the effect of reduced maternal placental blood flow is comparatively greater.

Figure 8 covers a very wide physiological range, and it will be noticed that as placental volume is increased (in terms of fetal weight), no allowance was made for increase in maternal placental blood flow. That is, it was assumed that maternal placental flow is solely dependent on fetal weight. This is approximately true later in gestation, but not earlier (Table 2). The effective time constants calculated from Dr. Bruce's observations on rabbits during the last third of gestation have been inserted as closed circles in Fig.

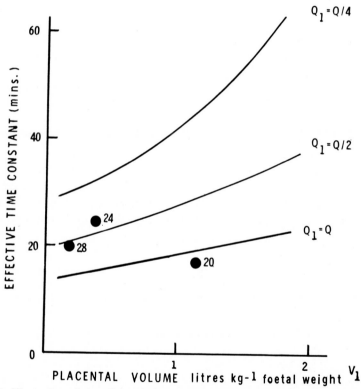

FIG. 8. Illustration of the effect of placental volume on the effective time constant for fetal drug equilibration, with changing proportions of maternal placental (Q_1) to umbilical (Q) blood flows. See text for other conditions. The closed circles (●) illustrate data from N. Bruce (*unpublished*) on rabbits at 28, 24, and 20 days of gestation, respectively.

TABLE 2. *Mean observations on pregnant rabbits.*

		28	24	20
	Gestational age (days)	28	24	20
(V_1)	Placental weight (g/kg fetus)	180	390	1140
(Q_1)	Maternal placental flow (ml/min/kg fetus)	94	115	254
	When $Q = 200$, Q_1/Q	0.47	0.57	1.27

Courtesy of Dr. N. Bruce (*unpublished observations*). Maternal placental flow was measured using the isotope-labeled microsphere method under pentobarbital anesthesia.

8, on the assumption that fetal umbilical and tissue flows are constant and equal at 200 ml/min/kg fetal weight. From this it would seem that the upper right quadrant of Fig. 8 may well be outside the physiological range.

The liver and the ductus venosus

We now examine the effect to be anticipated from the presence of the liver and ductus venosus, as depicted in Fig. 9. The effect of the placenta is assumed negligible. The general solution for Fig. 9 is identical with Eq. (2), i.e., as for Figs. 6 and 7, but with different values for τ_1 and τ_2 (see Appendix). As with Fig. 7, there is interaction between the effects of liver and ductus venosus, on the one hand, and of fetal tissues, on the other hand, on drug equilibration.

The effective time constant τ' [where $C_2/C = 0.63$ in Eq. (2)] has been calculated for the condition where $Q_1 = Q_2 = Q_3 = 200$ ml/min/kg fetal weight, where fetal fluid volume $V = 900$ ml/kg and where liver volume $= 50$ ml/kg (see Dawes, 1968, Table 4). The drug is assumed equally soluble in fetal liver as in blood and tissues. When ductus venosus flow is

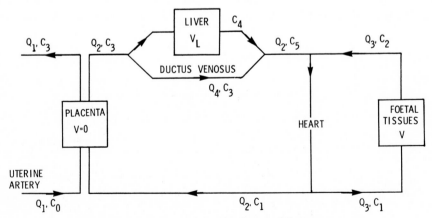

FIG. 9. The fetal circulation, with liver and ductus venosus.

zero (i.e., all umbilical flow passes through the liver), τ' is 14.5 min, as compared with 13.5 min when the liver is ignored. When ductus venosus flow is half the umbilical flow, τ' is intermediate in value, i.e., 13.9 min. This result suggests that the presence of the liver and ductus venosus has only a trifling effect on the fetal drug equilibration time when the affinity of the liver is no greater than that of other tissues.

The effect of increased hepatic drug affinity was examined by attributing to the liver a greater notional volume, e.g., by a factor of 10 when affinity is increased 10-fold. The liver acts as a "sink" interposed between the placenta and the rest of the fetal tissues. Figure 10 shows the effect of increasing hepatic drug affinity on the effective time constant for fetal tissue equilibration when ductus venosus flow is zero (———) or half umbilical blood flow (- - - -). When hepatic drug affinity is high (say, $\times$ 10) and hepatic sinusoid flow low (e.g., when half umbilical flow passes through the ductus venosus), then hepatic equilibration becomes a dominant factor and the effective time constant for fetal tissue equilibration is increased 50%.

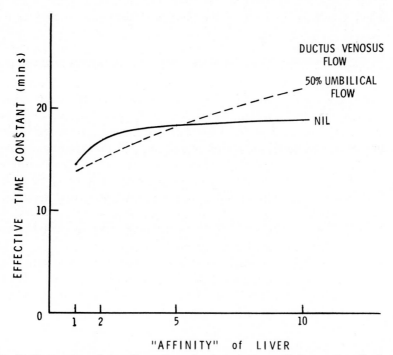

FIG. 10. Illustration of the effect of varying hepatic drug affinity on the effective time constant for fetal drug equilibration, with different ductus venosus blood flows. The affinity of fetal blood and extrahepatic tissues is assumed to be unity. See text for other conditions.

It is also interesting to consider the change in hepatic drug concentration with time, which can be predicted in such closely defined circumstances. When hepatic drug affinity is unity, liver volume is relatively small and hepatic flow relatively high; then hepatic drug concentration will rapidly approximate that in the umbilical vein. When hepatic drug affinity is 10, notional liver volume is large and, if the ductus venosus is widely open, flow is relatively less; then hepatic drug concentration will lag far behind that in the umbilical vein.

DISCUSSION

Qualifications

This analysis is subject to a number of qualifications. For instance, each variable (e.g., cardiac mixing, placental volume, ductus venosus and liver flow) has been considered separately rather than together. This is a desirable preliminary to a more thorough and very much more complex analysis.

It is assumed that not only the placental tissue but also the fetal tissues are homogeneous, so far as drug equilibration is concerned. Yet they are not homogeneous, and it is likely that the time course of drug equilibration in the fetus is not a simple exponential. Also, no account has been taken of equilibration in the fetal fluids—amniotic, allantoic, pulmonary, gastrointestinal, and urinary. The fetal circulation has been oversimplified. Yet, equilibration of the large variations in O_2 contents of bloodstreams entering the fetal heart is remarkably complete (Dawes, 1968), and ventricular volumes are normally small, so the simplication may be justified. No distinction is drawn between equilibration in the vascular bed and fetal tissues (however, see below). Also, we have assumed that umbilical flow is half the combined output of both ventricles in the fetus. In sheep this is roughly true from 0.4-1.0 of term, but is uncertain at an earlier age or in other species. Finally, we have assumed that fetal blood flows are invariant with time. They do vary considerably from time to time, especially with fetal breathing *in utero*. With these reservations, we may discuss the results first as to the equilibration of O_2, and then more generally.

The equilibration of oxygen

This is a special case. It has been known for a long while that a stepwise change in maternal oxygenation is followed by equilibration of O_2 con-

TABLE 3. *Relative O_2 contents of placenta and fetal tissues and blood of a lamb near term, weighing 3.5 kg.*

	Volume (ml)	Oxygen Content (ml)
Placenta	350	0.8 at 76 mm Hg[a]
Fetal tissues (80% of body)	2,800	2.1 at 25 mm Hg[b]
Fetal blood	500	30.0 at half-saturation[c]

[a] Calculated as dissolved O_2 at a PO_2 intermediate between maternal artery and uterine vein.

[b] Calculated as dissolved O_2 at a PO_2 near fetal arterial values.

[c] With an O_2 carrying capacity of 12 ml/100 ml.

tent in the fetal circulation within 6 to 8 min (Born, Dawes, and Mott, 1956; Dawes, Duncan, Lewis, Merlet, Owen-Thomas, and Reeves, 1969). Similarly during maternal hyperventilation, fetal carotid PCO_2 equilibrates rapidly (Baillie, Dawes, Merlet, and Richards, 1971). Yet other substances equally soluble in blood and tissues, equilibrate less rapidly. These include nitrous oxide (Metcalfe, Romney, Ramsey, Reid, and Burwell, 1955; Crenshaw, Huckabee, Curet, Mann, and Barron, 1968; Stenger, Blechner, and Prystowsky, 1969; Blechner, Makowski, Cotter, Meschia, and Barron, 1969; Marx, Joshi, and Orkin, 1970), urea (Meschia, Breathnatch, Cotter, Hellegers, and Barron, 1965), and antipyrine (Metcalfe, Romney, Swartwout, Pitcairn, Lethin, and Barron, 1959; Meschia, Cotter, Makowski, and Barron, 1966; Meschia, Battaglia, and Bruns, 1967), all of which take 30 to 40 min for full equilibration after maternal administration.

The solubility coefficient for O_2 in biological fluids is 0.023 at 39°C and 760 mm Hg. Hence, the O_2 contents of placental and fetal tissues are small compared with that of fetal blood (Table 3). Consequently, the time constant which is of predominant importance is that derived for the fetal blood vascular system, of a volume, for example, of 140 ml/kg fetal weight. The placental volume is neglected (as in Fig. 2). The time constant will be about 2.1 min when Q and Q_1 are 200 ml/min/kg, giving a 90% equilibration time of 4.8 min.

Nitrous oxide is almost equally soluble in blood and tissues, and is distributed between them in proportion to volume. The time constant for equilibration in the fetal tissues must therefore be calculated on the basis of total fetal fluid (say, 900 ml/kg) and is much larger (13.5 min) than that for equilibration in series-perfused placental tissue (0.5 min). If the latter is neglected (as in Fig. 2), the 90% equilibration time is 31 min.

We conclude that the different equilibration times for O_2 and NO_2 in the fetal circulation can be explained by the different partition of the two gases in fetal blood and tissue and by the physical characteristics of the fetal circulation. The equilibration times calculated agree well with the values observed experimentally.

Other models

The analysis presented differs in several respects from that of Goldstein et. al. (1968). They treated the placenta as a mixing chamber of finite volume, approximate to that of the intervillous space in man, in which umbilical and maternal arterial blood are equilibrated. There is no physiological evidence to support this design. Little of the placental blood, on maternal or fetal side, is actually in the exchange area at any one time. Successive boluses of blood pass through on either side, equilibrating with each other. In the jargon of placental physiology, there has never been any serious support for a pool-system; the exchange area is considered as a cross-current (rather than a counter-current or concurrent) system (Dawes, 1968; Rankin, 1972). If we have to deal with only one mixing chamber (in the fetal tissues), analysis is greatly simplified (as in Fig. 2).

On the other hand, we must take into account placental volume, not so much at term as earlier in gestation when it is of a proportionately greater size as compared with the fetus. For example, in the lamb, guinea pig, and human infant at term, the fetus is normally up to 10 times the weight of the placenta; at 0.4-0.6 of term, placental and fetal weights are approximately equal, and earlier in gestation the placenta can be many times the weight of the fetus. At term in a normal fetus, the effect of placental volume is small. For instance, with a lamb weighing 3.5 kg and placenta 350 g (approximately 100 ml/kg), the net effect of adding the placenta (Fig. 7 as compared with Fig. 2) is to increase τ from 13.5 to 14.0 min. (The effect of ignoring placental volume in the numerical example chosen by Goldstein et al., where placental intervillous blood volume was taken as 250 ml $= 71$ ml/kg, would be proportionally less).

Other variables

At term, there are variations in maternal placental blood flow between species (lamb estimated at approximately 200 ml/min/kg fetal weight; rabbit 60 to 100/ml/min/kg), with physiological conditions (e.g., hypoxemia reduces flow in the rabbit; Duncan, 1969), and with drug action (e.g., noradrenaline infusion, 1 μg/min/kg i.v., reduces flow in the rabbit; Leduc, *unpublished*). As Fig. 8 shows, this can substantially affect the time constant for drug equilibration.

The case of the immature fetus is of special interest to pharmacologists involved with drug trials to study teratological effects. When the placenta is relatively greater in size than the fetus, its volume (in relation to maternal placental flow) could become the dominant factor in determining the time constant for fetal drug equilibration. There is so little physiological evidence about maternal placental and fetal blood flow rates available in early fetal life that further analysis is hypothetical.

We must consider the case where a drug is injected intravenously into the mother and disappears rapidly from the circulation. Goldstein et al. (1968) suggested that in these circumstances "fetal equilibration will be speeded," from examining the shape of their numerically computed concentration curves. As the maternal drug concentration falls, so does the concentration gradient across the placenta (Fig. 3), and the umbilical concentration soon becomes so low that the arterio-venous difference is no longer measurable, as shown by Kosaka, Takahashi, and Mark (1969) after injection of thiobarbiturate in man. Yet the time constant of the system is independent of drug concentration, and true final equilibration time is infinite and unalterable when the fall in maternal drug concentration is exponential.

Finally, it might be supposed from Figs. 3 and 4 that the fetus would be relatively immune to the effects of many drugs administered as a single brief injection to the mother. Yet this depends on other factors as well as the kinetics of distribution in the fetal circulation. For instance, injection into a pregnant ewe of a dose of pentobarbital (4 mg/kg i.v.) leads to mild sedation of the mother, who remains on her feet, yet it causes an arrest of fetal intrauterine "rapid irregular" breathing and a change in its electrocorticogram within 2.5 min (K. Boddy, G. S. Dawes, and J. Robinson, *unpublished observations*). Evidently these fetal physiological systems are especially sensitive to the drug in question.

SUMMARY

A theoretical analysis of drug equilibration between mother and fetus is presented. (1) The geometry of the fetal circulation results in a time constant for equilibration three times that which would obtain if the fetal tissues were supplied directly by maternal blood. (2) The effect of incomplete cardiac mixing is considered. (3) The effects of an exponential fall in maternal arterial drug concentration are described. (4) The effect of placental tissue volume on the time constant for equilibration is estimated. This effect is small near term, in proportion to the small size of the placenta compared with the fetus. (5) The effect of changes in maternal-placental blood flow near term can be great. (6) The effects of the liver and the ductus venosus, and of differing hepatic drug affinities, are considered. (7) With O_2, equilibration in fetal blood is very rapid. This is attributed to the fact that the tissue content is much smaller than the blood content. (8) The applications and limitations of the analysis are discussed.

ACKNOWLEDGMENT

I acknowledge gratefully the advice and help of Dr. D. G. Wyatt. It was also a pleasure to have the benefit of discussions with Dr. M. Finster.

REFERENCES

Baillie, P., Dawes, G. S., Merlet, C. L., and Richards, R. (1971): Maternal hyperventilation and foetal hypocapnia in sheep. *Journal of Physiology*, 218:635-650.

Blechner, J. N., Makowski, E. L., Cotter, J. R., Meschia, G., and Barron, D. H. (1969): Nitrous oxide transfer from mother to fetus in sheep and goats. *American Journal of Obstetrics and Gynecology*, 105:368-373.

Born, G. V. R., Dawes, G. S., and Mott, J. C. (1956): Oxygen lack and autonomic nervous control of the foetal circulation in the lamb. *Journal of Physiology*, 134:149-166.

Crenshaw, C., Huckabee, W. E., Curet, L. B., Mann, L., and Barron, D. H. (1968): A method for the estimation of the umbilical blood flow in unstressed sheep and goats with some results of its application. *Quarterly Journal of Experimental Physiology*, 53:65-75.

Dawes, G. S. (1968): *Foetal and Neonatal Physiology*. Year Book Medical Publishers, Chicago.

Dawes, G. S., Duncan, S. L. R., Lewes, B. V., Merlet, C. L., Owen-Thomas, J. B., and Reeves, J. T. (1969): Hypoxaemia and aortic chemoreceptor function in foetal lambs. *Journal of Physiology*, 201:105-116.

Duncan, S. L. B. (1969): The partition of uterine blood flow in the pregnant rabbit. *Journal of Physiology*, 204:421-433.

Goldstein, A., Aronow, L., and Kalman, S. M. (1968): *Principles of Drug Action*. Harper & Row, New York, pp. 189-194.

Kosaka, Y., Takahashi, T., and Mark, L. C. (1969): Intravenous thiobarbiturate anaesthesia for caesarean section. *Anesthesiology*, 31:489-506.

Marx, G., Joshi, C. W., and Orkin, L. R. (1970): Placental transmission of nitrous oxide. *Anesthesiology*, 32:432-439.

Meschia, G., Battaglia, F. C., and Bruns, P. D. (1967): Theoretical and experimental study of transplacental diffusion. *Journal of Applied Physiology*, 22:1171-1178.

Meschia, G., Breathnatch, C. S., Cotter, J. R., Hellegers, A., and Barron, D. H. (1965): The diffusibility of urea across the sheep placenta in the last 2 months of gestation. *Quarterly Journal of Experimental Physiology*, 50:23-41.

Meschia, G., Cotter, J. R., Makowski, E. L., and Barron, D. H. (1966): Simultaneous measurement of uterine and umbilical blood flow and oxygen uptakes. *Quarterly Journal of Experimental Physiology*, 52:1-18.

Metcalfe, J., Romney, S. L., Ramsey, L. H., Reid, D. E., and Burwell, C. S. (1955): Estimation of uterine blood flow in normal human pregnancy at term. *Journal of Clinical Investigation,* 34:1632-1638.

Metcalfe, J., Romney, S. L., Swartwout, J. R., Pitcairn, D. M., Lethin, A. N., and Barron, D. H. (1959): Uterine blood flow and oxygen consumption in pregnant sheep and goats. *American Journal of Physiology,* 197:929-934.

Rankin, J. H. G. (1972): The effects of shunted and unevenly distributed blood flows on crosscurrent exchange in the sheep placenta. In: *Gas Exchange in the Placenta,* edited by L. D. Longo (*in press*).

Stenger, V. G., Blechner, J. N., and Prystowsky, H. (1969): A study of prolongation of obstetric anesthesia. *American Journal of Obstetrics and Gynecology,* 103:901-910.

APPENDIX

For both Figs. 7 and 9, the appropriate time constants required for Eq. (2) are given by:

$$\tau_1 = \frac{2}{a - \sqrt{a^2 - 4\beta}} \text{ and } \tau_2 = \frac{2}{a + \sqrt{a^2 + 4\beta}}$$

For Fig. 7,

$$a = \frac{V(Q_1Q_2 + Q_2Q_3 + Q_3Q_1) + V_1Q_2Q_3}{VV_1(Q_2 + Q_3)}$$

$$\beta = \frac{Q_1Q_2Q_3}{VV_1(Q_2 + Q_3)}$$

For Fig. 9,

$$a = \frac{V(Q_1Q_2 + Q_2Q_3 + Q_3Q_1)(Q_2 - Q_4) + V_LQ_2Q_3(Q_1 + Q_2 - Q_4)}{VV_L[(Q_1 + Q_2)(Q_2 + Q_3) - Q_2Q_4]}$$

$$\beta = \frac{Q_1Q_2Q_3(Q_2 - Q_4)}{VV_L[(Q_1 + Q_2)(Q_2 + Q_3) - Q_2Q_4]}$$

DISCUSSION

CALDEYRO-BARCIA: The injection of 10 to 20 mg of diazepam to parturient women is followed by a reduction in the amplitude of the irregularities which are normally present in the electrocardiographic tracing of fetal heart rate. Have you observed if diazepam reduces the respiratory movements in the lamb (or human) fetus *in utero*?

DAWES: We have begun to study diazepam. We have not yet enough observations to answer your question.

DRABKOVA: In late pregnancy there are rhythmic changes in uterine activity. I suppose this occurs also in pregnant sheep. Have you noted such changes when measuring the amniotic fluid pressure? Isn't the fetal rhythmicity induced exogenously by the mother?

DAWES: In fetal sheep changes in intrauterine pressure, apart from those at term (such as Braxton-Hicks contractions), are small. They do not affect fetal blood gas tensions or blood pressure or fetal breathing *in utero*. There is no evidence that changes in the rhythm of fetal breathing is dependent on physiological changes in the mother.

BRADBURY: In your mathematical analysis, you assumed equality of drug concentration in the maternal and fetal bloods leaving the placenta. Presumably this is true of highly lipid-soluble drugs. Do you have any knowledge of how low the oil-water partition coefficient of a drug has to be before this ceases to be true?

DAWES: No, I have no knowledge from personal experiment. You will find good reviews of many aspects of placental physiology in the proceedings of a symposium on "Gas Exchange in the Placenta," held in Hannover in August 1971. It looks as if it will be necessary to perfuse the fetal side of the placenta, so that the complication introduced by equilibration within the fetal circulation can be removed, in order to obtain quantitative information on the placental exchange of drugs with different physico-chemical characteristics.

JOST: I wish to ask a question concerning the *in vivo* perfusion of the placenta after removal of the fetus. In rats or in rabbits when the uterine chamber is opened, when the fetus is removed and the fluids lost, the uterus shrinks. If the surface of the uterine wall on which the placenta is inserted diminishes, the geometry of the system is altered and the circulation on both the maternal and the fetal sides could be changed. This might also apply to the human placenta under similar circumstances. Could you, Dr. Dawes, comment upon that?

DAWES: Certainly. The morphology of the cotyledonary placenta of the sheep is such that it is peculiarly well suited to such experiments as Huggett showed many years ago. The uterus does not contract, as does the primate uterus when the fetus is removed. Dr. Maureen Young also has used the guinea pig placenta, perfused from the umbilical (fetal) side while remaining *in situ*, with satisfactory results.

SAUNDERS: What volume of fluid is moved in and out of the trachea during a single breathing movement *in utero?*

DAWES: Very little, about 0.5 ml on average, because although the intratracheal pressure changes may exceed 30 mm Hg, the density and viscosity of the tracheal fluid are so very much greater than those of air. The tidal flow of tracheal fluid *in utero* is about one-fiftieth that of the tidal volume after birth.

SAUNDERS: Does the smallness of this volume mean that there is relatively little mixing of alveolar and amniotic fluid?

DAWES: Yes and no. There are relatively larger expiratory effects, occurring less frequently in which 2 to 3 ml of fluid are expelled. It is reported that the net flow of tracheal fluid amounts to about 5 ml per kg fetal weight per hour.

MIRKIN: Since the uptake of pharmacologically active molecules by the liver does not appear to influence the equilibration time as much as one might predict (according to Fig. 9), do you feel that this is a reflection of the extent to which a drug is retained in the liver, which will vary with each compound, rather than an indication that this mechanism is unimportant in modulating tissue levels of drug?

DAWES: It is true (Fig. 10) that the effect of the liver appears less than has been supposed. The model suggests that the liver is less important because it is only about 4 to 5% of body weight. If liver affinity for a drug is high, the hepatic concentration of a drug can be very large. If the drug is sequestered in the liver (in other words, remains there for a very long while), then the result of its presence will indeed be large. But if the drug is released as umbilical venous concentration falls, the presence of the liver will not greatly affect equilibration time.

Fetal Pharmacology, edited by L. Boréus
Raven Press, New York © 1973

Contributions of Teratology to Fetal Pharmacology

K. Sune Larsson

Laboratory of Teratology, Karolinska Institutet, Stockholm, Sweden

INTRODUCTION

The urgent need for a better understanding of the possible side effects of drugs on the unborn became evident to scientists and laymen as well when McBride (1961) and Lenz (1961) independently showed that thalidomide ingestion during pregnancy could cause severe fetal malformations. The discovery of this unexpected adverse drug effect has been a major stimulus of the current interest in fetal pharmacology. Other recent contributions of teratology to fetal pharmacology have been:

(1) Establishment of basic principles for studies of adverse drug effects on the embryo and fetus;

(2) Development of special experimental techniques for studies of the embryo and fetus; and

(3) Collection of information on drug effects in order to prevent fetal damage.

Teratology and fetal pharmacology are both closely related to developmental pharmacology which has been interpreted (Done, 1966; Yaffe, 1968) as both the study of the *effect* of drugs at different developmental stages from the fertilized egg to maturity, and the study of the *fate* of drugs at different developmental periods.

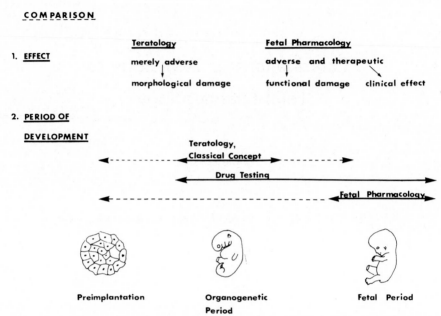

FIG. 1. Comparison between teratology and fetal pharmacology with regard to effect of treatment and period of development.

It is important to note that teratology deals with side effects of drugs whereas fetal pharmacology also encompasses therapeutic effects during different periods of development (Fig. 1) (Catz and Yaffe, 1962). Teratogenesis means, according to the classic concept, interference with the organogenesis, the end result of which is *morphological* damage, a malformation. An impairment during the fetal period would instead result in *functional* defects detected by biochemical and physiological methods. In clinics these differences in effects might be used to distinguish between the diagnostic responsibilities of teratology and fetal pharmacology. However, both the organogenetic period and the fetal period are dealt with in the same guidelines for testing new drugs, which are the practical consequences of experimental teratology.

The chapters in this volume show that the fate of drugs administered during the prenatal period has been intensively studied by the pharmacologists and to some extent also by the teratologists. In many countries, material from legal abortions has been used, and for practical and legislative reasons the specimens have been restricted to the fetal period. Teratologists have now more and more adopted pharmacological methods in their experiments during the organogenetic period.

TERATOLOGICAL PRINCIPLES

Teratological principles were developed during early experimental studies mainly designed to elucidate the mechanism behind congenital malformations (Wilson, 1959; Wilson and Warkany, 1965). The teratogenic effect is dependent on the following four important factors: (1) the *time* in embryonic development when organogenesis is disturbed; (2) the *agent* causing the disturbance; (3) the *dose* of the teratogen; and (4) the *genetic constitution* of the animal.

These generalizations have been found valid and practical and are used when guidelines and protocols for the evaluation of the new drugs are drawn up (Food and Drug Administration, 1966; World Health Organization, 1967).

The stage of organogenesis at the time of disturbance determines mainly the type of malformation

This rule is based on animal experiments and has been transferred to the scheme for human development. Examples of timing of some malformations are given in Table 1. Some authors have determined from the type of malformation very precisely when the damage occurred. Lenz and Knapp (1962) have demonstrated a very close correlation between day of thalidomide intake and the type of malformation. However, Nishimura, Takano, Tanimura, and Yasuda (1968) showed in a study on about 1,200 early Japanese therapeutic abortions a great individual variation in rate of morphological development.

The type of damage is different during embryonic and fetal life, but intra-uterine death is a common end result in both periods (Nishimura, 1970). Experimental work with salicylate as the model substance in mice demonstrates a higher fetal mortality when the drug is given later in gestation (Larsson and Eriksson, 1966). During the organogentic period, the salicylate treatment also caused skeletal and vessel malformations; during the fetal period, liver and subcutaneous bleedings were observed with increased prothrombin time and decreased glycogen concentration in liver and heart (Eriksson, 1971). These results stress the need of extended testing for side effects of drugs during the fetal period.

TABLE 1. *Relative timing of certain malformations.*

Malformation	Caused prior to
Anencephaly	26 days
Meningomyelocele	28 days
Cleft lip	36 days
Cleft palate	8 to 9 weeks
Esophageal atresia plus tracheo- esophageal fistula	30 days
Rectal atresia with fistula	6 weeks
Duodenal atresia	7 to 8 weeks
Omphalocele	10 weeks
Diaphragmatic hernia	6 weeks
Extroversion of bladder	30 days
Bicornuate uterus	10 weeks
Hypospadias	12 weeks
Cryptorchidism	7 to 9 months
Transposition of great vessels	34 days
Ventricular septal defect	6 weeks
Aplasia of radius	38 days
Syndactyly, severe	6 weeks
Sirenomelia	23 days

(Data from D. W. Smith: *Recognizable Patterns of Human Malformation,* W. B. Saunders Company, Philadelphia, 1970).

The same agent can cause different types of malformations but different agents can cause the same type of malformation

Many different malformations can be induced by A-hypervitaminosis in the mouse, e.g., cleft lip, microstomia, fusions in ribs and vertebrae, exophthalmus, exencephalia, and spina bifida (Fig. 2), even if such effects are not very typical for A-hypervitaminosis (Kalter and Warkany, 1961). It is also well known that different external agents such as hyper- and hypo-vitaminosis and alkylating agents can give the same type of malformation, e.g., malformed extremities in different species (Millen, 1962). It is evident that we are not allowed to draw conclusions from the type of malformation as to which external agent caused it. This is probably also true for other types of damage caused in the fetal period, such as fetal bleeding or re-duced glycogen content. The possibilities for the fetus to recover from such damages need to be further studied.

Teratology is now more and more focused on possible *teratogenic mechanisms.* Neubert and Köhler (1970) studied the inhibition of proto-collagen prolinhydroxylase by hydrolysis products of thalidomide. This ascorbate-dependent oxidase is responsible for the formation of hydroxyproline residues in collagen and thus represents a key enzyme in collagen synthesis. The enzyme prepared from mouse or chicken embryos was variably inhibited in the *in vitro* tests by thalidomide itself in contrast to a reproducible inhibition by phtalylglutamic acid. A variability in the rate of hydrolysis and rate of elimination in different species is suggested as an

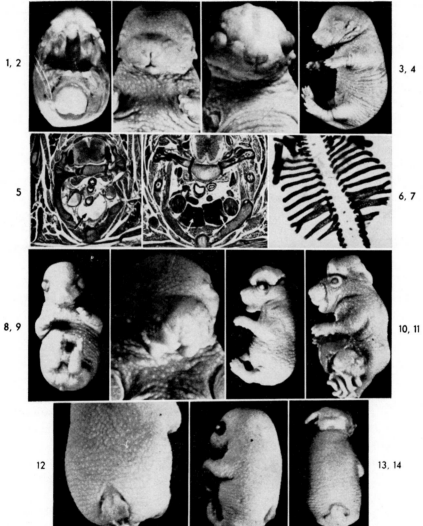

FIG. 2. Different types of malformations in mice induced by A-hypervitaminosis (Kalter and Warkany, 1961).

explanation of the species difference in teratogenic susceptibility to thalido-mide.

The mechanism of the teratogenic effect of sodium salicylate in mice has been demonstrated in a series of studies from our laboratory (Larsson, 1962; Larsson, Boström, and Ericson, 1963a; Larsson, Ericson, and Boström, 1963b). Induced congenital defects consisted of severe disturbances in the skeletal and vascular development thus affecting essentially mesenchymal organs. When A/Jax and CBA mice were given a single intra-muscular injection of sodium salicylate, p-hydroxybenzoic acid, or acetyl-salicylic acid in doses of up to 500 mg/kg on day 9 or 12 of gestation, the incidence of fetal death and vessel and skeletal malformations in the fetuses was increased in the A/Jax strain with salicylic acid but not with the other two drugs (Larsson and Boström, 1965). A reasonably good agreement was found between the teratogenic action of these drugs and their ability to depress the biosynthesis of acid mucopolysaccharides. This will be discussed in more detail.

Since sodium salicylate is most active in producing depression of polysaccharide synthesis as well as skeletal and vessel anomalies, the effect of this drug has been investigated on several enzyme systems involved in mucopolysaccharide synthesis (Whitehouse, 1965). It has been suggested that the salicylate inhibition of mucopolysaccharide synthesis is due to the interference of the drug with oxidative phosphorylation (Boström, Berntsen, and Whitehouse, 1964). However, studies by Kalbhen and Domenjoz (1967) on the failure of salicylate to reduce the ATP-level in rat paw edema seem to contradict this theory. Moreover, Jacobson, Boström, and Larsson (1964) could show that the synthesis of glucosamine-6-phosphate by L-glutamine-D-fructose-6-phosphate amino transferase prepared from mouse fetal tissue is inhibited by sodium salicylate. It is interesting to note that the structural isomer of salicylate, p-hydroxybenzoic acid, has no anti-inflammatory effect, does not produce fetal damage when given in the same concentration as salicylate, has no effect on sulfate incorporation in mucopolysaccharide, and does not inhibit L-glutamine-D-fructose-6-phosphate amino transferase from mouse fetal tissue.

Additional support has been obtained from our *in vitro* studies on ^{35}S-sulfate incorporation in calf cartilage, that glucosamine-6-phosphate formation from fructose-6-phosphate and glutamine is inhibited by salicylate since a stimulatory effect by 0.1 mM glutamine is abolished by salicylate in 6 mM concentration (Beaudoin, Boström, Friberg, and Larsson, 1969; Larsson, Boström, and Jutheden, 1968). The alternative pathway for glucosamine-6-phosphate formation from glucosamine and ATP is apparently much less affected by salicylate since salicylate does not markedly interfere with a stimulatory effect of glucosamine (Beaudoin et al., 1969).

The teratogenic dose is found between that dose which does not cause permanent fetal damage and that dose which causes fetal death

In experimental studies, it is not easy to determine the proper dose range which produces many surviving but malformed embryos and at the same time very few deaths. Similarly, it is difficult to select the proper dose range in testing teratogenicity of new drugs. The role of individual differences in drug metabolism is now receiving increased attention from fetal pharmacologists. Results of such studies should be important in teratological experiments (Gibson and Becker, 1968).

Genetic factors modify the effect of exogenous factors so that the teratogenic effect varies between individuals, strains, and species

The variation in *individual* sensitivity is best illustrated by the fact that only 20% of the women who had taken thalidomide during the critical stage of fetal development gave birth to children with congenital malformations (Lenz and Knapp, 1962). It is also interesting to note that the low frequency of hearing defects among children to mothers who have had rubella during early pregnancy may be explained by the interaction of hereditary and exogenous factors (Andersen, Barr, and Wedenberg, 1970).

The role of the genetic constitution for the risk of intrauterine damage has been thoroughly studied in experimental teratology (Smithberg, 1967). The principles are given in Fig. 3. It is well known that the *strain difference* in genetic constitution modifies the effect of teratogenic agents. Such a difference in susceptibility to several teratogens, e.g., cortisone, galactoflavin, 6-amino-nicotinamide, and salicylates, has been demonstrated in many laboratories in mice (Walker and Fraser, 1954; Kalter, 1954; Larsson, 1962; Larsson and Eriksson, 1966; Davidson, Fraser, and Schlager, 1969). The strain difference in frequency of cortisone-induced cleft palate has been used for further analysis and will serve as an example in the following discussion. Thus, in the A/Jax strain, cleft palate is produced in 100% of living embryos if embryos with cleft lip-palate are excluded (Larsson, 1962; Walker and Fraser, 1954). This latter type of malformation occurs spontaneously in about 10% in the A/Jax strain. Isolated cleft palate can be

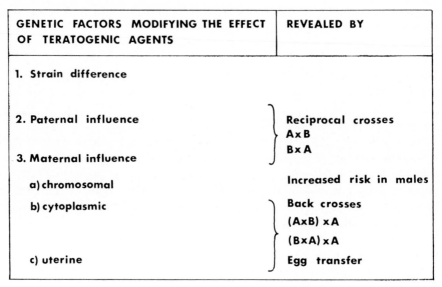

FIG. 3. Scheme of interactions between genetic and environmental teratogenic agents.

induced with cortisone only in about 20% in two other strains, C57Bl and CBA (Kalter, 1954; Larsson, 1962).

A paternal or a maternal influence can be demonstrated by reciprocal crosses. Reciprocal cross differences demonstrated in the frequency of cortisone-induced cleft palate or salicylate-induced fetal death have been shown to be matroclinous (Kalter, 1957; Larsson and Eriksson, 1966). The maternal influence could be chromosomal, cytoplasmic, or uterine.

Reciprocal crosses have revealed that fetuses growing in the A/Jax mother still get a higher percent of cortisone-induced cleft palate than those in the CBA mother (Kalter, 1954; Marsk, Theorell, and Larsson, 1971). There was no male dominance in the cleft palate groups, thus excluding a pure X-linked inheritance (Kalter, 1954). Since the autosomal genome must be considered identical in the two crosses, there remain two probable alternatives: cytoplasmic factors, inherited through the egg, or a uterine influence. Back-crosses did not show any difference, which seems to exclude a cytoplasmic influence (Kalter, 1954).

McLaren and Michie (1958) showed that a specific morphogenetic modification, a detail of form rather than the promotion or inhibition of overall growth, was brought about by the mother through the uterine environment. They introduced the elegant method of egg-transfer and demonstrated that the maternal effect on the number of lumbar vertebrae in mice was uterine. It seems justified to investigate further the possibilities of transferring eggs and blastocysts in experimental teratology (Runner, 1965).

Instead of doing the back-cross experiments we (Marsk et al., 1971) have used the nonsurgical blastocyst transfer technique (Beatty, 1951). No cleft palate was found in 25 implanted A/Jax x A/Jax embryos transferred to 13 CBA foster mothers. Homozygous A/Jax blastocysts were transferred to A/Jax foster mothers and homozygous A/Jax blastocysts to CBA foster mothers. Since the recipients were mated with fertile males of their own strain, we obtained a control to the transferred fetuses within the same mother. Because of differences in eye pigmentation, it is easy to differentiate between the two strains. The results clearly demonstrate that transferred A/Jax x A/Jax fetuses are not protected in the CBA uterus; they still show 100% cortisone-induced cleft palate. The CBA x CBA fetuses in CBA mothers had cleft palates only in 20%. Even though we had only a small number of transferred living CBA x CBA fetuses to the A/Jax foster mothers, it was clear that there was no real increase in frequency of cleft palate above the original 20%. The A/Jax fetuses had cleft palate in 100%. Thus, the maternal influence observed in the reciprocal crosses cannot be interpreted as uterine.

The technique of blastocyst transfer seems to be promising not only for studying the effect on the isolated blastocyst and the morphological malformations in the orthodox sense of teratology but also for study of problems more related to fetal pharmacology.

Concerning the *species difference,* it is well known that isolated cleft palate can be induced with cortisone in the mouse and in the rabbit but not in the rat.

In looking for species similarities, nonhuman primates have been used in teratological studies during the last few years. It is understandable that the studies have dealt with production of the thalidomide syndrome, establishing the fact that three simian forms show the same malformations at dosages comparable to those used in man (Delahunt and Lassen, 1964; Hendrickx, Axelrod, and Clayborn, 1966; Wilson and Gavan, 1967; Barrow, Steffek, and King, 1969). It has also been shown that radiation (Rugh, Duhamen, Skaredoff, and Somogyi, 1966) and androgenic hormones (van Wagenen and Hamilton, 1943; Wharton and Scott, 1964) produce similar teratological manifestations in rhesus monkeys and man. Other agents are known to produce some degree of embryotoxicity in both man and other higher primates but the parallel is less striking. For example, massive doses of aspirin given to pregnant rhesus monkeys between days 18 and 21 of gestation caused both abortion and malformation of the offspring (Wilson, 1969, 1971), and folic acid antagonists have at least abortifacient action in macaque monkeys (Delahunt, 1966; Wilson, 1971). Finally, rubella virus, an established teratogen in man, has been reported to cause cataracts and a high rate of abortion in monkeys (Delahunt, 1966). Thus, although all agents known to be teratogenic or otherwise embryotoxic in man have not been shown to be embryotoxic to the same extent in other primates, there are indications that higher primates are usually affected in one way or another by the same agents at comparable dosages and times in development.

SPECIAL EXPERIMENTAL TECHNIQUES

In some instances we would like to study the embryo directly as an entity separate from the mother's influence during development. There are three approaches for direct observations: opening the uterus to remove the embryo, opening the uterus to study the embryo *in situ,* and removing the uterus and the embryo for study. These methods have been worked out by embryologists in order to study normal developmental processes and have, moreover, been valuable tools in studying teratogenic mechanisms (Thomas, 1970; Daniel, 1971).

The influence upon blastocysts by suspected teratogenic agents was early studied *in vitro* by Lutwak-Mann and Fabro and is discussed by them elsewhere in this volume. For the fetal pharmacologist, it must also be of interest to adapt the methods for culture of post-implantation embryos worked out by New (1966). The direct influence of a drug on the fetus can then be studied under highly standardized conditions. Even the methods of organ culture, e.g., those used for studies of the teratogenic influence on limb development (Shepard, Tanimura, and Robkin, 1971), can be used for studies of a specific drug action on developmental processes.

The exposed guinea pig or lamb fetus with the placenta still attached to the uterus is a good system for pharmacological and teratological studies on the development of patent ductus arteriosus (Dawes, 1968; Hörnblad, 1969; Hörnblad, Boréus, and Larsson, 1971; Hörnblad and Larsson, 1972). Direct observation of head movements of the embryo at the stage of palate closure has been used in studies of the possible role by muscle relaxants causing cleft palate (Walker, 1969). It seems justifiable to correlate direct observations of functional impairment with results obtained by pharmacological studies on isolated organ *in vitro.*

In an attempt to elucidate the teratogenic mechanism of the commonly used teratogenic substance trypan blue, Lloyd, Beck, Williams, and Davies (1971) have studied particularly the lysosomal activity in the yolk sac placenta. According to these authors, several teratogens might act via a block of the normal degradation of proteins and thereby cause nutritional deprivation of the embryo which might lead to a malformation. It seems to me that the method for culture of the rat visceral yolk sac on a defined liquid medium would be of great value for studies on drug effects late in pregnancy.

I will give some examples of methods for direct studies on the effect on the fetus *in situ* at a later stage in the continued pregnancy. Jost (1951) early worked out methods for surgery and micro-injections on fetuses and was able to study the effect of vasopressin on the distal part of the extremities with severe injuries as an end result. Micro-methods for intra-amniotic injections have been refined by teratologists since leak of fluid can cause cleft palate (Dostal, 1971).

Böving's design of a method with which it is possible to make observations inside the living uterus and expose the living blastocyst to different agents seems to be an excellent method for studies on the local influence of drugs upon the newly implanted embryo (Daniel, 1971).

PREVENTION OF FETAL DAMAGE BY INCREASED KNOWLEDGE OF DRUG EFFECTS

Collection of information on drug effects for prevention of fetal damage can be obtained by: (1) monitoring registers of malformation; (2) literature information service; and (3) arranging research training, symposia, and workshops. I will briefly discuss the last two items.

In order to retrieve the pertinent literature on the fetal damage caused by exogenous agents, teratologists have utilized modern data techniques. This has evidently also helped the fetal pharmacologists. The databases MEDLARS, Bioses, and CAC have been used for 2 years at the Biomedical Documentation Center of the Karolinska Institute. In collaboration with the European Teratology Society, a "Teratology Lookout" containing about 250 references is produced and distributed monthly. We have been able to send it free of charge to 1,000 persons who are members of teratology societies.

The Committee for Environmental Control has suggested to the Swedish Government that the teratological effects of environmental agents should be recorded in a special data bank. Of course the bank should include also the fetal period, and we hope that this will be another important contribution from teratologists to fetal pharmacologists in our common effort to organize information and documentation systems.

The need of interdisciplinary contacts between teratologists and fetal pharmacologists was early evident. Several societies have been founded with the aim to study the etiology and pathogenesis of birth defects. A great deal of the time at meetings and congresses has been devoted to problems within the field of fetal pharmacology, and people with this special interest have been brought together. Also special foundations have been created to support prenatal research. The Association for the Aid of Crippled Children has for many years supported research and arranged workships in teratology. Such support has given inspiration to the present symposium in fetal pharmacology. It is my sincere hope that fetal pharmacology will gain as much public attention as teratology and, of course, that the two disciplines will have a mutual exchange of ideas.

ACKNOWLEDGMENT

This study was supported by grants from the Swedish Medical Research Council (B72-14P-993-07 and B72-14X-993-07) and from the Association for the Aid of Crippled Children, New York.

REFERENCES

Andersen, H., Barr, B., and Wedenberg, E. (1970): Genetic disposition–a prerequisite for maternal rubella deafness. *Archives of Otolaryngology*, 91:141-147.

Barrow, M. V., Steffek, A. J., and King, C. T. G. (1969): Thalidomide syndrome in rhesus monkeys (*Macaca mulatta*). *Folia Primatologica*, 10:195-203.

Beatty, R. A. (1951): Transplantation of mouse eggs. *Nature*, 168:995.

Beaudoin, A. R., Boström, H., Friberg, U., and Larsson, K. S. (1969): The effect of sodium salicylate on the glutamine- and glucosamine-induced stimulation of S^{35}-sulfate incorporation *in vitro*. *Arkiv för Kemi*, 30:523-527.

Boström, H., Berntsen, K., and Whitehouse, M. W. (1964): Biochemical properties of anti-inflammatory drugs. II. Some effects on sulphate-^{35}S metabolism *in vivo*. *Biochemical Pharmacology*, 13:413-420.

Catz, L., and Yaffe, S. J. (1962): Pharmacological modification of bilirubin conjugation in the newborn. *American Journal of Diseases of Children*, 104:116-117.

Daniel, J. C. (1971): *Methods in Mammalian Embryology*. W. H. Freeman and Company, San Francisco.

Davidson, J. G., Fraser, F. C., and Schlager, G. (1969): A maternal effect on the frequency of spontaneous cleft lip in the A/J mouse. *Teratology*, 2:371-376.

Dawes, G. S. (1968): *Foetal and Neonatal Physiology. A Comparative Study of the Changes at Birth*. Year Book Medical Publishers, Inc., Chicago.

Delahunt, C. S. (1966): Rubella-induced cataracts in monkeys. *Lancet*, 7441:825.

Delahunt, C. S., and Lassen, L. J. (1964): Thalidomide syndrome in monkeys. *Science*, 146:1300-1305.

Done, A. K. (1966): Perinatal pharmacology. *Annual Review of Pharmacology*, 6:189-208.

Dostal, M. (1971): Morphogenesis of cleft palate induced by exogenous factors. III. Intraamniotic application of hydrocortisone in mice. *Teratology*, 4: 63-68.

Eriksson, M. (1971): Salicylate-induced foetal damage late in pregnancy. An experimental study in mice. *Acta Paediatrica Scandinavica*, suppl. 211.

Gibson, J. E., and Becker, B. A. (1968): Effect of phenobarbital and SKF 525-A on the teratogenicity of cyclophosphamide in mice. *Teratology*, 1:393-398.

Guidelines for Reproduction Studies for Safety Evaluation of Drugs for Human Use. (1966). Food and Drug Administration (FDA), USA.

Hendrickx, A. G., Axelrod, L. R., and Clayborn, L. D. (1966): "Thalidomide" syndrome in baboons. *Nature*, 210:958-959.

Hörnblad, P. Y. (1969): Experimental studies on closure of the ductus arteriosus utilizing whole-body freezing. *Acta Paediatrica Scandinavica*, suppl. 190.

Hörnblad, P. Y., Boréus, L. O., and Larsson, K. S. (1970): Studies on closure of the ductus arteriosus. VIII. Reduced closure rate in guinea pigs treated with phenoxybenzamine. *Cardiology*, 55:237-241.

Hörnblad, P. Y., and Larsson, K. S. (1972): Studies on closure of the ductus arteriosus. IX. Transitory effect of phenoxybenzamine on ductal closure in the guinea pig. *Acta Pharmacologica et Toxicologica*, 31:149-152.

Jacobson, B. J., Boström, H., and Larsson, K. S. (1964): The effect of sodium salicylate on hexosamine synthesis in eviscerated mouse fetuses. *Acta Chemica Scandinavica*, 18:818-821.

Jost, A. (1951): Sur le rôle de la vasopressine et de la corticostimuline (A.C.T.H.) dans la production expérimentale de lésions des extrémités foetales (hémorragies, nécroses, amputations congénitales). *Comptes Rendus des Séances de la Société de Biologie et de ses Filiales*, 145:1805-1809.

Kalbhen, D. A., and Domenjoz, R. (1967): The effect of phenylbutazone and sodium salicylate on the adenosin-triphosphate level in rat paw edema. *Bulletin de Chimi Therapeutique*, 5:375-377.

Kalter, H. (1954): Inheritance of susceptibility to the teratogenic action of cortisone in mice. *Genetics*, 39:185.

Kalter, H. (1957): Factors influencing the frequency of cortisone-induced cleft palate in mice. *Journal of Experimental Zoology*, 134:449-467.

Kalter, H., and Warkany, J. (1961): Experimental production of congenital malformations in strains of inbred mice by maternal treatment with hypervitaminosis A. *American Journal of Pathology*, 38:1-21.

Larsson, K. S. (1962): Closure of the secondary palate and its relation to sulphomucopolysaccharides. *Acta Odontologica Scandinavica*, 20: suppl. 31.

Larsson, K. S., Boström, H., and Ericson, B. (1963a): Salicylate-induced malformations inhibition of mucopolysaccharide synthesis. *Acta Paediatrica Scandinavica*, 54:43-48.

Larsson, K. S., Boström, H., and Ericson, B. (1963a): Salicylate-induced malformations in mouse embryos. *Acta Paediatrica Scandinavica*, 52:36-40.

Larsson, K. S., Boström, H., and Jutheden, G. (1968): Influence of *in vivo* salicylate treatment on S^{35}-sulfate *in vitro* incorporation in mesenchymal tissue. *Arkiv för Kemi*, 29:389-394.

Larsson, K. S., Ericson, B., and Boström, H. (1963b): Salicylate-induced skeletal and vessel malformations in mouse embryos. *Acta Morphologica Neerlando-Scandinavica*, 6:35-44.

Larsson, K. S., and Eriksson, M. (1966): Salicylate-induced fetal death and malformations in two mouse strains. *Acta Paediatrica Scandinavica,* 55:569-576.

Lenz, W. (1961): Diskussion, Tagung der Rhein-Westf. Kinderätze. *Deutsche Medizinische Wochenschrift,* 86:2555-2556.

Lenz, W., and Knapp. K. (1962): Die Thalidomid-Embryopathie. *Deutsche Medizinische Wochenschrift,* 87:1232-1242.

Lloyd, J. B., Beck, F., Williams, K. E., and Davies, M. (1971): Biochemical data on teratogenic mechanisms. In: *Malformations Congénitales des Mammifères,* edited by H. Tuchmann-Duplessis. Masson et Cie, Paris, pp. 315-332.

Marsk, L., Theorell, M., and Larsson, K. S. (1971): Transfer as applied in experimental teratology. *Nature,* 234:358-359.

McBride, W. G. (1961): Thalidomide and congenital abnormalities. *Lancet,* II:1358.

McLaren, A., and Michie, D. (1958): Factors affecting vertebral variation in mice. 4. Experimental proof of the uterine basis of a maternal effect. *Journal of Embryology and Experimental Morphology,* 6:645-659.

Millen, J. W. (1962): Thalidomide and limb deformities. *Lancet,* II:599-600.

Neubert, D., and Köhler, E. (1970): Hypothetical explanation of the embryotoxic action of thalidomide. Eine Hypothese zur Erklärung der embryotoxischen Wirkung von Thalidomid. *Naunyn-Schmiedeberg's Archiv für experimentelle Pathologie und Pharmakologie,* 266:408-409.

New, D. A. T. (1966): *The Culture of Vertebrate Embryos.* Logos Press, London.

Nishimura, H. (1970): Fate of human fertilized eggs during prenatal life: Present status of knowledge. *Okajimas Folia Anatomica Japonica,* 46:297-305.

Nishimura, H., Takano, K., Tanimura, T., and Yasuda, M. (1968): Normal and abnormal development of human embryos: First report of the analysis of 1,213 intact embryos. *Teratology,* 1:281-290.

Rugh, R., Duhamen, L., Skaredoff, L., and Somogyi, C. (1966): Gross sequelae of fetal X-irradiation of the monkey (*Macaca mulatta*). I. Effect on body and organ weights at 23 months. *Atompraxis,* 12:468-472.

Runner, M. N. (1965): Transplantation of mammalian ova: Blastocyst and earlier stages. In: *Teratology. Principles and Techniques,* edited by J. G. Wilson and J. Warkany. University of Chicago Press, Chicago, pp. 95-111.

Shepard, T. H., Tanimura, T., and Robkin, M. (1971): *In vitro* studies for analysis of teratogenic events. In: *Malformations Congénitales des Mammifères,* edited by H. Tuchmann-Duplessis. Masson et Cie, Paris, pp. 54-64.

Smithberg, M. (1968): Teratogenesis in inbred strains of mice. In: *Advances in Teratology II,* edited by D. H. M. Woollam. Academic Press, London, pp. 258-288.

Thomas, J. A. (1970): *Organ Culture.* Academic Press, New York.

Van Wagenen, G., and Hamilton, J. B. (1943): The experimental production of pseudohermaphroditism in the monkey. *Essays in Biology,* University of California Press, pp. 583-607.

Walker, B. E. (1969): Correlation of embryonic movement with palate closure in mice. *Teratology,* 2:191-198.

Walker, B. E., and Fraser, F. C. (1954): The embryological basis for a strain difference in susceptibility to a teratogenic action of cortisone. *Genetics,* 39:1000.

Wharton, L. R., and Scott, R. B. (1964): Experimental production of genital lesions with norethindrone. *American Journal of Obstetrics and Gynecology,* 89:701-715.

Whitehouse, M. W. (1965): Some biochemical and pharmacological properties of anti-inflammatory drugs. *Fortschritte der Arzneimittelforschung,* 8:321-429.

Wilson, J. G. (1959): Experimental studies on congenital malformations. *Journal of Chronic Diseases,* 10:111-130.

Wilson, J. G. (1969): Teratological and reproductive studies in non-human primates. In: *Methods for Teratological Studies in Experimental Animals and Man,* edited by H. Nishimura and J. R. Miller. Igaku Shoin Ltd., Tokyo, pp. 16-31.

Wilson, J. G. (1971): Use of primates in teratological research and testing. In: *Malformations Congénitales des Mammifères,* edited by H. Tuchmann-Duplessis. Masson et Cie, Paris, pp. 273-290.

Wilson, J. G., and Gavan, J. A. (1967): Congenital malformations in non-human primates: Spontaneous and experimentally induced. *Anatomical Record,* 158:99-110.

Wilson, J. G., and Warkany, J. (1965): *Teratology. Principles and Techniques.* University of Chicago Press, Chicago.

World Health Organization (WHO) (1967): Principles for the testing of drugs for teratogenicity. Report of a WHO scientific group. *World Health Organization. Technical Report Series,* 364.

Yaffe, S. J. (1968): Fetal and neonatal toxicity of drugs. *Canadian Medical Association Journal,* 98:301-306.

DISCUSSION

NISHIMURA: We believe that the critical period in man for a certain teratogen is hard to define if the age of the embryo is determined on the basis of LMP. In our studies on several hundred human embryos from mothers with fairly regular menstrual cycles, there was a remarkable individual variation of developmental stage at any given calendar age. The reported critical period for limb defects by thalidomide, 26 to 40 days after fertilization, are not in accord with our results.

SWINYARD: Dr. Larsson has very adequately presented the contributions of teratology to fetal pharmacology. The fine papers we have heard here from biochemical pharmacologists and fetal physiologists suggest that biochemical pharmacology as applied to maternal-fetal drug distribution and metabolism holds the greatest promise for future resolution of many of the human malformation problems.

I should like to call your attention to the existence of the Japanese, American, and European Teratology Societies. The Journal of the American Teratology Society has expanded its scope to include clinical and biochemical pharmacology. Dr. Neubert will be one of the editors. I urge you to look at the expanded journal which may serve as a very appropriate journal for publication of data on malformations.

KARCZMAR: This is a comment rather than a question. You described the type of teratological drug-induced change and you specified the extent of time (embryonic and fetal time) during which the tests of teratogenicity are carried out. To the morphological change (teratology in the strict sense of the word), the behavioral change should be added as another parameter to be tested. Moreover, the test time should be extended to postnatal life, particularly with regard to the behavioral changes which may be due to pharmacological challenge during pregnancy. In our laboratory, we have found a number of drugs, hormones, food preservatives, and pollutants the exposure to which during pregnancy caused behavioral changes of the offspring at adulthood (mice experiments). Moreover, in some cases this "behavioral teratology" occurred without appreciable changes in a number of biochemical parameters that were studied, and certainly in the absence of morphological teratology.

ELIS: The teratogenic tests should be extended to more than one generation. We performed several "multigeneration experiments" in which drugs such as 6-azauridine, actinomycin D, urethane, and others were administered to experimental animals for several generations. We observed qualitative and quantitative changes in teratogenic effect in each generation.

JOST: Dr. Larsson, looking at the title of your presentation, I wonder whether you would not even extend the ambition of teratology for the future. When the effect of teratogenic agents will be studied at the cellular and biochemical level, teratology will become a very useful tool in exploring the mechanism of normal and abnormal development, and of many pharmacological effects.

LARSSON: Teratology is going in the direction toward biochemistry and pharmacology-toxicology with regard to methodology used. It is important that we can arrange the training so that the methods in these disciplines can be used optimally.

MANN: The experiments of Dr. Larsson, involving blastocyst transfer between mice of two different strains (A/Jax and CBA), provide a particularly clear-cut illustration of the great value which the transfer method has in determining the influence of uterine environment specifically and in teratological studies generally. I wonder, however, if the same difference between the two strains (A/Jax and CBA) which Dr. Larsson observed would have been equally apparent if the donor and recipient mouse had been not of the same but of different ages. Age of the pregnant animal has, after all, a very important influence on the behavior of the uterine environment toward the conceptus, and two strains of the same species may very well differ in that respect, in the same way as two strains of a single species are known to differ in respect of the age at which they reach puberty and become fertile. A classical example of an age-dependent process is provided by the well-known experiment by Adams in our Unit who demonstrated that although an old rabbit doe produces a nearly normal number of fertilized ova, these zygotes are incapable of developing further in that animal. However, the same zygotes, when transferred to the uterus of a young doe, undergo normal development there. Conversely, zygotes produced by a young doe, although capable of developing normally in that doe, are incapable of development after transfer to the old doe.

FUCHS: In relation to the comment about behavioral changes, I would like to point out that we also have to consider changes that are not present at birth but occur later in life. I am thinking of the recent finding that intake of diethylstilbestrol by the mother predisposes of the development of cancer of the vagina in young women. There is also the suggestion that chorioretinitis developing later in life may be due to congenital toxoplasmosis; although this is not a drug effect, it does indicate that even late changes may be traced back to pregnancy with the use of registries and case records.

ELIS: I think this is a very important remark. We studied the effect of N-hydroxy-urethan, applied to pregnant mouse females 24 to 48 hours before delivery, and we found that about 53% of the offspring from injected mothers 6 months after birth developed lung adenomas. In control offspring, when mothers were injected by saline only, the incidence of lung adenomas was only 6%.

NEUBERT: The problem of extrapolating data from animal studies to man is as old as pharmacology and toxicology. Research within the last decades has shown that the problem may be solved at least partially.

I personally feel that, at the moment, good experiments which stand on solid statistical grounds can only be performed in mice, rats, rabbits or similar small experimental animals, the metabolism of which, in many respects, is much better known than that of the primates. As soon as we have more basic knowledge on the biochemistry and micromorphology of embryonic development in these species, we have to compare our results with metabolic pathways in human tissues, and I feel that this is possible today.

With regard to experiments with nonhuman primates, I feel that such studies are valuable but they should be restricted to special problems because of the fact that statistically adequate experiments can hardly be performed today. The value of such studies in primates should not be overestimated.

LEVY: Teratogenic studies in animals should be carried out with drug doses which match free drug concentrations in the plasma or produce multiples of therapeutic free drug concentrations used in man. Similar studies should be done with the drug metabolites formed in man.

LARSSON: This is true and should be considered during revisions of guidelines for teratology tests of new drugs.

KARCZMAR: Studies on "behavioral teratology" are difficult in man, but not impossible. Subtle behavioral tests (of memory, conditioning, etc.) are available. Insofar as animal material is concerned, let me say a word or two in defense of mice. These are "man-like" animals in the behavioral and evolutionary sense, successful in evolution and exhibiting a wide range of individual, social, and ethological behavior, and all these types of behavior can be readily and relatively cheaply quantified (see Karczmar, Scudder, and Richardson: *Neurosciences Research*, 1972, 5:*in press*).

MANN: The rabbit zygote, as already pointed out, is capable of further development either when transferred to another rabbit (synchronized) or when left in a suitable culture medium for a day or two. I may add perhaps in relation to that phenomenon, that a zygote of one species may even survive for a few days after transfer to the uterus of another species. As shown by Rowson and his colleagues in our Unit, a sheep zygote, for example, originating from an English Border-Leicester ewe, can be inserted in Cambridge into a live rabbit, and that rabbit, which acts as a living incubator, can be sent by air to South Africa. There, the sheep embryo, after recovery from the rabbit, can be transferred successfully into the uterus of a South-African Dorper ewe. In due course, the Dorper ewe will produce an English Border-Leicester lamb.

MCBRIDE: Dr. Larsson mentioned that we had been studying drugs for 10 years. Ten years ago, 1961, I postulated that thalidomide affected developing mesenchyme by acting as a glutamic acid antagonist. Now, 10 years later, I cannot prove that I was right and no one can say that I am wrong because no one is working on the problem of thalidomide.

Fetal Pharmacology, edited by L. Boréus
Raven Press, New York © 1973

Drugs and the Blastocyst

C. Lutwak-Mann

Unit of Reproductive Physiology and Biochemistry, Department of Applied Biology, University of Cambridge, Cambridge, England

INTRODUCTION

This chapter needs little historical introduction. One can safely assert that 15 or even 10 years ago, the conveners of a symposium on fetal pharmacology would not have bothered to include in their proceedings a section devoted to the effect of drugs on the mammalian blastocyst. What were the reasons for such a negative attitude? One was simply the lack of sufficient information on the early stages of embryonic development. The other, rather more weighty and arising directly from that deficiency, was the generally held conviction that, until implantation and maternal-fetal blood links become fully established, the conceptus cannot be a target for maternally conveyed noxious agents: the dictum "safe, as in the mother's womb" amounted to an article of faith among obstetricians, gynecologists, and pediatricians alike. The notion that anything *detrimental* to the progress of the early free-lying embryo could emanate from the mother appeared so heretical as to be wholly unacceptable. Another view, supporting the former, and entrenched among anatomists and embryologists, was that the zygote relies exclusively on its own preformed supplies, and is inherently incapable of taking up any materials, nutrient or otherwise, from its tubal environment. This concept virtually ruled out the possibility that medication of the mother at the zygote stage could have deleterious repercussions on simultaneous or subsequent embryonic growth.

Today these views strike one as preposterous, but their prevalence until fairly recently can readily be verified by perusal of older literature. While reminiscing, I may as well add a more personal note: the intransigence alluded to above, dismissing as it did the value of pharmacological experimentation at the blastocyst stage, made me wonder if this line of investigation was worth pursuing as an end in itself.

Ultimately, however, these controversies only served to strengthen my determination to press on with the study of the physiology and biochemistry of the blastocyst. Parallel with research on embryos, and in order to provide the necessary background, some properties of the maternal environment were also being studied. As an integral part of these basic investigations on blastocyst-uterine relationships, an enquiry was made into the action upon the blastocyst of various agents, including pharmacologically active substances, transmitted by the maternal route; this work was later extended to observations on the effect of embryonic exposure in vitro.

Research on all these problems was proceeding quietly and unobtrusively in a few laboratories in addition to our own when, rather unexpectedly, in the early sixties, it gained immensely in popularity and therefore multiplicity of endeavor, owing to the unprecedented upsurge of interest in the pharmacology of the early conceptus stirred up by the thalidomide disaster. This boost to experimentation in hitherto neglected areas of pharmacology yielded a considerable amount of heterogeneous information. Looking back, one can say that, although some of it has since proved to be of permanent value, much has turned out to be useless and is already practically forgotten. In a small way, we, too, have been able to contribute to the store of knowledge concerning the action of thalidomide. But because thalidomide and its effects at various stages of development will be discussed by more than one contributor in this volume, comments in this chapter are restricted to experiments which pertain to this drug chiefly in relation to the free-lying rabbit blastocysts.

In order to understand and be able to assess the results that have been obtained over the years in studies with a vast number of "embryo-seeking" agents, it is essential to view the findings in their proper setting. Therefore, a brief synopsis will be given of developmental, physiological, and biochemical properties peculiar to the blastocyst stage, as well as some of the processes which are concomitantly underway in the maternal environment. Although the main emphasis will be on blastocysts, reference will be made to the zygote and the immediate post-blastocyst stages. Some methodological aspects and requirements of experimentation will also be briefly discussed.

SOME PROPERTIES OF THE EARLY MAMMALIAN EMBRYO

The recent widespread interest and intense research activity in the pre-implantation stages of embryonic growth are reflected in the contents of two multidisciplinary symposia which cover the manifold aspects of this sector of developmental biology. The first, *The mammalian oviduct* (Hafez and Blandau, 1969), deals with the zygote stage, and the second, *The biology of the blastocyst* (Blandau, 1971), is directly linked to our particular subject matter. These two volumes may be consulted by the expert for detailed information and references concerning the zygote and the blastocyst stage, respectively; they are a *must* for beginners in this field.

Developmental characteristics of the blastocyst

For clarity it may be convenient in the discussion of mammalian embryos to use the following terminology to denote developmental stages: "oocyte" (secondary oocyte at metaphase II) for the cell type that undergoes ovulation; "egg" (ovum) for the oocyte after ovulation but before fertilization; "fertilized egg" or "zygote" for cleavage stages up to the morula; and "blastocyst" for the stage that begins with cavitation, leading to the formation of the blastocoele, and terminates in implantation. In certain species, for example, the rabbit, before implantation the blastocyst first undergoes endometrial attachment, which represents a type of transient placentation, functional for a limited period only, until implantation proper has been completed. The term "embryo" will be restricted to the pre-implantation conceptus only, and "fetus" used for the post-implantation stages.

The blastocyst is an obligatory phase of embryonic development. It is as yet uncertain exactly how the cells of the morula sort themselves out so that some proceed to form the embryo and others become extraembryonic tissues. It is conceivable that when the morula-into-blastocyst development is in progress, at least two cell layers are formed, an inner and an outer one, bounded by the unyielding zona pellucida; the cells that find themselves in the interior, and are thus cut off from the maternal environment, evolve into the embryo, whereas the peripheral layer, exposed directly to maternal elements, develops into the trophoblast. This is an attractive hypothesis (Tarkowski and Wróblewska, 1967), but a great deal of experimental evidence will have to be accumulated before it can be accepted.

Blastocysts show innumerable species-dependent variations in size, cell number, degree of differentiation, and timing, as well as type of uterine attachment and implantation. What must be stressed about the blastocyst is that, regardless of the many diverse attributes, all blastocysts represent a complex entity, made up of morphologically as well as physiologically distinct regions, *viz,* the embryo proper (inner cell mass, embryonic disc), and the trophoblast, which forms the layer of cells that lines the blastocoelic cavity. The latter contains a fluid which qualitatively and quantitatively has a very special composition. The mechanism whereby the blastocyst fluid accumulates and the various solutes are held by the trophoblast, often against a concentration gradient, is not yet clearly understood. Some of the constituents of the blastocyst fluid are probably common to all species, but others are likely to be species-characteristic.

So long as the blastocyst lies free in the uterine lumen, it is encased in the zona pellucida, the external surface of which is heavily coated with a secretory deposit produced by the endometrial glands. During the time preceding attachment or nidation, the zona pellucida becomes greatly attenuated, and is finally shed in a manner which is typical for each species.

Physiological and biochemical aspects of the blastocyst

From this oversimplified description of the blastocyst, it is immediately obvious that before any exogenous, maternally transmitted agent can reach the embryonic cells within the blastocyst, it must be able to traverse several "barriers." These are operative partly within the surrounding maternal tissues (that is, the endometrial mucosa) and partly in the vestments of the embryo itself. Thus, the initially blood-borne substance first passes from the epithelial cells of the endometrium into the endometrial secretion, which at the blastocyst stage usually consists of a thick and scanty material, abounding in cellular debris. From there it penetrates, through the external coating laid down on the zona pellucida, into the zona itself, and reaches the highly selective trophoblast.

It has been hitherto believed that only relatively small molecules are capable of surmounting all these barriers, and especially the trophoblast. In the light of more recent evidence, however, it seems likely that certain proteins (e.g., uteroglobin, carbonic anhydrase, molecular weight about 30,000) and even large molecules such as ferritin (molecular weight about 500,000) can enter at any rate the rabbit blastocyst (A. C. Enders, *personal communication*). That there is a high degree of regulatory power at the blastocyst level can be demonstrated in various ways, but perhaps most simply and convincingly in experiments with trypan blue. This azo-dye, when administered to the rabbit maternally, quickly reaches the endometrium and its secretion, both of which it stains a deep blue, but it is unable to enter free-lying blastocysts; on the other hand, it passes into blastocyst fluid readily once the uterine attachment of these embryos has been accomplished. Altogether, some of the observations on the transmissibility of exogenous agents in relation to molecular size, appear somewhat contradictory; therefore, for the time being, it seems safest not to generalize but to judge each case on its own merits. Doubtless, a great deal depends upon the chemical configuration of the agent; it is the chemical nature of the substance which will, to a considerable extent, facilitate or hinder blastocyst penetration.

Having found access into the inner space of the blastocyst, the foreign substance and/or its breakdown products must duly return to the peripheral circulation by the same intricate pathway if elimination is to take place at the blastocyst stage. In this context, however, one must realize that because of the extremely rapid rate of growth, even if the hypothetical agent had entered the embryonic compartment at the blastocyst stage, by the time it has been metabolized, a different and more advanced embryonic phase will have been attained, which of course, would possess physiological properties more highly evolved than the blastocyst.

The biochemistry of the mammalian zygote and blastocyst, the understanding of which is mandatory for pharmacological experimentation, has been studied recently with great vigor, and several review articles which discuss in detail various aspects of the biochemical properties of the pre-implantation embryo, chiefly mouse and rabbit, are included in the two monographs referred to above.

The lines of biochemical investigation pursued consist of compilation of data on the chemical composition of the embryos, the type and rate of metabolism at the zygote and blastocyst stage, respectively, and the ability to utilize certain key substrates. In addition, the presence of a variety of enzymes has been studied, at stages ranging from the oocyte to the blastocyst.

The study of the chemical composition of the zygote is rudimentary. But a fair amount is known about the chemical constituents of the blastocyst (Lutwak-Mann, 1966, 1971). The available information indicates that the blastocysts are equipped in all the coenzymes needed to catalyze and sustain an advanced type of metabolism. Of the more recent findings, perhaps the most intriguing one is the detection in blastocysts of hormones, namely, progesterone and its derivatives and corticosterone (Seamark and Lutwak-Mann, 1972), confirming the earlier preliminary report of the occurrence of progesterone in rabbit blastocyst fluid (Lutwak-Mann, 1971).

It is as yet unknown what role, if any, these hormones play in blasto-cyst metabolism. It would be useful in this respect to find out if cyclic AMP occurs in blastocysts. So far, information is available only with respect to ATP in the blastocysts of the rabbit (Brooks and Lutwak-Mann, 1971) and of the mouse (Quinn and Wales, 1971).

The main points that have emerged from the biochemical researches on embryonic metabolism are that, whereas the zygote chiefly utilizes pyruvate and lactate, the metabolism of the blastocyst is more like that of adult tissue, and its main energy-yielding substrate is glucose. This at any rate is the situation in the two species generally studied, the mouse and the rabbit. It remains as yet to be seen if in other species, and especially in the human, there is this much emphasized dependence of zygotes on pyruvic and lactic acid. The doubt in this respect is due to the fact that the blood levels of these two acids are much higher in the laboratory animals than in man; on the other hand, the blood glucose levels are the same.

As an inseparable part of studies on the chemistry of the embryos, at-tention has been devoted by our laboratory to blastocyst-uterine links, within the wider problem of maternal-embryonic exchange mechanisms. These ex-periments included the investigation of the entry and clearance from the blastocysts of certain sugars (Lutwak-Mann, 1954), labeled ions (Lutwak-Mann, Boursnell, and Bennett, 1960; Lutwak-Mann and McIntosh, 1971). and drugs (Lutwak-Mann, 1962a). In addition, a large variety of agents, which will be discussed later, was examined by the application of purely morphological criteria.

Concerning quantitative aspects of maternal-blastocyst exchange mecha-nisms, it is evident that these are carefully adjusted, for native as well as foreign substances, by specialized but as yet unidentified, regulatory systems, active at the level of the endometrium and the blastocyst itself. The experi-mental results available indicate that the flux in the blastocyst compartment is low. In practical terms, it means that following penetration of the blasto-cyst space by an exogenous agent, the embryo shows only a small fraction (in terms of concentration) of the load present in the maternal bloodstream; this disparity is, of course, most striking in the early post-treatment interval. Furthermore, there is a delay in the rate of clearance of maternally intro-duced substances from the embryonic compartment, which lags significantly behind the rate of elimination from the mother's circulation. Owing to this delay, a noxious agent or its breakdown products are likely to persist, often for an unpredictable length of time, in the growing embryos.

Among the many processes and problems that impinge upon blastocyst biology are: the formation of certain endometrial proteins (Krishnan and Daniel, 1967; Beier, 1968) and nucleic acids (Vittorelli, Harrison, and Lutwak-Mann, 1967), concomitantly with the development of blastocysts; the accumulation in uterine tissue of certain trace metals such as zinc (Lutwak-Mann and McIntosh, 1969); and the role of calcium and zinc in blastocyst metabolism (Lutwak-Mann and McIntosh, 1971; McIntosh and Lutwak-Mann, 1972). As yet, it has not been possible to link any of these processes directly with the action of drugs on blastocysts.

THE ACTION OF VARIOUS AGENTS ON THE MAMMALIAN EMBRYO

Methodology

Thorough knowledge of reproductive physiology and biochemistry, at least of the animal species that the investigator proposes to work with, is essential in studies with agents administered so as to induce effects at embryonic level. No matter how sophisticated the approach, no scientifically sound advance can be made in ignorance of basic facts concerning embryonic development as well as the accompanying situation in the maternal environment. In other words, one must at least know what may be expected to happen and where and how to look for it. The points made below follow from the above statement.

The first requirement in experiments involving the action of pharmacodynamically active agents upon embryos is to ensure the availability of high-fertility animal donors, preferably from a colony with a well-established record of reproductive performance. This is obviously necessary if the effect of drug treatment is to be judged, for instance, by the occurrence of malformations: without determining the incidence of spontaneously occurring malformations, one cannot assess the teratogenic potency of the chemical under examination.

The choice of a suitable provider of experimental material is another requirement in biochemical or pharmacological experiments dealing with an object of study as small and delicate, and scarce, as the early mammalian embryo. For studies on the zygote, the superovulated mouse has become the standard donor of material, mainly because its low cost permits the sacrifice of the vast numbers of animals that are needed for experiments at this early developmental stage. Quite a lot of work is also being done on zygotes of other animals, e.g., the rat and rabbit.

Insofar as blastocysts are concerned, the tiny mouse or rat blastocysts are often inadequate and awkward to cope with, so that a good many investigators, including the author, have preferred to use rabbit blastocysts. The advantages that the rabbit blastocyst offers as an experimental object have been fully discussed (Lutwak-Mann, 1971); they can be summarized as follows.

The rabbit is one of the few laboratory species in which the time of ovulation, and therefore the age of the conceptus, is predictable; the numerical availability enables the investigator to subdivide embryos within each batch into directly comparable groups; free-lying rabbit blastocysts can be lifted directly off the endometrial surface, which makes it possible to preserve intact the important secretory deposit on the surface of the zona pellucida; the large size enables the application of histological techniques, such as the flat-mount procedure (Moog and Lutwak-Mann, 1958); the relatively prolonged duration of the blastocyst stage, consisting of 2 days in the free state and (roughly) 3 days in the attached condition, gives opportunity for long-term experimentation; and, finally, the rabbit uterus and the endometrium especially lend themselves particularly well to the biochemical study of the blastocysts' maternal environment. The one serious disadvantage in the use of the rabbit lies in the fact that the endometrial secretion is scarce at the progestational, that is, the blastocyst, stage; thus, it is impractical to use this material for quantitative analysis, even by adopting sophisticated methods. As a substitute, however, we have often used the abundant estrous uterine fluid (Lutwak-Mann, 1962a; Leone, Libonati, and Lutwak-Mann, 1963; Lutwak-Mann and McIntosh, 1971).

Of the three basic requirements of any "pharmacological" experimentation—route, dosage, and timing—dosage and timing take precedence over route of administration in experiments with embryos. Whereas the route of administration is mostly a question of expediency or dependent upon the nature of the agent, dosage matters a great deal. It cannot be stressed too strongly that if dosage is stepped up so as to interfere with maternal health in pregnancy, this will deprive of all significance observations subsequently made with embryos (always provided they survive), because, to an unpredictable extent, the results will be due to the upheaval in the maternal organism and not to the action of the examined agent on the embryo itself. Even a relatively minor effect, e.g., moderate maternal hyperglycemia, which can be produced (in the rabbit) by disparate agents such as certain sulfonamides, alloxan, or cortisone, may be sufficient to inflict serious damage on the embryo.

With regard to timing, if one wishes to act on the oocyte, treatment must start before or, at the latest, at the time of mating; if on the zygote, then treatment must be spaced to coincide with the well-defined progress of cleavage. Among criteria of a deleterious action on the oocyte will be absence of ovulation or fertilization; the effect on the zygotes would express itself as arrest of cleavage.

In experiments with blastocysts as potential targets (using the rabbit embryo as a convenient model), the options open to the experimenter are that administration of the active substance can begin at any point before, or be limited to, the blastocyst stage. Criteria of effects induced in blastocysts are rather more diverse than in zygotes. Upon autopsy of the treated female, we may be confronted with (1) total absence or (2) diminished number, of blastocysts, as judged by comparison with the number of corpora lutea found, (3) grossly substandard blastocysts, (4) interference with the chronology of uterine attachment and/or implantation, in which case deficiencies in placental structure will probably also be obvious; minor, but significant, signs of interference are (5) irregularity in blastocyst spacing (very pronounced, e.g., after suitably timed estrogen treatment), and (6) excess free fluid in the uterine lumen, the presence of which, at the blastocyst stage, is unphysiological and denotes leakage from the blastocoele of dying embryos.

The handling of the embryos for morphological or chemical or any other type of experiment will depend on the species and the developmental stage. Irrespective of species, the zygotes can be recovered only by washing through the oviduct with a suitable wash-fluid. The same treatment applies to the small rat or mouse blastocysts; in the rabbit, however, washing is unnecessary, and individual blastocysts are scooped up from the endometrium with a glass or steel spoon. The scanty uterine secretion is best taken up by capillary suction in filter or lens paper, and subsequently eluted; care must be taken to ensure that chemicals contained in filter paper do not interfere with assays. From attached blastocysts, the fluid is withdrawn by aspiration across the attachment dome; this is the only material available for study at this stage, unless one resorts to the freezing procedure (Brambell, 1948) which permits collection of the entire conceptus, albeit no longer suitable for morphological examination or culture *in vitro*.

The scope of embryonic pharmacology

What type(s) of experiment do we envisage when we speak of embryonic pharmacology? Presumably, we have in mind experiments which involve the action upon embryos of maternally transmitted agents, supposed to possess some pharmacodynamic properties capable of inducing clearly recognizable changes in the embryos. This means a wide spectrum of experimental approaches, ranging from routine testing of known or newly synthesized "pharmaceuticals" to maternal exposure to radiation, pathogenic virus, acute or chronic nutritional deprivation, endocrine interference, and the like.

A fairly recent extension of this well-tried approach is the experiments in which various agents are made to act on embryos directly, under conditions *in vitro*. Probably their inclusion under the heading of embryonic pharmacology is justifiable, if we insist that the free-lying embryo represents an individual finite entity, capable under chosen conditions of continuous orderly development, at any rate for a limited length of time—usually long enough, however, to permit assessment of pharmacological action. Since so much interesting information has been obtained from experiments with embryos *in vitro,* this type of study certainly merits our consideration. As a more esoteric upshot of the *in vitro* incubation, we might also mention experiments in which embryos are transferred into certain extrauterine sites (e.g., kidney capsule, eye, testis), where they also manage to survive for some time. However, the weakness of this approach is that embryonic growth tends to be disorganized, and consists almost exclusively of trophoblastic tissue which proliferates under these conditions.

How is one to assess "pharmacological" action on early embryos? Insofar as effects on the zygote are concerned, these have routinely been evaluated under conditions *in vitro* by observing the formation of the blastocoelic cavity in control and treated embryos. This is a weak criterion, since it is perfectly possible that a blastocoele will develop in a purely trophoblastic vesicle, completely devoid of proper embryonic elements.

A more complex method, which we attempted in the past (Adams, Hay, and Lutwak-Mann, 1961), is to expose the zygotes *in vivo* to the tubal environment of a host that had been treated with a pharmacologically active agent, while control zygotes from the same litter are made to spend an equally long time in the oviduct of an untreated host. After this preliminary exposure, usually lasting a few hours, both the treated and the untreated control zygotes are retransferred to the oviducts of normal, hormonally synchronized hosts and permitted to proceed to term. This is admittedly a roundabout way, which, nevertheless gave us clear-cut results: we were able to prove that zygotes that had been temporarily exposed to a noxious maternal environment (caused by administration of mercaptopurine), failed to develop to term upon transfer to normal hosts; in contrast, a high percentage of control zygotes progressed normally to term.

In experiments with blastocysts, there is a wider choice of methods by which to judge what has happened to the embryos. First, one can apply a histological method, such as the flat-mount technique (Adams et al., 1961; Lutwak-Mann and Hay, 1965a,b, 1967), which throws light on the condition of the blastocyst. A variant of this approach is to remove (at laparotomy) the free-lying blastocysts from one uterine horn for histological study, and, for comparison, let the embryos in the contralateral horn go on to term. One can also do blastocyst transfers in the manner outlined above for zygotes, but this is more convenient with the small blastocysts of the rat or mouse than with the large rabbit blastocysts. Furthermore, one can recover blastocysts after various periods of maternal exposure, and transfer them to a culture medium known to support their growth. We have tried this method (Lutwak-Mann, Hay, and New, 1969) and found that, provided the blastocysts had not been excessively damaged by the preceding maternal exposure, they were capable of recovery under conditions *in vitro*. To obtain a convincing proof of recovery in this type of experiment, however, one would have to transfer the cultured blastocysts back to suitable hosts in order to check their ability to develop normally to term.

Recently we attempted to utilize the ATP/ADP ratio as an indicator of blastocyst integrity and viability (Brooks and Lutwak-Mann, 1971), in experiments in which the blastocysts had been exposed to well-defined conditions both *in vivo* and *in vitro*. We found that there was only a minor change in the ATP/ADP ratio after brief, and therefore ineffective, exposures; however, in response to treatment known to result in serious disorganization of blastocyst structure, such as, e.g., anoxia, the ATP/ADP ratio showed a significant decrease.

Yet another approach has recently been gaining ground, namely, the chemical followup of the maternally administered agent, preferably labeled isotopically for easy identification, in the blastocyst and sometimes also in the endometrial secretion. This was first successfully attempted in experiments with (^{14}C)-thalidomide (Fabro, Schumacher, Smith, and Williams, 1964; Fabro, Smith, and Williams, 1965; Keberle, Loustalot, Maller, Faigle, and Schmid, 1965) and has since been further extended (Sieber and Fabro, 1971) to several other substances.

The chemical followup, leading to the identification of the substance and its metabolites within the embryo, is scientifically purposeful and rewarding, and should be energetically pursued. However, by itself it gives us no idea as to what, if anything, has happened to the blastocysts during or after the treatment. It is rather frustrating to read that this or that drug manages to enter rabbit blastocysts, without information on the response of the embryos, because penetration *per se* is not tantamount to pharmacological action. Another requirement in this type of experiment is that the data must be validated statistically if any significance is to be ascribed to the results. This is due to the variability encountered within and between blastocyst litters in perfectly normal animals. In our experiments with maternally administered labeled ions, we have repeatedly found a high degree of variability in the results. We therefore insist that statistical appraisal is essential in all experiments involving maternally administered agents. Otherwise, erroneous impressions may be obtained concerning the potency of the agent examined.

Survey of agents studied in experiments with zygotes and blastocysts

An attempt has been made to compress into two tables the information on the numerous agents that have been shown to produce effects in embryos. Table 1 is an annotated list of selected agents, the action of which has been investigated at the zygote as well as the blastocyst stage, under conditions *in vivo* and *in vitro*. Table 2 compares certain agents acting both by the maternal route and in the course of incubation in a culture medium; the localization of the damage resulting from such exposures, in different areas of the blastocyst, is also indicated.

The criteria that have been applied by investigators to evaluate the condition of the embryos after exposure were as follows. In experiments with zygotes, the percentage of those that manage to proceed to the blastocyst stage has been routinely used as an expression of embryonic survival.

The condition of the blastocysts in experiments done in our laboratory was assessed by histological and cytological examination of flat-mounts in coded batches. This included: determination of the developmental stage; observations on the configuration, size, and incidence and degree of degeneration in the embryonic disc and trophoblast; mitotic activity; presence and degree of development of trophoblastic knobs; maintenance (or collapse) of the blastocoelic cavity.

In an evaluation relating to the experiments *in vitro*, the following points merit discussion. The culture of embryos under simple reproducible conditions has now become a routine laboratory procedure. It is clear from the numerous modifications published that more than one kind of nutrient medium can be used for any given stage of embryonic development. Basically, all the media in common use involve the standard, commercially available mixtures, made up of salts, various organic metabolites such as amino

TABLE 1. *Some agents the action of which on embryos (zygote[z], blastocyst[B]) has been studied under conditions* in vivo[1] *and/or* in vitro[2]. *(Figures in parentheses refer to authors.)*

Metabolites	glucose-6-phosphate[B,1] (19); 2-deoxyribose[B,1] (19); galactose[B,1] (19); DNA[B,1] (19); nucleosides[Z,2] (23)
Vitamins	vitamin B_{12}[B,1] (1,19); pyridoxine[B,1] (1,19); vitamin A[B,1] (1)
Hormones	estrogens [estradiol benzoate[B,1] (1), diethylstilbestrol[B,1] (1), polyestriol phosphate[B,1,2] (1,19)]; gestagens [progesterone[B,1] (1), deoxycorticosterone acetate[B,1] (1)]; gonadotrophin[B,1] (1,21); growth hormone[B,1,2] (16,19)
Antimetabolites	2-deoxyglucose[Z,2,B,1,2] (17,24); 2-deoxyglucose-6-phosphate[B,2] (19); 2-deoxygalactose[B,1,2] (17,19); 6-mercaptopurine[Z,1,B,1] (1,19); 6-mercaptopurine riboside[B,1] (19); 8-azaguanine[B,1] (1); 5-bromouracil[B,1] (1); DL-ethionine[B,1,2] (19); isoniazid[B,1,2] (16,16); vitamin B_{12} analogs[B,1,2] (1,19)
Enzymic and metabolic inhibitors	inhibitors of carbohydrate metabolism [iodoacetate, phloridzin, etc.[Z,2] (24)]; inhibitors of protein synthesis [actinomycin[Z,2,B,2] (26, 19), puromycin[Z,2] (26), mitomycin[Z,2] (26)]; DL-glyceraldehyde[B,1,2] (19); salicylates[B,1,2] (1,19); bromoacetylcarnitine[B,1,2] (19); p-chloromercuribenzoate[B,2] (19); fluoride[Z,2,B,2] (24,19)
Antimitotic agents	colchicine derivatives: colcemid[Z,1,B,1] (1); thiolcolciran[B,1] (1); aminopterin[B,1,2] (1,19); amethopterin[B,1] (1)
Alkylating agents	thiotepa, triethylene-thiophosphoramide[B,1] (1); TEM, triethylenemelamine[B,1] (1); myleran, 1,4-dimethane sulfonoxybutane[B,1] (1); E 39, *bis*-ethyleneimino-methoxyethoxybenzoquinone[B,1] (1); degranol, bis-chloroethylamino-D-mannitol[B,1] (1)
Thalidomide	thalidomide and its breakdown products[B,1] (7,8,12,13,16,20)
Oxygen deprivation	anoxia[B,2] (19)
Hormone deprivation	ovariectomy[B,1] (5,6,18)
Radiation	X-rays[Z,1,B,1] (1,11); radiocobalt[B,1] (10)
Miscellaneous agents	cytochalasin[B,2] (1); sulfonamides[B,1] (1); thiocyanates[B,1] (1); alloxan[B,1] (15); barbiturates[B,1] (21,22); antifertility agents[Z,1,2,B,1] (4, 25); trypan blue[B,1] (1,9); carbon tetrachloride[B,1] (1); carbutamide[B,1] (1); virus[Z,1] (2,3); uteroglobin, blastokinin[B,2] (14)

1. Adams et al. (1961)
2. Baranska et al. (1971)
3. Brackett et al. (1971)
4. Chang (1964)
5. Dickson (1966a)
6. Dickson (1966b)
7. Fabro et al. (1964)
8. Fabro et al. (1965)
9. Ferm (1958)
10. Harvey and Chang (1962)
11. Harvey and Chang (1963)
12. Hay (1964)
13. Keberle et al. (1965)
14. Krishnan and Daniel (1967)
15. Lutwak-Mann (1954)
16. Lutwak-Mann and Hay (1962)
17. Lutwak-Mann and Hay (1965a)
18. Lutwak-Mann et al. (1962)
19. Lutwak-Mann et al. (1969)
20. Marin-Padilla and Benirschke (1963)
21. Moog and Lutwak-Mann (1958)
22. Sieber and Fabro (1971)
23. TenBroeck (1968)
24. Thomson (1967)
25. Thomson (1968)
26. Thomson and Biggers (1966)

acids, sugar, lactate, pyruvate, vitamins, and supplemented by a small a-
mount of protein. Embryos are usually cultured at 37°C, but they can withstand low temperatures, down to 4°C. The blastocysts are sensitive to lack
of oxygen, especially at elevated temperature (Lutwak-Mann et al., 1969).
The commonly used gas mixture is 5% CO_2 + 95% O_2; developmentally advanced stages are sensitive to alterations in partial pressure of oxygen (New
and Coppola, 1970a,b).

Concerning the duration of experiments *in vitro*, we have found that a
period of 6 to 8 hr is sufficient for most of the agents tested to display their
effect in a recognizable fashion. A shorter period might be insufficient, as some
ultimately very potent substances showed little effect before the lapse of 2 to
3 hr.

The comparative aspect of tests carried out with the same substance
acting under both conditions is of major interest, because it shows that, according to type of experiment, different results may be obtained with the
same substances. Table 2 gives some examples from our own experiments.
Speaking generally, agents seemed to fall into several distinct categories:
some, such as mercaptopurine riboside, colcemid, and deoxyglucose, were
toxic both ways; others, such as deoxygalactose, DNA, or glyceraldehyde,
showed high toxicity *in vitro*, but were metabolized in such a way as to become innocuous *in vivo*; some substances, for example, the amino acid analog ethionine, known to be toxic at the fetal stage, produced no effect what-
soever on blastocysts. A hormone such as polyestriol phosphate was inert
in culture; under conditions *in vivo*, it was inactive in strictly short-duration
experiments, but it would, of course, interrupt pregnancy if allowed to act
for an extended period of time.

With regard to the localization of damage within morphologically distinct blastocyst regions, and disregarding finer gradation due to dosage, we
can say that, perhaps with the exception of glyceraldehyde, in all the other
experimental situations the area most affected was the embryonic disc. Some
agents induced recognizable damage, of differing extent, in both blastocyst
regions; but, for instance, deoxyglucose, when acting *in vivo* produced damage only in the disc, whereas under conditions *in vitro* the effect of this
antimetabolite was visible also in the trophoblast.

Thalidomide as a special case in blastocyst pharmacology

Thalidomide, endowed with properties that put it in a class of its own,
deserves special mention for the following reasons. It was at first generally
believed, on the basis of human case histories, that to exert its embryopathic

TABLE 2. *Comparison of effects produced in 6-day-old rabbit blastocysts by certain agents under conditions in vivo and in vitro.*

Agent	Effect Demonstrable in Blastocysts		Localization of Damage in Blastocysts	
	following administration to pregnant animal	under conditions *in vitro*	embryonic disc	trophoblast
6-Mercaptopurine riboside	+	+	+ *(in vivo)*	± *(in vivo)*
2-Deoxyglucose	+	+	+ *(in vivo)* / + *(in vitro)*	− *(in vivo)* / ± *(in vitro)*
2-Deoxygalactose	−	+	+	±
Ethionine	−	−	−	−
Colcemid	+	+	++	±
DNA	−	+	+	±
DL-Glyceraldehyde		+	±	+
Polyestriol phosphate (short duration)	−	−	−	−
(long duration)	+	0	0	0

+ and ±, recognizable damage, differing in extent; −, absence of recognizable damage; 0, condition not examined.

effect, thalidomide action must be limited to the post-implantation period. However, in 1962, we were able to prove beyond doubt that in the rabbit thalidomide produces unmistakable effects at the blastocyst stage of gestation, that is, before implantation. The effects seen in the blastocysts and illustrated at the time (Lutwak-Mann and Hay, 1962) was quite unlike the changes produced by other drugs.

In conformity with numerous drugs, thalidomide also acted predominantly upon the embryonic disc. But the type of response in the disc differed: the degeneration, which is the familiar response, e.g., to maternally administered alkylating agents or antimetabolites, was absent; instead, the thalidomide blastocysts exhibited a very characteristic disorganization in the configuration of the discs (see Plate 4, Lutwak-Mann and Hay, 1967). The occurrence of this readily identifiable pathology (or malformation) in the embryonic disc was checked in a large number of thalidomide-treated rabbits, showing a high degree of incidence and reproducibility. In contrast to disc degeneration, which is irreparable, the condition arising in the blastocysts from thalidomide treatment was not lethal. In spite of a temporary delay in uterine attachment, such blastocysts were viable and went on to term, with a small percentage of the young showing typical malformations (Hay, 1964). It may be added that chemical constituents such as DNA, RNA, protein, amino acids, lactic acid, and bicarbonate showed no appreciable change in concentration in the thalidomide blastocysts.

For the time being, and for lack of a better explanation, we assume that the peculiar thalidomide-induced embryopathy in blastocysts described above was due to the interference by thalidomide or its products with the active cell movement that is known to accompany the differentiation of the embryonic disc at the time of primitive streak formation.

Our histological findings gained greatly in significance when it was later shown by chemical methods (Keberle et al., 1965) that thalidomide and its metabolites do, in fact, reach the free-lying rabbit blastocysts. In this way additional proof was provided of the accessibility, and thereby potential vulnerability, of the conceptus at the pre-implantation stage. The entry and slow clearance of thalidomide at a more advanced stage of rabbit pregnancy was also demonstrated (Fabro et al., 1964, 1965).

These and many other researches concerned with thalidomide have all succeeded in confirming that this unusual drug readily penetrates the embryos at a time when it could produce a specific reaction. But how and why thalidomide acts the way it does has remained unsolved. Among the causes of this failure may be, that while biologists engaged in experiments with thalidomide lacked biochemical expertise, the biochemists were rather deficient in embryological experience. But the root cause surely was that we were all hampered by the meager amount of basic knowledge relating to embryonic physiology and pharmacology.

While on the subject of thalidomide, a passing mention may be made of findings obtained with this drug acting on the progeny by the paternal route. It was shown (Lutwak-Mann, 1964, 1965) that when male rabbits of proven fertility were dosed with thalidomide for extended periods of time, and subsequently mated to fertile females who had not been treated with thalidomide, a high percentage of such matings resulted in numerically small, underweight litters, many of which failed to survive. Some of the young from these matings exhibited skeletal and visceral malformations, such as absence of tail, hemorrhages on paws, spina bifida, and absence of one kidney.

In an attempt to elucidate the mode of action of thalidomide propagated by the male route, we have followed the entry of orally administered [^{14}C]-thalidomide into the blood and semen of male rabbits (Lutwak-Mann, Schmid, and Keberle, 1967). We found that (1) the drug quickly penetrated into rabbit semen, (2) it became firmly bound to the spermatozoa, from which it could not be dislodged by washing with saline, and (3) the label was still detectable in the sperm fraction several days after the ingestion of thalidomide by the bucks.

Certain recent observations lend new interest to these results. Morphological studies indicate that remnants of spermatozoa can persist for a long time and still be present in embryos, as late as the blastocyst stage (rat, Tachi and Kraicer, 1967; mouse, McReynolds and Hadek, 1970; guinea pig, Blandau, 1971). It is therefore conceivable that, following protracted feeding of males with thalidomide (as in the author's experiments with rabbits), the drug itself or its products in semen could be conveyed to the females at mating; thalidomide bound to spermatozoa could become incorporated in oocytes, remain with sperm remnants in the embryos until the blastocyst or an even later stage has been attained, and then induce its embryopathic effect. That this is a valid speculation is shown by observations made with estrogens, which, if given to male rats, are transported at copulation into females, and in this way cause pregnancy wastage by the paternal route (Ericsson and Baker, 1966).

CONCLUDING REMARKS

Probably the most outstanding achievement to date in the pharmacology of the blastocyst is the fact that the existence of this fascinating sector of developmental pharmacology has at last been formally recognized! Profiting from experience gained over the years from morphological, physiological, and biochemical studies, we can now enumerate certain characteristic traits of the blastocysts and briefly comment on their significance in relation to pharmacology.

Embryonic variability and natural wastage

Attention has previously been drawn to the blastocyst features of embryonic variability and natural wastage. Presumably they are responsible for the variability seen in response to exogenous agents, both under conditions *in vivo* and *in vitro*. Because of this inherent inequality among blastocysts even within the same litter, the only way to avoid erroneous results is to aim at maximum reproducibility in highly standardized experimental conditions. Unfortunately, the lack of quantifiable, that is, metabolic, parameters of blastocyst viability (such as perhaps the ATP/ADP ratio) hinders meaningful expression of the extent and range of variability in drug response; for the time being, histological and cytological assessment (as, e.g., in the flat-mount procedure) of large numbers of embryos in coded batches remains the most practical means open to investigators.

Regulatory mechanisms operative at blastocyst level

Studies on maternal-embryonic exchanges indicate that, while penetration of embryos occurs promptly, the clearance from the blastocyst compartment for most agents hitherto examined is slow. An outcome of this delayed clearance, at a stage of rapid growth, may be the carry-over of deleterious materials into the more highly differentiated, and thus more susceptible, fetal stage.

This situation puts the onus upon the investigator to compare drug distribution and action at several time intervals after administration in both the maternal body fluids and in the embryonic system. It also accentuates the inadequacy of limiting the monitoring of drugs (e.g., in the pharmaceutical industry) to maternal peripheral fluids alone.

Type of response to the action of exogenous agents

Many agents that have been tested were selected by investigators from among those drugs and other substances and conditions that could be expected to bring development to a halt by causing degeneration and consequently break-up of embryonic tissues. But one ought not to forget that a significant, and ultimately detrimental, disruption of the orderly progress of development can also arise from over-stimulation and premature enhancement of growth, such as we have seen in blastocysts recovered from rabbits pre-treated, for example, with estrogens, growth hormone, or DNA.

Differential sensitivity

We have first demonstrated the existence of differential sensitivity in morphologically disparate regions of the blastocyst in our early experiments quoted above. This phenomenon is, of course, more strikingly obvious in the large rabbit blastocysts than in the small blastocysts of other species. It is one of the most marked features and biologically important facts brought out by studies on exogenous factors. It is equally evident in experiments *in vivo* and *in vitro*.

The vast majority of the substances tested affect the cells of the embryo proper much more severely than those of the extra-embryonic tissue (trophoblast, endoderm, trophoblastic knobs). The trophoblast emerges as a particularly tough tissue: about the only substance that exhibited a marked anti-trophoblastic effect in our experiments was DL-glyceraldehyde, a metabolic inhibitor known to interfere with tumor tissue glycolysis. There is some indication of trophoblast stratification into the very resistant abembryonic pole region, and the gradually more sensitive equatorial and near-disc zones.

Why there should be this difference in degree of sensitivity between the embryo proper and trophoblast is unknown. Provisionally we interpret this phenomenon as being due to a fundamentally different type and rate of metabolism in these two regions of the blastocyst.

Adaptational and recuperative capacity

Two more qualities need to be mentioned, namely, the exceptional adaptational and recuperative capacity of the young mammalian embryo. Survival and continuation of development *in vitro* and in certain extrauterine sites testify to the adaptability of zygotes and blastocysts. Experiments with mouse chimeras (Tarkowski, 1961; Mintz, 1965) further underline the potency, of the mouse zygotes at any rate, to withstand a wide range of manipulation without significant impairment of their developmental ability.

Blastocysts are also capable of overcoming *in vivo* and *in vitro* the effects of damage or developmental delay, as we have observed in experiments with certain antimitotics, thalidomide, and other agents. Because of the emphasis placed on embryonic sensitivity, the natural resilience of the young embryo needs to be constantly stressed.

There is, however, an element of risk in this embryonic resistance. From the purely experimental angle, there is the danger that because embryonic adaptability enables us to place the embryos in environments completely divorced from physiological situations, our conclusions drawn from observations made in such unnatural conditions, may be completely wrong. From the developmental viewpoint, there is the hazard that if embryos incur minor or moderate damage, and subsequently there is only partial repair, such incomplete healing may escalate into gross or discrete structural derangement or other aberrations; these may not become manifest until some advanced stage of fetal or even postnatal life has been attained.

From what has been said above, one can see that a modest beginning has been made, but if we are to understand better the action of drugs on the blastocyst, a further concentration of research endeavor is needed in fundamental aspects of blastocyst physiology and biochemistry, such as the chemical composition of the embryos, the mechanisms operative in maternal-blastocyst exchange, and the metabolic properties of the embryo proper as opposed to those of extra-embryonic tissue such as the trophoblast.

ACKNOWLEDGMENT

The investigations on the physiology and biochemistry of the mammalian blastocyst, published by the author and her co-workers, were carried out on behalf of the Agricultural Research Council of Great Britain.

REFERENCES

Adams, C. E., Hay, M. F., and Lutwak-Mann, C. (1961): The action of various agents upon the rabbit embryo. *Journal of Embryology and Experimental Morphology,* 9:468-491.

Baranska, W., Sawicki, W., and Koprowski, H. (1971): Infection of mammalian unfertilized and fertilized ova with oncogenic viruses. *Nature,* 230:591-592.

Beier, H. B. (1968): Biochemisch-entwicklungssphysiologische Untersuchungen am Proteinmilieu für die Blastozystenentwicklung des Kaninchens (*Oryctolagus cuniculus*). *Zoologischer Jahresbericht,* 85:72-190.

Blandau, R. J. (1971): *The Biology of the Blastocyst.* University of Chicago Press, Chicago.

Brackett, B. G., Baranska, W., Sawicki, W., and Koprowski, H. (1971): Uptake of heterologous genome by mammalian spermatozoa and its transfer to ova through fertilization. *Proceedings of the National Academy of Sciences,* 68:353-357.

Brambell, F. W. R. (1948): Studies on sterility and prenatal mortality in wild rabbits. 2. *Journal of Experimental Biology,* 23:332-345.

Brooks, D. E., and Lutwak-Mann, C. (1971): Content of ATP and ADP in rabbit blastocysts. *Nature,* 229:202-203

Chang, M. C. (1964): Effects of certain antifertility agents on the development of rabbit ova. *Fertility and Sterility*, 15:97-106.

Dickson, A. D. (1966a): Observations on blastocysts recovered from ovariectomized mice. *International Journal of Fertility*, 11:227-230.

Dickson, A. D. (1966b): The size of the inner cell mass in blastocysts recovered from normal and ovariectomized mice. *International Journal of Fertility*, 11:231-234.

Ericsson, R. J., and Baker, V. F. (1966): Transport of oestrogens in semen to the female rat during mating and its effect on fertility. *Journal of Reproduction and Fertility*, 12:381-384.

Fabro, S., Schumacher, H., Smith, R. L., and Williams, R. T. (1964): Identification of thalidomide in rabbit blastocysts. *Nature*, 201:1125-1126.

Fabro, S., Smith, R. L., and Williams, R. T. (1965): The persistence of maternally administered (^{14}C)-thalidomide in the rabbit embryo. *Biochemical Journal*, 97:14P.

Ferm, V. H. (1958): Teratogenic effects of trypan blue on hamster embryos. *Journal of Embryology and Experimental Morphology*, 6:284-287.

Hafez, E. S. E., and Blandau, R. J. (1969): *The Mammalian Oviduct*. University of Chicago Press, Chicago.

Harvey, E. B., and Chang, M. C. (1962): Effects of radiocobalt irradiation of pregnant hamsters on the development of embryos. *Journal of Cellular and Comparative Physiology*, 59:293-306.

Harvey, E. B., and Chang, M. C. (1963): Effects of X-irradiation of ovarian ova on the morphology of fertilized ova and development of embryos. *Journal of Cellular and Comparative Physiology*, 61:133-144.

Hay, M. F. (1964): Effects of thalidomide on pregnancy in the rabbit. *Journal of Reproduction and Fertility*, 8:59-76.

Keberle, H., Loustalot, P., Maller, R. K., Faigle, J. W., and Schmid, K. (1965): Biochemical effects of drugs on the mammalian conceptus. *Annals of the New York Academy of Sciences*, 123:252-262.

Krishnan, R. S., and Daniel, J. C., Jr. (1967): "Blastokinin": Inducer and regulator of blastocyst development in rabbit uterus. *Science*, 158:490-492.

Leone, E., Libonati, M., and Lutwak-Mann, C. (1963): Enzymes in the uterine and cervical fluid and in certain related tissues and body fluids of the rabbit. *Journal of Endocrinology*, 25:551-552.

Lutwak-Mann, C. (1954): Some properties of the rabbit blastocyst. *Journal of Embryology and Experimental Morphology*, 2:1-13.

Lutwak-Mann, C. (1962a): Some properties of uterine and cervical fluid in the rabbit. *Biochimica et Biophysica Acta*, 58:637-639.

Lutwak-Mann, C. (1962b): Glucose, lactic acid and bicarbonate in rabbit blastocyst fluid. *Nature*, 193:653-654.

Lutwak-Mann, C. (1964): Observations on progeny of thalidomide-treated male rabbits. *British Medical Journal*, 1:1090-1091.

Lutwak-Mann, C. (1965): Experimental embryopathy as a tool in research on animal reproduction. In: *Embryopathic Activity of Drugs*, Biological Council Symposium, edited by J. M. Robson, F. Sullivan, and R. L. Smith. J. and A. Churchill Ltd., London, pp. 261-274.

Lutwak-Mann, C. (1966): Some physiological and biochemical properties of the mammalian blastocyst. *Bulletin of the Swiss Academy of Medical Sciences*, 22:101-122.

Lutwak-Mann, C. (1971): The rabbit blastocyst and its environment: Physiological and biochemical aspects. In: *The Biology of the Blastocyst*, edited by R. J. Blandau. University of Chicago Press, Chicago, pp. 243-260.

Lutwak-Mann, C., Boursnell, J. C., and Bennett, J. P. (1960): Blastocyst-uterine relationships: Uptake of radioactive ions by the early rabbit embryo and its environment. *Journal of Reproduction and Fertility*, 1:169-185.

Lutwak-Mann, C., and Hay, M. F. (1962): Effect on the early embryo of agents administered to the mother. *British Medical Journal*, 2:944-946.

Lutwak-Mann, C., and Hay, M. F. (1965a): Effect of 2-deoxy-D-glucose on the rabbit blastocyst. *Journal of Reproduction and Fertility*, 10:133-135.

Lutwak-Mann, C., and Hay, M. F. (1965b): Maternally transmitted embryotropic agents. In: *Agents Affecting Fertility*, Biological Council Symposium edited by C. R. Austin and J. S. Perry. J. A. Churchill Ltd., London, pp. 138-151.

Lutwak-Mann, C., and Hay, M. F. (1967): The blastocyst flat-mount technique in studies on embryotropic agents. In: *Advances in Teratology*, Vol. II, edited by D. H. M. Woollam. Academic Press, London, pp. 229-238.

Lutwak-Mann, C., Hay, M. F., and Adams, C. E. (1962): The effect of ovariectomy on rabbit blastocysts. *Journal of Endocrinology*, 24:185-197.

Lutwak-Mann, C., Hay, M. F., and New, D. A. T. (1969): Action of various agents on rabbit blastocysts *in vivo* and *in vitro*. *Journal of Reproduction and Fertility*, 18:235-257.

Lutwak-Mann, C., and McIntosh, J. E. A. (1969): Zinc and carbonic anhydrase in the rabbit uterus. *Nature*, 221:1111-1114.

Lutwak-Mann, C., and McIntosh, J. E. A. (1971): Calcium content and uptake of ^{45}Ca in rabbit blastocysts and their environment. *Journal of Reproduction and Fertility*, 27:471-475.

Lutwak-Mann, C., Schmid, K., and Keberle, H. (1967): Thalidomide in rabbit semen. *Nature*, 214:1018-1020.

Marin-Padilla, M., and Benirschke, K. (1963): Thalidomide induced alterations in the blastocyst and placenta of the armadillo, *Dasypus novemcinctus mexicanus*, including a choriocarcinoma. *American Journal of Pathology*, 43:999-1016.

McIntosh, J. E. A., and Lutwak-Mann, C. (1972): Transport of zinc in rabbit tissues. Zinc content and transport in rabbit reproductive tract tissues, liver and blood in early pregnancy. *Biochemical Journal*, 126:869-876.

McReynolds, H. D., and Hadek, R. (1970): A study on sperm tail elements in mouse blastocysts. *Journal of Reproduction and Fertility*, 24:291-295.

Mintz, B. (1965): Nucleic acid and protein synthesis in the developing mouse embryo. In: *Preimplantation Stages of Pregnancy*, Ciba Foundation Symposium, edited by G. E. W. Wolstenholme and M. O'Connor. J. and A. Churchill Ltd., London, pp. 145-159.

Moog, F., and Lutwak-Mann, C. (1958): Observations on rabbit blastocysts prepared as flat-mounts. *Journal of Embryology and Experimental Morphology*, 6:133-135.

New, D. A. T., and Coppola, P. T. (1970a): Development of explanted rat fetuses in hyperbaric oxygen. *Teratology*, 3:153-160.

New, D. A. T., and Coppola, P. T. (1970b): Effects of different oxygen concentrations on the development of rat embryos in culture. *Journal of Reproduction and Fertility*, 21:109-118.

Quinn, P., and Wales, R. G. (1971): ATP content of preimplantation mouse embryos. *Journal of Reproduction and Fertility*, 25:133-135.

Seamark, R. F., and Lutwak-Mann, C. (1972): Progestins in rabbit blastocysts. *Journal of Reproduction and Fertility*, 29:147-148.

Sieber, S. M., and Fabro, S. (1971): Identification of drugs in the preimplantation blastocyst and in the plasma, uterine secretion and urine of the pregnant rabbit. *Journal of Pharmacology and Experimental Therapeutics*, 176:65-75.

Tachi, S., and Kraicer, P. F. (1967): Studies on the mechanism of nidation. XXVII. Sperm-derived inclusions in the rat blastocyst. *Journal of Reproduction and Fertility*, 14:401-405.

Tarkowski, A. (1961): Mouse chimeras developed from fused eggs. *Nature*, 190:857-860.

Tarkowski, A., and Wróblewska, J. (1967): Development of blastomeres of mouse eggs isolated at the 4- and 8-cell stage. *Journal of Embryology and Experimental Morphology*, 18:155-180.

TenBroeck, J. T. (1968): Effect of nucleosides and nucleoside bases on the development of pre-implantation mouse embryos *in vitro*. *Journal of Reproduction and Fertility*, 17:571-573.

Thomson, J. L. (1967): Effect of inhibitors of carbohydrate metabolism on the development of preimplantation mouse embryos. *Experimental Cell Research*, 46:252-262.

Thomson, J. L. (1968): Effect of two non-steroidal antifertility agents on pregnancy in mice. I. Comparison of *in vitro* and *in vivo* effects on zygotes. *Journal of Reproduction and Fertility*, 15:223-231.

Thomson, J. L., and Biggers, J. D. (1966): Effect of inhibitors of protein synthesis on the development of preimplantation mouse embryos. *Experimental Cell Research*, 41:411-427.

Vittorelli, M. L., Harrison, R. A. P., and Lutwak-Mann, C. (1967): Metabolism of ribonucleic acid in the endometrium of the rabbit during early pregnancy. *Nature*, 214:890-892.

DISCUSSION

WEISS: How long can the blastocyst be kept viable under *in vitro* conditions such as in tissue culture? And secondly, what factors (for example, hormones and other endogenously occurring substances) are necessary for the growth and development of these cells?

LUTWAK-MANN: The blastocysts of laboratory animals can be kept under conditions *in vitro* for 24 to 48 hours, during which time their development and differentiation appear fairly normal. Thereafter, there is a tendency for the embryonic elements to die off, while the extra-embryonic tissues (trophoblast, etc.) may continue to proliferate.

The commercially available media such as, for example, TC 199, supplemented with protein, seem to be all that the young embryos require during such limited periods of exposure. The addition of hormones, in appropriately low concentrations, does not produce recognizable effects during short periods of explantation; the situation might change radically on longer incubation.

We have just found that rabbit blastocysts at any rate contain progesterone, 20αHP, and 17αHP, possibly also cortisone, in relatively large amounts. But we are as yet uncertain, what role, if any, to ascribe to the occurrence of these hormones in blastocyst development or metabolism.

NEUBERT: Just a brief comment to the problem Dr. Weiss has raised. It is always astonishing that so few hormones are needed for embryonic development, even at late states of development. You can hypophysectomize rats and just supplement with progesterone and estrone and you get a perfect embryonic development over all the stages of organogenesis with a lack of growth hormone, thyroid hormone, and glucocorticoids. Professor Köhler in our laboratory has shown this clearly and has even made bichemical studies which revealed only minor differences when compared with controls.

ELIS: According to your opinion, is it better when the donor-host are synchonized or when they are 24 hours apart?

LUTWAK-MANN: To obtain the best results in embryo transfer experiments, it is advisable to use recipients that, from the endocrine point of view, are fully synchronous with the embryo donors. A difference of 24 hours in synchrony is the most that is still tolerable; if asynchrony exceeds that interval, then upon transfer the embryo encounters an entirely out-of-phase maternal environment, and under such conditions only very few embryos manage to survive to term.

FUCHS: Dr. Lutwak-Mann, you mentioned that very few agents seen to affect the trophoblastic cells, in contrast to the embryonic cells. Does this apply also to drugs which are used against trophoblastic tumors such as methotrexate?

LUTWAK-MANN: The rabbit happens to be an animal that is remarkably resistant to folic acid analogs, probably owing to the high level of folic acid in this species. Therefore, the rabbit blastocyst is a rather unsuitable object of study when one wishes to investigate the effect of either methotrexate or aminopterin, and, indeed, we have found that excessively high concentrations of aminopterin must be used (*in vitro*) to produce clearly recognizable effects on blastocyst mitosis. Similarly, aminopterin and methotrexate were ineffective *in vivo* toward the rabbit conceptus, both at the early and advanced stages.

FUCHS: Can your technique be applied to human blastocysts as well?

LUTWAK-MANN: As to the applicability of our investigational approach in general and the blastocyst flat-mount procedure in particular, I believe that if only one had a supply of human blastocysts, the basic findings established by observations made on rabbit or other animal blastocysts, would be equally true of the human embryo.

PAOLETTI: I wonder if the role of prostaglandin on blastocysts before and during implantation has been investigated; PGF_2 and PGE_2 are likely to act not only at the blastocyst level but also by modifying the uterine wall conditions, being a rather unique agent in this respect.

LUTWAK-MANN: I have had no opportunity so far to experiment with any of the prostaglandins. It is highly probable that, as you say, these substances would exert an effect on the free-lying blastocysts not primarily but secondarily, that is, by altering the function of the myometrium.

Fetal Pharmacology, edited by L. Boréus
Raven Press, New York © 1973

Passage of Drugs and Other Chemicals into the Uterine Fluids and Preimplantation Blastocyst

Sergio Fabro

*Departments of Obstetrics & Gynecology, and Pharmacology,
The George Washington University, Washington, D.C.*

Some of the first indications that substances can pass from the maternal circulation into the preimplantation blastocyst derived from observations by Greenwald and Everett (1959) and Lutwak-Mann, Boursnell, and Bennett (1960). The former workers demonstrated the uptake and incorporation of ^{35}S-methionine by preimplantation blastocysts of mice treated parenterally with this compound. Lutwak-Mann's group showed passage of $^{32}PO_4$, ^{42}K, $^{35}SO_4$, ^{24}Na, and ^{131}I into endometrial fluids and preimplantation blastocysts of rabbits receiving these ions parenterally.

Research in our laboratory has been directed toward a fuller understanding of the extent to which foreign chemicals reach the preimplantation blastocyst and the mechanism(s) by which this process takes place. Our approach to this problem has been to examine (1) the means by which drugs and other chemicals pass from the maternal circulation into the uterine fluids, and (2) how these compounds pass from the uterine fluid into the preimplantation blastocyst.

METHODOLOGY

The radioactive compounds used in our studies were obtained from commercial sources, and their purity checked by paper or thin-layer chromatography before use. The compounds were administered orally or parenterally to New Zealand White rabbits. When experiments with pregnant rabbits were performed, the does were treated at 144 to 156 hr after mating. Uterine secretions were obtained by the method of Krishnan and Daniel (1967); preimplantation blastocysts were collected by a method similar to that described by Hafez (1971). The radioactivity in the plasma, uterine fluid, and preimplantation blastocysts was measured by the method previously described (Sieber and Fabro, 1971). Identification of the radioactivity in samples of plasma, urine, uterine fluid, and blastocysts was carried out by an inverse isotope dilution technique after thin-layer or paper chromatographic separation (Fabro, Smith, and Wiliams, 1967a,b; Sieber and Fabro, 1971).

PASSAGE OF COMPOUNDS INTO UTERINE FLUIDS

Following the administration of (1-methyl-^{14}C)-caffeine, G-(^{3}H)-nicotine, (7-^{14}C)-salicylate, (carbonyl-^{14}C)-isoniazid, (2-^{14}C)-antipyrine, (2-^{14}C)-barbital, (2-^{14}C)-thiopental, and (phenyl-^{14}C)-DDT, the unchanged compounds as well as some of their metabolites have been identified in significant amounts in the uterine fluid of rabbits, rats, and mice (McLachlan, Sieber, and Fabro, 1969; Sieber and Fabro, 1971).

For example, after the administration of (1-methyl-^{14}C)-caffeine to

TABLE 1. *Distribution of radioactivity between plasma and uterine fluid following the intravenous administration to rabbits of some radioactive compounds differing in molecular weight.*

Compound	Molecular Weight	Relative amount of Radioactivity in Uterine Fluid[a] at 1 hr
(N-Methyl-^{14}C)-antipyrine	188	1.21 ± 0.07
(Phenyl-^{14}C)-DDT	355	0.67 ± 0.08
(Carboxyl-^{14}C)-inulin	5,500	0.28 ± 0.02
(Carboxyl-^{14}C)-dextran	15,000-17,000	0.08 ± 0.02
(Carboxyl-^{14}C)-dextran	60,000-90,000	0.04 ± 0.02

(N-Methyl-^{14}C)-antipyrine (4.5 mg/kg; 5 μC/kg); (phenyl-^{14}C)-DDT (0.7 mg/kg; 5 μC/kg); (carboxyl-^{14}C)-inulin (2.7 mg/kg; 5 μC/kg); (carboxyl-^{14}C)-dextran, m.w. 15,000-17,000 (1.1 mg/kg; 5 μC/kg); and (carboxyl-^{14}C)-dextran, m.w. 60,000-90,000 (4.9 mg/kg; 5 μC/kg) were given intravenously to nonpregnant adult female rabbits.

[a] As expressed by the uterine fluid (DPM/g)/plasma (DPM/ml) radioactivity ratio. Figures represent means ± SEM of 3 to 5 experiments in duplicate. The percent of radioactivity identified as unchanged compound in the uterine fluid and plasma, respectively, was as follows: ^{14}C-antipyrine 87.2, 90.1; ^{14}C-DDT 96.4, 98.1; ^{14}C-inulin and ^{14}C-dextran were not metabolized by 1 hr after their injection, since all the radioactivity in plasma was identified as the unchanged compound (McLachlan and Fabro, 1971, *unpublished*).

adult nonpregnant does, the uterine fluid/plasma radioactivity ratio ranged between 0.78 and 1.54 at all of the times examined during the 6 hr of the experiment. Unchanged caffeine contributed in proportional amounts to the radioactivity in both tissues. Other foreign chemicals did not pass into the uterine fluid as readily as caffeine. Table 1 shows that there is an inverse relationship between the molecular weight of a radioactive compound and its uterine fluid/plasma radioactivity ratio; the correlation between these two parameters is statistically significant ($p < 0.001$). Moreover, human serum proteins (molecular weight 41,000 to 1,000,000) were not detectable immunologically in the uterine fluid of rabbits 1 hr after the administration of 4 ml of human serum.

However, factors other than molecular weight are likely to influence the passage of foreign chemicals into the uterine fluid. This is suggested by the fact that in a series of small molecular weight compounds, the degree of this transfer into the uterine fluid was statistically correlated ($p < 0.05$) to their degree of ionization (Table 2).

These results were not unexpected, since the uterine fluid is primarily a product of the exocrine glands of the endometrium. It has long been known that foreign chemicals can pass into the secretion of several other exocrine glands, including saliva, bile and other gastrointestinal secretions, sweat, tears, milk, and seminal fluid (Table 3). Furthermore, the pH of the secretion (Shore, Brodie, and Hogben, 1957; Schanker, 1959), the molecular weight (Martin and Burgen, 1962) and the degree of ionization of the compound (Thaysen and Schwartz, 1953; Sisodia and Stowe, 1964; Miller, Banerjee, and Stowe, 1967) can influence the penetration of drugs into these exocrine secretions.

In another series of experiments, we further explored an earlier observation that pregnancy may modify the degree to which drugs pass into the uterine fluid. For most of the radioactive compounds examined, including barbital, isoniazid, thiopental, and caffeine, the amount of radioactivity in the uterine secretion of 6-day pregnant rabbits was not significantly different from that of nonpregnant animals (Fabro and Sieber, 1968). This, however, was not the case following administration of ^{3}H-nicotine. Table 4 shows that in nonpregnant rabbits the uterine fluid/plasma radioactivity ratio ranged between 0.78 and 1.75. In the 6-day pregnant animals, however, there was 5 to 10 times more radioactivity in the uterine fluid than in the plasma.

In the nonpregnant rabbits, nicotine reaches a concentration in the uterine fluid which parallels that in the plasma. Thus, at 30 min after dosing, the concentration of unchanged nicotine in the uterine fluid and plasma averaged 0.034 μg/g and 0.028 μg/ml, respectively. On the other hand, cotinine, a

TABLE 2. Relationship between the passage of radioactivity into the uterine fluid and degree of ionization of some radioactive compounds given intravenously to rabbits.

Compound	Dose (mg/kg; μC/kg, i.v.)	Relative Amount of Radioactivity in Uterine Fluid at 1 Hr[a] (Mean ± SEM)	Molecular Weight	pK$_a$ Values	% Ionized at pH 7.2
(1-Methyl-^{14}C)-caffeine	3.5; 5	1.14 ± 0.15	194	0.8[1]	<0.01
(N-Methyl-^{14}C)-antipyrine	4.5; 5	0.91 ± 0.12	188	1.4[1]	<0.01
(7-^{14}C)-Salicylic acid	17.0; 5	0.69 ± 0.18	138	3.0[2]	99.98
(Phenyl-^{14}C)-DDT	0.7; 5	0.67 ± 0.08	355	—	<0.01
(Methyl-^{14}C)-hexamethonium	0.6; 5	0.20 ± 0.04	273	cation	99.99
		correlation[b]	r^2	0.51 ($p < 0.05$)	

Compounds were given i.v. to nonpregnant adult rabbits.

[a] As expressed by the uterine fluid (DPM/gm)/plasma (DPM/ml) radioactive ratio.

[b] According to Snedecor (1959). References: (1) Shore et al. (1957), (2) Weast (1962). Figures are means ± SEM obtained using 3 to 8 does for each compound. The percent of radioactivity identified as unchanged compound in the uterine fluid and plasma, respectively, was as follows: ^{14}C-caffeine 65.2, 63.8; ^{14}C-antipyrine 80.1, 97.2; ^{14}C-salicylic acid 91.3, 88.7; ^{14}C-DDT 96.4, 98.1 (McLachlan and Fabro, 1971, unpublished).

TABLE 3. *Foreign compounds which have been identified in some exocrine secretions.*[a]

Secretion	Compounds Identified (reference)
Sweat	Methylurea (1), acetamide (1), thiourea (1), ethanol (1), antipyrine (1-3), phenol (2), salicylic acid (2), methylene blue (2), thiocyanate (3), barbital (4), quinine (5), fluorescein (5), nicotinamide (6), sulfanilamide (7), sulfapyridine (7), sulfathiazole (7), sulfadiazine (7)
Tears	Sulfonamides (8)
Saliva	Mannitol (9), sucrose (9), N-ethyl-urea (9), chloramphenicol (9), 4-acetamido-antipyrine (9), thiourea (9), p-aminohippurate (10), inulin (10), sulfonamides (10), barbiturates (10), penicillin (11), tetracyclines (11), dihydrostreptomycin (11), diphenylhydantoin (12), aureomycin (13), ethanol (14)
Milk	Antipyrine (15), chloroform (15), salicylate (15), caffeine (15), morphine (15), nicotine (15), strychnine (15), sulfathiazole (16), sulfanilamide (16), sulfapyridine (16), sulfamethazine (16), sulfamerazine (16), sulfadiazine (16), sulfamethoxine (16), sulfacetamide (16), tetracycline (16), quinine (16), salicylic acid (17), benzoic acid (17), phenol (17), p-aminohippurate (17), ephedrine (17), penicillin (18), erythromycin (18), ethanol (19), phenobarbital (20), thiopental (21), atropine (22), codeine (23), DDT (24)
Semen	Ethanol (25), sulfonamides (26), thalidomide (27)

[a] This list is not comprehensive. Bile and other gastrointestinal secretions have not been included in this table. The reader is referred to Smith (1966) and Shore et al. (1957) for discussions of the transfer of foreign compounds into bile and gastric secretion, respectively.

References: (1) Brusilow and Gordes, 1966; (2) Tachau, 1911; (3) Koch, 1938; (4) Weinig and Jahn, 1954; (5) Comaish and Shelley, 1965; (6) Sargent et al., 1944; (7) Thaysen and Schwartz, 1953; (8) Balik, 1965; (9) Burgen, 1956; (10) Killman and Thaysen, 1955; (11) Borzelleca and Cherrick, 1965; (12) Noach et al., 1958; (13) Bender et al., 1953; (14) Friedemann et al., 1938; (15) Dreyfus-Seé. 1934; (16) Sisodia and Stowe, 1964; (17) Miller et al., 1967; (18) Rasmussen, 1959; (19) Fantus and Dyneiwicz, 1936; (20) Tyson et al., 1938; (21) Mayo and Schlicke, 1942; (22) Reed, 1908; (23) Kwit and Hatcher, 1935; (24) Zweig et al., 1961; (25) Farrell, 1938; (26) Farrell et al., 1938; (27) Lutwak-Mann et al., 1967.

more polar metabolite of nicotine, does not appear to pass into the uterine fluid as readily as unchanged nicotine. Mean values at 30 min were 0.010 μg/g for the uterine fluid and 0.055 μg/ml for plasma. This is in accordance with the thesis that metabolites tend to be confined to the extracellular compartment and more rapidly excreted (Smith and Williams, 1966).

In the 6-day pregnant rabbit, unchanged nicotine accumulated in the uterine fluid; average values at 30 min were 1.050 μg/g and 0.029 μg/ml for the uterine fluid and plasma, respectively. Radioactive cotinine also ac-

TABLE 4. *Distribution of radioactivity between plasma and uterine secretion of non-pregnant and 6-day pregnant rabbits treated with ^3H-nicotine.*

Time after Treatment (min)	Relative Amount of Radioactivity in the Uterine Fluid[a] of	
	Nonpregnant Does	6-Day Pregnant Does
5	0.78 ± 0.12	6.51 ± 1.96
15	n.d.	10.85 ± 2.04
30	0.96 ± 0.08	9.76 ± 1.67
60	1.75 ± 0.10	8.35 ± 2.45
120	1.01 ± 0.07	5.71 ± 2.66

G-(^3H)-nicotine (50 μg/kg; 60 μC/kg) was given intravenously.
[a] As expressed by the uterine fluid (DPM/g)/plasma (DPM/ml) radioactivity ratio. Figures represent mean values ± SEM obtained with 3 or 4 animals. n.d. = not determined (McLachlan, Sieber, and Fabro, 1970, *unpublished*).

cumulated in the uterine fluid of these animals, but to a smaller extent than unchanged nicotine (Fig. 1). This cotinine accumulation may result from the ability of the pregnant endometrium to accumulate not only nicotine but also other compounds structurally similar to nicotine, such as cotinine. Alternatively, this accumulation of cotinine may be secondary to the accumulation of nicotine, which is subsequently metabolized to cotinine by the endometrial glands. It would not really be surprising if the pregnant uterus provides a site for the breakdown of nicotine, since Miller and Larson (1953) and Hansson and Schmiterlöw (1962) have shown that, besides the liver, other organs (e.g., lung, kidney, and small intestine) can metabolize nicotine.

The mechanism by which nicotine accumulates in the uterine fluid of pregnant rabbits has been puzzling us for some time. We first attempted to determine if a pH gradient between the uterine fluid and plasma of 6-day pregnant rabbits could be responsible for the accumulation of nicotine in the uterine fluid, since this mechanism has been used to explain the accumulation of ephedrine in the milk (Sisodia and Stowe, 1964) and quinine in the gastric fluid (Shore et al., 1957). However, the pH of uterine fluid of 6-day pregnant does (pH 7.68) is not significantly different from that of non-pregnant animals (pH 7.61) (McLachlan, Sieber, Cowherd, Straw, and Fabro, 1970), ruling out this postulated mechanism for the accumulation of nicotine in the pregnant uterine fluid (McLachlan et al., 1969). Others have reported accumulation of foreign chemicals in the secretion of exocrine glands which cannot be explained by a pH gradient. For example, the milk/plasma concentration ratio for quinine and erythromycin has been reported to be 4.8 and 8.7, respectively (Sisodia and Stowe, 1964; Rasmussen,

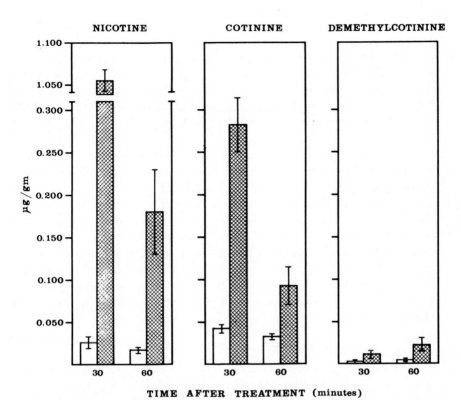

FIG. 1. Radioactive compounds in uterine secretion and plasma of 6-day pregnant rabbits after the intravenous administration of G-(^{3}H)-nicotine (50 μg/kg; 60 μC/kg). The open bars correspond to plasma values; the shaded bars correspond to uterine secretion values. Bars represent mean values of duplicate determinations with two animals; lines represent the ranges (McLachlan, Sieber and Fabro, 1970, *unpublished*).

1959); urea reaches levels in human sweat two to four times that of plasma (Bulmer, 1957).

Furthermore, there was no difference in physiological disposition of nicotine between 6-day pregnant and nonpregnant does which could account for the accumulation of nicotine in the pregnant uterine fluid. Following the intravenous administration of ^{3}H-nicotine to both nonpregnant and 6-day pregnant rabbits, the volume of distribution and plasma half-life of either radioactivity or unchanged nicotine were equal. In addition, rate of metabolism, urinary excretion, and plasma protein binding of either total radioactivity or of unchanged nicotine were similar in pregnant and nonpregnant animals. In view of the well-known pharmacological actions of nicotine, it is possible that nicotine may affect the blood flow of the pregnant uterus, thereby increasing the passage of any foreign chemical into the uterine lumen. Therefore, ^{14}C-caffeine, a compound which is not accumulated in the uterine fluid of 6-day pregnant rabbits, was injected simultaneously with ^{3}H-nicotine into the lateral ear veins of 6-day pregnant rabbits. The average uterine fluid/plasma radioactivity ratio for ^{14}C-activity was 0.88 at 30 and 0.79 at 120 min, whereas that for ^{3}H-activity was 9.41 at 30 and 14.14 at 120 min.

It appears, therefore, that neither factors related to the physiological disposition of nicotine nor those related to its pharmacological action are responsible for the accumulation of this compound in the fluid of the 6-day pregnant uterus. On the other hand, these findings may well indicate that the endometrial tissue in the functional stage of pregnancy influences the active transfer of nicotine into the uterine fluid. This hypothesis is supported by the fact that the accumulation of nicotine seen in the 6-day pregnant rabbit can be reproduced by treating nonpregnant rabbits with either human chorionic gonadotrophin or progesterone. We are presently attempting to determine if this accumulation of nicotine in the uterine fluid is energy-dependent and if it occurs with other bases which are chemically related to nicotine.

PASSAGE OF COMPOUNDS FROM THE UTERINE FLUID INTO THE PREIMPLANTATION BLASTOCYST

Parenterally and orally administered drugs and other chemicals not only enter the endometrial fluid but also penetrate the free-lying blastocyst. Sodium thiocyanide, sulfonamide and salicylate (Lutwak-Mann, 1954, 1962), thalidomide (Fabro, Schumacher, Smith, and Williams, 1964; Keberle, Loustalot, Maller, Faigle, and Schmid, 1965; Fabro et al., 1965, 1967a), caffeine and nicotine (Fabro and Sieber, 1969), as well as DDT, isoniazid, barbital, and thiopental (Fabro and Sieber, 1968; Sieber and Fabro, 1971) have been identified in the pre- and post-implantation blastocysts of the rabbit. Austin and Lovelock (1958) found that rat, hamster, and rabbit eggs were permeable to toluidine blue, digitonin, and alcian blue, but not to heparin. Glass (1963), however, has demonstrated by immunofluorescent methods that macromolecules such as serum proteins can pass into the eggs of the mouse *in vivo.* In our experiments *in vitro,* dextran of 60,000 to 90,000 molecular weight did not penetrate the 6-day rabbit blastocyst, whereas 12 other compounds of smaller molecular weight, including 16,000 to

19,000 molecular weight dextran, salicylate, sulfanilamide, antipyrine, and hexamethonium enter the blastocyst at a rate which seems dependent upon their lipid solubility and degree of ionization (Sieber and Fabro, 1971).

Although it is clear from these findings that the preimplantation blastocyst is permeable to numerous foreign compounds, there is no clear picture available on the mechanism by which these substances enter the free-lying blastocyst. If one views the uterine fluid and the blastocyst as two compartments separated by a semipermeable membrane, the zona-coated trophoblast, then the question of passive diffusion may be considered first. There is an absence of a marked gradient in the level of free amino acids between the uterine and blastocyst fluid which suggests that these amphoteric compounds penetrate the blastocyst by a process of diffusion rather than by a more complex form of transport (Lutwak-Mann, 1971). It is likely that this also applies for antipyrine, caffeine, and isoniazid, which are largely uncharged at physiological pH. Thus, for these compounds, we found that there was an approximately equal concentration in the uterine fluid and in the preimplantation blastocyst (Sieber and Fabro, 1971). *In vitro* experiments also showed that neutral molecules such as tritiated water and gluthetimide reach approximately the same concentration in the blastocyst and in the medium (Keberle, Schmid, Faigle, Fritz, and Loustalot, 1966).

Since there is a marked difference in hydrogen ion concentration of the 6-day pregnant rabbit uterine fluid (pH 7.6) (McLachlan et al., 1970) and the blastocoelic fluid (pH 9.0) (Gottschewski, 1962), molecules may attain a different concentration in the uterine and blastocoelic fluids. Thus, unequal distribution of foreign chemicals can be explained with the pH partition hypothesis (Brodie, 1964). Nicotine, being a base ($pK_{b1} = 6.16$; $pK_{b2} = 10.96$), would be expected to attain at equilibrium much smaller concentrations in the compartment at pH 9.0 (i.e., blastocoelic fluid) than in that with a pH of 7.6 (i.e., the uterine fluid). We found that, following administration of ^{3}H-nicotine to 6-day pregnant animals, the amount of ^{3}H-activity reaching the blastocoelic fluid at 15 to 120 min after dosing was about 4 to 25 times less than that of the uterine fluid (Table 5).

According to this hypothesis, acids would be expected to accumulate in the blastocyst. Six hr after oral administration of (2-^{14}C)-barbital to 6-day pregnant rabbits, this compound was found in a concentration 1.5 to 2.3 times greater in the preimplantation blastocyst than in the uterine fluid. Keberle et al. (1966) also reported results on the accumulation of acids (e.g., tolbutamide and some sulfanilamide derivatives) in the preimplantation blastocysts of the rabbit which are consonant with the pH partition hy-

TABLE 5. Distribution of radioactivity between plasma, uterine and blastocyst fluids of 6-day pregnant rabbits treated with ³H-nicotine.

Doe No.	Time After Treatment (min)	Radioactivity in:			Blastocyst Fluid (DPM/ml) / Uterine Fluid (DPM/g)
		Plasma (DPM/ml)	Uterine Fluid (DPM/g)	Blastocyst Fluid (DPM/ml)	
364	15	138,380	1,492,101	93,318	0.06
365	15	133,100	1,752,635	98,049	0.06
444	15	228,438	1,160,493	130,380	0.11
					(0.08 ± 0.02)
96	30	145,033	1,868,798	77,341	0.04
372	30	133,732	1,038,990	116,775	0.11
373	30	129,486	1,584,520	106,935	0.07
					(0.07 ± 0.02)
374	120	95,163	1,296,195	70,441	0.05
376	120	107,506	354,429	95,253	0.27
					(0.16)

G-(³H)-Nicotine (50 μg/kg; 60 μC/kg) was given intravenously (McLachlan and Fabro, 1971, *unpublished*). Figures in parentheses represent means ± SEM, where appropriate.

pothesis. They also state that for this accumulation to take place, the acidic compound must be relatively lipophilic.

An accumulation of radioactivity in the preimplantation rabbit blastocyst has been observed after incubation in a medium containing ^{14}C-thalidomide (Keberle et al., 1965; Keberle et al., 1966; Fabro, 1968, *unpublished*). This accumulation is likely to be related to the instability of thalidomide at physiological pH; in solution at a pH above 6, thalidomide undergoes spontaneous hydrolysis at a rate which is proportional to the pH value of the medium (Williams, Schumacher, Fabro, and Smith, 1965). At least 11 acidic hydrolysis products are formed which are more polar than is unchanged thalidomide. Some of these acid metabolites of thalidomide have been identified in pre- and post-implantation rabbit blastocysts (Keberle et al., 1966; Fabro et al., 1967*a*). It is conceivable, therefore, that unchanged thalidomide is more rapidly broken down in the more alkaline blastocoelic fluid than in the uterine fluid, with a resultant accumulation of its metabolic products in the preimplantation blastocyst.

Recently, we have begun an investigation of the distribution of compounds within the blastocyst itself. When 6-day preimplantation rabbit blastocysts were incubated for 60 min in a medium containing ^{14}C-DDT, the zona-coated trophoblast with its associated embryonic disc contained a concentration of DDT which was approximately five times that of the blastocoelic fluid, which by this time had equilibrated with the medium (Dames and Fabro, 1971, *unpublished*). In view of these results, it would be interesting to know whether compounds such as 6-mercaptopurine, actinomycin D, and thalidomide, which have been shown to cause abnormalities of the embryonic disc and trophoblast (Lutwak-Mann et al., 1969), do indeed preferentially accumulate in these tissues.

THE TOXICOLOGICAL SIGNIFICANCE OF THE PENETRATION OF FOREIGN CHEMICALS INTO THE UTERINE FLUID AND PREIMPLANTATION BLASTOCYST

The presence of a number of foreign chemicals in the preimplantation blastocyst following maternal exposure has raised the obvious question of the toxicological significance of these findings. The reader is referred to the chapter by Cecelia Lutwak-Mann where this subject is discussed in detail. Here we will confine ourselves to a discussion of some results obtained recently in our laboratory (McLachlan, Dames, and Fabro, 1971, *unpublished*).

We have administered daily doses of caffeine (25 mg/kg, orally), salic-

TABLE 6. *Effects of some drugs and other chemicals given before implantation on the outcome of pregnancy in the New Zealand White rabbit.*

| Treatment | Litter Size | Weight (g) of: | |
		Whole Fetus	Fetal Brain
Control	6.4 ± 0.5	37.4 ± 1.4	0.93 ± 0.03
DDT	8.2 ± 0.6	28.0 ± 2.1[a]	0.83 ± 0.05[a]
Nicotine	6.6 ± 1.9	29.0 ± 2.1[a]	0.87 ± 0.06
Salicylate	5.0 ± 1.5	35.5 ± 2.3	0.90 ± 0.04
Caffeine	6.8 ± 1.8	34.0 ± 2.5	0.91 ± 0.03

Drugs and other chemicals were administered in the following doses and routes: DDT (1 mg/kg, p.o.), nicotine (0.1 mg/kg, i.v.), sodium salicylate (100 mg/kg, p.o.), or caffeine (25 mg/kg, p.o.); in each case, the animals were treated on days 4, 5, 6, and 7 of gestation and killed on day 28; out of 365 fetuses removed from 52 pregnant rabbits, only one fetus found in a litter of a DDT-treated mother was grossly malformed (ectopia viscerum). Figures represent means ± SEM.

[a] Significantly ($p < 0.05$) different from control values.

ylate (100 mg/kg, orally), DDT (1 mg/kg, orally), and nicotine (0.1 mg/kg, intravenously) to pregnant New Zealand White rabbits on days 4 through 7 of gestation. The effects of this treatment were assessed by measuring the implantation ratio and volume of the conceptus at 8 days, as well as by evaluating the outcome of pregnancy at 28 days according to the methods previously described (Fabro and Smith, 1966). None of these treatments can be considered teratogenic, since out of 365 fetuses removed from 52 28-day pregnant rabbits, only one fetus found in a litter of a DDT-treated mother was grossly malformed (ectopia viscerum) (Table 6). The administration of caffeine or salicylate to rabbits during the preimplantation stages of pregnancy failed to show any toxicity. Nicotine did not affect either the number of implantations or the volume of the conceptus at 8 days, although the average weight of the offspring recovered at 28 days of pregnancy was statistically lower than control fetuses. It has been shown that women who smoke have a higher spontaneous abortion rate (O'Lane, 1963); the babies they deliver are more likely to be premature (Peterson, Morese, and Kaltreider, 1965), and have relatively lower birth weights (Mulcahy, Murphy, and Martin, 1970). Whether this type of human toxicity has any relationship to exposure to nicotine during the preimplantation stages of pregnancy remains to be assessed.

Treatment with DDT during the preimplantation stages of pregnancy did not decrease the number of implantations, but the average volume of the implanted embryos at 8 days of pregnancy was significantly less than that of the controls. As in the case of nicotine, the 28-day fetuses of the DDT-treated rabbits were significantly smaller than those of the control group. In addition, brain weights of the DDT-exposed fetuses were significantly lower than the brain weights of the control animals. These effects were not seen with caffeine, salicylate, or nicotine. Since Wigglesworth (1964) and Harding and Shelley (1967) have reported that during intrauterine life the increasing brain weight of rat and rabbit fetuses parallels gestational age and is relatively independent of the total body weight of the conceptus, the decrease in fetal brain weight of DDT-treated animals may be of significance. It may very well be that this decreased brain weight represents a specific toxic effect of DDT.

An interesting finding was the observation that the yolk-sac fluid of implanted 8-day embryos whose mothers had been treated with DDT during the preimplantation stages of pregnancy possesses an abnormal protein electrophoretic pattern. Thus, three additional bands were present, two pre-albumin bands as well as a post-albumin band (Fig. 2). These bands were

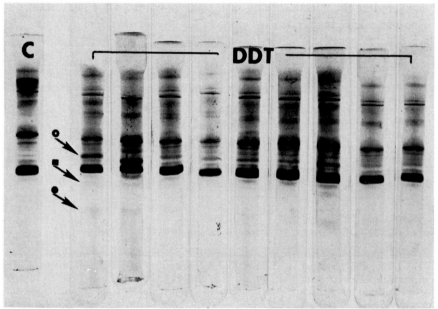

FIG. 2. Gel electrophoretic patterns of yolk-sac fluid from embryos of 8-day pregnant rabbits given DDT during the preimplantation stages of pregnancy. The protein profiles were obtained by discontinuous gradient polyacrylamide gel electrophoresis according to the method of Wright et al. (1971), followed by staining with Coomassie Brilliant Blue. The arrows denote bands which are not found in the yolk-sac fluid protein profiles of control (C) embryos: (○) post-albumin, (■) pre-albumin, (●) fast pre-albumin. Protein profiles of 8-day yolk-sac fluid are results obtained with a representative litter from a doe treated with DDT (1 mg/kg, p.o.) on days 4, 5, 6, and 7 of gestation and killed on day 8 (McLachlan, Dames and Fabro, 1971, unpublished).

identified by R_f values and color reactions as proteins which are characteristic of the preimplantation blastocyst fluid (Dames, McLachlan, and Fabro, 1970, *unpublished*).

Thus, DDT treatment during the preimplantation stages of pregnancy resulted in a decreased size of the conceptus at 8 and 28 days of gestation, and produced an alteration in the 8-day yolk-sac fluid suggestive of biochemical immaturity. This may well be an indication that, at least in the rabbit, DDT exerts a toxic action which is manifested by intrauterine growth retardation. Hart, Adamson, and Fabro (1971) showed that DDT causes prematurity and intrauterine growth retardation when given in large amounts to pregnant rabbits during morphogenesis. O'Leary, Davies, Edmundson, and Feldman (1970) have reported that low birth weights in human infants could be correlated with high serum levels of DDE, a major metabolite of DDT. Thus, our results in the rabbit seem to indicate that exposure of the mother during the preimplantation stages of pregnancy to some commonly encountered environmental agents such as nicotine and DDT may result in a type of toxicity manifested by intrauterine growth retardation in the absence of teratogenesis.

ACKNOWLEDGMENTS

It is a pleasure to acknowledge the help of my graduate students, N. M. Dames, J. A. McLachlan, P. Skolnick, and S. M. Sieber, who carried out most of these experiments. This research was supported by U.S. Public Health Service Research Grant GM-13749 from the National Institute of General Medical Sciences.

REFERENCES

Austin, C. R., and Lovelock, J. E. (1958): Permeability of rabbit, rat and hamster egg membranes. *Experimental Cell Research,* 15:260-261.

Balik, J. (1965): Method for the biochemical study of tears. *Acta Ophthalmologica,* 43:190-198.

Bender, I. B., Pressman, R. S., and Tashman, S. G. (1953): Studies on excretion of antibiotics in human saliva. Aureomycin. *Journal of Dental Research,* 32:435-439.

Borzelleca, J. F., and Cherrick, H. M. (1965): The excretion of drugs in saliva. Antibiotics. *Journal of Oral Therapy and Pharmacology,* 2:180-187.

Brodie, B. B. (1964): Physico-chemical factors in drug absorption. In: *Absorption and Distribution of Drugs,* edited by T. B. Binns. The Williams and Wilkins Co., Baltimore, Md., pp. 16-48.

Brusilow, S. W., and Gordes, E. H. (1966): The permeability of the sweat gland to non-electrolytes. *American Journal of Diseases of Children,* 112:328-333.

Bulmer, M. G. (1957): The concentration of urea in thermal sweat. *Journal of Physiology,* 137:261-266.

Burgen, A. S. V. (1956): The secretion of non-electrolytes in the parotid saliva. *Journal of Cellular and Comparative Physiology,* 40:113-138.

Comaish, J. S., and Shelley, W. B. (1965): Fluorometric determination of quinine and fluorescein excretion in human sweat. *Journal of Investigative Dermatology,* 36:279-281.

Dreyfus-Seé, G. (1934): Le passage dans le lait des aliments ou médicaments absorbés par les mourrices. *Revue de medecine* (Paris), 51:198-213.

Fabro, S., Schumacher, H., Smith,, R. L., and Williams, R. T. (1964): Identification of thalidomide in rabbit blastocysts. *Nature,* 201:1125-1126.

Fabro, S., and Sieber, S. M. (1968): Penetration of drugs into the rabbit blastocyst before implantation. *Excerpta Medica International Congress Series* No. 183. The Foeto-Placental Unit Symposium, Milan, pp. 313-411.

Fabro, S., and Sieber, S. M. (1969): Caffeine and nicotine penetrate the pre-implantation blastocyst. *Nature,* 223:410-411.

Fabro, S., and Smith, R. L. (1966): The teratogenic activity of thalidomide in the rabbit. *Journal of Pathology and Bacteriology,* 91:511-519.

Fabro, S., Smith, R. L., and Williams, R. T. (1965): The persistence of maternally administered ^{14}C-thalidomide in the rabbit embryo. *Biochemical Journal,* 97:14P.

Fabro, S., Smith, R. L., and Williams, R. T. (1967a): The fate of (^{14}C) thalidomide in the pregnant rabbit. *Biochemical Journal,* 104:565-569.

Fabro, S., Smith, R. L., and Williams, R. T. (1967b): The fate of the hydrolysis products of thalidomide in the pregnant rabbit. *Biochemical Journal,* 104:570-574.

Fantus, B., and Dyniewicz, J. M. (1936): Phenolphthalein administration to nursing women. *American Journal of Digestive Diseases,* 3:184-185.

Farrell, J. I. (1938): Secretion of alcohol by the genital tract; experimental study. *Journal of Urology,* 40:62-65.

Farrell, J. I., Lyman, Y., and Youman, G. P. (1938): The rationale of sulfanilamide in gonococcic urethriuis. *Journal of the American Medical Association,* 110:1176-1177.

Friedemann, T. E., Motel, W. G., and Necheles, H. (1938): The excretion of ingested ethyl alcohol in saliva. *Journal of Laboratory and Clinical Medicine,* 23:1007-1014.

Glass, L. E. (1963): Transfer of native and foreign serum antigens to oviducal mouse eggs. *American Zoology,* 3:135-156.

Gottschewski, H. M. (1962): Probleme der Früheutwicklung beim Säugetier, *Naturwiss. Rundschau,* 15:257-264.

Greenwald, G. S., and Everett, N. B. (1959): The incorporation of S^{35} methionine by the uterus and ova of the mouse. *Anatomical Record,* 134:171-184.

Hafez, E. S. E. (1971): Some maternal factors affecting physicochemical properties of blastocysts. In: *The Biology of the Blastocyst,* edited by R. J. Blandau. University of Chicago Press, Chicago, pp. 139-191.

Hansson, E., and Schmiterlöw, C. G. (1962): Physiological disposition and fate of C-^{14}-labelled nicotine in mice and rats. *Journal of Pharmacology and Experimental Therapeutics,* 137:91-102.

Harding, P. G. R., and Shelley, H. J. (1967): Some effects of intrauterine growth retardation in the foetal rabbit. In: *Intrauterine Dangers to the Foetus,* edited by J. Horsky and Z. K. Stembera. Excerpta Medica Foundation, Amsterdam, pp. 529-531.

Hart, M. M., Adamson, R. H., and Fabro, S. (1971): Prematurity and intrauterine growth retardation induced by DDT in the rabbit. *Archives Internationales de Pharmacodynamie de Thérapie,* 192:286-290.

Keberle, H., Loustalot, P., Maller, R. K., Faigle, J. W., and Schmid, K. (1965): Biochemical effects of drugs on the mammalian conceptus. *Annals of the New York Academy of Sciences,* 123:252-262.

Keberle, H., Schmid, K., Faigle, J. W., Fritz, H., and Loustalot, P. (1966): Über die Penetration von Korperfremden Stoffen in den jungen Wirbeltierkeim. *Bulletin der*

Schweizerschen Akademie der Medizinischen Wissenschaften, 22:134-152.

Killman, S. A., and Thaysen, J. H. (1955): The permeability of the human parotid glands to a series of sulfonamide compounds, para-aminohippurate and inulin. *Scandinavian Journal of Clinical and Laboratory Investigation,* 7:86-91.

Koch, F. (1938): Über exkretorische Fähigkeiten des Schweisses. *Archiv für Dermatologie und Syphilis,* 177:163-166.

Krishnan, R. S., and Daniel, J. C., Jr. (1967): "Blastokinin": inducer and regulator of blastocyst development in the rabbit uterus. *Science,* 158:490-492.

Kwit, N. T., and Hatcher, R. A. (1935): Excretion of drugs in milk. *American Journal of Diseases of Children,* 49:900-904.

Lutwak-Mann, C. (1954): Some properties of the rabbit blastocyst. *Journal of Embryology and Experimental Morphology,* 2:1-13.

Lutwak-Mann, C. (1962): Glucose, lactic acid and bicarbonate in rabbit blastocyst fluid. *Nature,* 193:653-654.

Lutwak-Mann, C. (1971): The rabbit blastocyst and its environment: Physiological and biochemical aspects. In: *The Biology of the Blastocyst,* edited by R. J. Blandau. University of Chicago Press, Chicago, pp. 243-260.

Lutwak-Mann, C., Boursnell, J. C., and Bennett, J. P., (1960): Blastocyst-uterine relationships: Uptake of radioactive ions by the early rabbit embryo and its environment. *Journal of Reproduction and Fertility,* 1:169-185.

Lutwak-Mann, C., Hay, M. F., and New, D. A. T. (1969): Action of various agents on rabbit blastocysts *in vivo* and *in vitro. Journal of Reproduction and Fertility,* 18:235-257.

Lutwak-Mann, C., Schmid, K., and Keberle, H. (1967): Thalidomide in rabbit semen. *Nature,* 214:1018-1020.

McLachlan, J. A., Sieber, S. M., Cowherd, C. M., Straw, J. A., and Fabro, S. (1970): The pH values of the uterine secretions and pre-implantation blastocyst of the rabbit. *Fertility and Sterility,* 21:84-87.

McLachlan, J. A., Sieber, S. M., and Fabro, S. (1969): Studies on the transfer of drugs into the uterine secretion. *Federation Proceedings,* 28:744.

Martin, K., and Burgen, A. S. V. (1962): Changes in the permeability of the salivary gland caused by sympathetic stimulation and by catecholamines. *Journal of General Physiology,* 46:225-243.

Mayo, C. W., and Schlicke, C. P. (1942): Appearance of a barbiturate in human milk. *Proceedings Staff Meeting Mayo Clinic,* 17:87-88.

Miller, A. W., Jr., and Larson, P. S. (1953): Observations on the metabolism of nicotine by tissue slices. *Journal of Pharmacology and Experimental Therapeutics,* 109:218-222.

Miller, G. E., Banerjee, N. C., and Stowe, C. M. (1967): Diffusion of certain weak organic acids and bases across the bovine mammary gland membrane after systemic administration. *Journal of Pharmacology and Experimental Therapeutics,* 157:245-253.

Mulcahy, R., Murphy, J., and Martin, F. (1970): Placental changes and maternal weight in smoking and non-smoking mothers. *American Journal of Obstetrics and Gynecology,* 104:703-704.

Noach, E. L., Woodbury, D. M., and Goodman, L. S. (1958): Studies on the absorption, distribution, fate and excretion of 4-C^{14}-labeled diphenylhydantoin. *Journal of Pharmacology and Experimental Therapeutics,* 122:301-314.

O'Lane, J. M. (1963): Some fetal effects of maternal cigaret smoking. *Obstetrics and Gynecology,* 22:181-184.

O'Leary, J. A., Davies, J. E., Edmundson, W. F., and Feldman, M. (1970): Correlation of prematurity and DDE levels in fetal whole blood. *American Journal of Obstetrics and Gynecology,* 106:939.

Peterson, W. F., Morese, K. N., and Kaltreider, D. F. (1965): Smoking and prematurity.

A preliminary report based on study of 7740 Caucasians. *Obstetrics and Gynecology,* 26:775-779.

Rasmussen, F. (1959): Mammary excretion of benzyl-penicillin, erythromycin and penethamate hydrochloride. *Acta Pharmacologica et Toxicologica,* 16:194-200.

Reed, C. B. (1908): A study of the conditions that require the removal of the child from the breast. *Surgery, Gynecology and Obstetrics,* 6:514-527.

Sargent, F., Robinson, P., and Johnson, R. E. (1944): Water-soluble vitamins in sweat. *Journal of Biological Chemistry,* 153:285-294.

Schanker, L. S. (1959): Absorption of drugs from the rat colon. *Journal of Pharmacology and Experimental Therapeutics,* 126:283-290.

Shore, P. A., Brodie, B. B., and Hogben, C. A. M. (1957): The gastric secretion of drugs: a pH partition hypothesis. *Journal of Pharmacology and Experimental Therapeutics,* 119:361-369.

Sieber, S. M., and Fabro, S. (1971): Identification of drugs in the preimplantation blastocyst and in the plasma, uterine secretion and urine of the pregnant rabbit. *Journal of Pharmacology and Experimental Therapeutics,* 176:65-75.

Sisodia, C. S., and Stowe, C. M. (1964): The mechanism of drug secretion into bovine milk. *Annals of the New York Academy of Sciences,* 111:650-661.

Smith, R. L. (1966): The biliary excretion and enterohepatic circulation of drugs and other organic compounds. *Progress in Drug Research,* 9:299-360.

Smith, R. L., and Williams, R. T. (1966): Implication of the conjugation of drugs and other exogenous compounds. In: *Glucuronic Acid-Free and Combined,* edited by G. J. Dutton. Academic Press, New York, pp. 457-491.

Snedecor, G. W. (1959): *Statistical Methods,* Iowa State College Press, Ames.

Tachau, H. (1911): Über den Ubergang von Arzneimitteln in den Schweiss. *Archiv für Experimentelle Pathologie und Pharmacologie,* 66:334-346.

Thaysen, J. H., and Schwartz, I. L. (1953): The permeability of human sweat glands to a series of sulfonamide compounds. *Journal of Experimental Medicine,* 98:261-268.

Tyson, R. M., Schrader, E. A., and Perlman, H. H. (1938): Drugs transmitted through breast milk. II. Barbiturates. *Journal of Pediatrics,* 13:86-90.

Weast, C R. (1962): *Handbook of Chemistry and Physics.* The Chemical Rubber Publishing Co., Cleveland.

Weinig, E., and Jahn, G. (1954): Die kriminalistische Bedeutung der Ausscheidung von Arzneimitteln im Schweiss. *Deutsche Zeitschrift für die gesamte gerichtliche Medizin,* 43:370-373.

Wigglesworth, J. S. (1964): Experimental growth retardation in the foetal rat. *Journal of Pathology and Bacteriology,* 88:1-13.

Williams, R. T., Schumacher, H., Fabro, S., and Smith, R. L. (1965): The chemistry and metabolism of thalidomide. In: *Embryopathic Activity of Drugs,* edited by J. M. Robson, F. M. Sullivan, and R. L. Smith. J. & A. Churchill Ltd., London, p. 167-182.

Wright, G. L., Jr., Farrell, K. B., and Roberts, D. B. (1971): Gradient polyacrylamide gel electrophoresis of human serum: Improved discontinuous gradient technique and identification of individual serum components. *Clinica Chemica Acta,* 32:285-296.

Zweig, G., Smith, L. M., Peoples, S. A., and Cox, R. (1961): DDT residues in milk from dairy cows fed low levels of DDT in their daily rations. *Journal of Agriculture and Food Chemistry,* 9:481-484.

DISCUSSION

MIRKIN: Nicotine appears to be retarded in its passage across the placenta (Tjälve, Hansson, and Schmiterlöw: *Acta Pharmacologica et Toxicologica, 26,*

539, 1965) so that the fetal concentrations are rather low. In contrast, cotinine appears to cross the placenta very rapidly. Your data suggest that nicotine enters the uterine lumen fluid quite readily.

FABRO: This apparent discrepancy probably arises from the fact that we are talking about two entirely different transport processes. The aim of my research has been to define the passage of compounds from the maternal circulation into the endometrial secretion. It is possible that the two systems are not identical.

JOST: The blastocyst is not only a membrane around fluid, it is also composed of important cells and I should like to know if these cells accumulate some drugs.

FABRO: This is a very good point. We have begun some experiments designed to localize radioactivity within the various compartments of blastocysts from rabbits treated with radioactive DDT. It appears that radioactivity associated with DDT is distributed unequally among these compartments. *In vitro* experiments have also shown that after incubating 6-day preimplantation blastocysts in a medium containing ^{14}C-DDT, the zona-coated trophoblast with its associated embryonic disc contained a concentration of DDT which was approximately five times that of the blastocyst fluid which by this time had equilibrated with the medium.

LUTWAK-MANN: It is not particularly surprising that pseudopregnant rabbits, such as used in some of your experiments, showed results that were analogous with those observed in the embryo-bearing animals. Equally, it is only to be expected that there would be marked differences in the levels of exogenous agents as between the watery uterine fluid produced by the nonpregnant estrous endometrium, and the scanty thick progestational secretion, typical of the blastocyst stage (day 6 of gestation in the rabbit). I think it would perhaps be more interesting either to ovariectomize or treat with estrogen some of the pregnant rabbits, or, alternatively, study days of pseudopregnancy earlier or later than day 6, and investigate the behavior of the drugs in your systems under such special endocrine conditions.

I rather doubt that one could ascribe to pH values the interesting differences that you have described concerning the partition of various drugs, as between the endometrial secretion and the blastocyst fluid. Under physiological conditions, the pH of the rabbit blastocyst fluid is the same as that of other biological fluids. But, owing to its high bicarbonate content, rabbit blastocyst fluid from which, on standing, CO_2 has been allowed to escape, will, of course, show increasing pH values, until all the bicarbonate has been converted to carbonate.

I also doubt if it is practicable to withdraw from the free-lying rabbit blastocyst, by means of micropipettes, samples of blastocyst fluid that would really be entirely free of cellular contaminants. These would inescapably form a contamination, as they are found on the blastocyst surface, or would enter the

Fetal Pharmacology, edited by L. Boréus
Raven Press, New York © 1973

The Future of Fetal Pharmacology

Fritz Fuchs

*Department of Obstetrics and Gynecology, Cornell University Medical College,
New York, New York 10021*

Obstetricians are notorious for being either therapeutic nihilists or igno-
rants, and I belong to the first category. In fact, I usually tell my residents
that the most important tool for an obstetrician is a stool. Why, then, was
an obstetrician asked to look into the crystal ball and discuss the future of
fetal pharmacology?

As a Dane I am keenly aware of the aphorism coined by the Danish
humorist Storm Petersen who said: "It is difficult to predict, particularly
about the future!" Why, then, did I accept the invitation to try to make predictions of the future of a new field of medicine which had hardly been defined before we got together at this symposium?

Well, trying to look into the future has a fascination to all of us, including myself. And the risk is probably not as great as it may seem. If the
weather forecast is wrong, the public will blame the meteorologist, but if my
predictions turn out to be false, who will remember what I said? If only
some of them turn out to be correct, I can point to the proceedings and
remind you that I told you so. I can then even try to share some of the
glory of those who *did* the things instead of just predicting that they *could*
be done. In fact, after all the excellent work presented here, it would seem
impossible not to be able to outline some of the developments which can be
expected.

Although some pharmacologists may take issue with this view, most clinicians consider the purpose of pharmacology to be to provide the scientific basis for pharmacotherapy. Any attempt at rational therapy requires an exact diagnosis, and it is precisely the rapid progress with regard to diagnosis of fetal diseases in recent years which led us to consider the possibilities of intrauterine treatment.

Treatment of fetal disease, however, is but one, and a minor one at that, of the areas of fetal pharmacology. Whenever the maternal organism is exposed to drugs, the fetus must be considered. Such exposures may conveniently be divided into four categories: (1) therapy of maternal disease directly related to pregnancy and delivery-obstetric complications with other words; (2) therapy of maternal disease unrelated to but coinciding with pregnancy; (3) maternal use or abuse of drugs for nontherapeutic purposes; and finally (4) incidental exposure of the pregnant woman to pharmaca and chemicals. I shall briefly consider some aspects of each of these areas.

Until 20 years ago, we had very limited means to assess the condition of the fetus—essentially nothing but palpation of the fetal size, auscultation of the fetal heart rate, and X-rays to detect gross malformations. Then it was found that there is some correlation between maternal blood and urine levels of certain feto-placental hormones, particularly estriol, and enzymes such as aminopeptidase and diamino oxidase and the growth rate and general condition of the fetus during pregnancy. About the same time, amniocentesis came into the picture, first introduced by Bevis in 1952 to assess the fetal condition in Rh-isoimmunization. Later, Riis and Fuchs (1960) used genetic information obtained through amniocentesis in the management of certain inherited disorders, and in the last few years studies of amniotic fluid constitutents have made it possible to detect a variety of genetic disorders, mainly those classified as inborn errors of metabolism (Fuchs and Cederqvist, 1970). At the end of 1970, Milunsky, Littlefield, Kaufer, Kolodny, Shih, and Atkins were able to list 44 genetic disorders which either have been or can be expected to be detected *in utero* by amniotic fluid studies. With the exception of erythroblastosis fetalis, which is usually not considered a genetic disease, although certainly due to a constellation of genetic factors, only one of these disorders has so far been treated *in utero,* namely the adrenogenital syndrome, and the rationale in this instance is debatable. But it is very likely that attempts will be made to treat other inborn errors of metabolism before birth. It is not even inconceivable that attempts will be made to correct genetic defects of the fetus in the future. The recent demonstrations that genetic material can be transferred into living cells by virus infection (Merril, Geirer, and Petricciani, 1971) or hybridization (Schwartz,

Cook, and Harris, 1971) indicate that "genetic manipulation" is already within reach. Promising as this may be, genetic manipulation of human embryos is not around the corner; it is deplorable when the public is given the impression that it is and that this will give rise to so many ethical problems that it might be better to stop the development before the corner.

Intrauterine infections are obvious targets for drug therapy. Such infections generally occur late in pregnancy due to rupture of the membranes. Prophylaxis and treatment with antibiotics have not been particularly effective, although most antibiotics are able to pass the placental barrier. This is probably due to the poorly developed immunological defense of the fetus. Induction of delivery is usually better than intrauterine treatment. In the maternal infections associated with high incidence of severe fetal damage such as rubella and toxoplasmosis, little attention has been given to the possibility of treatment of the fetal infection. Although prophylaxis through preconceptional immunization is preferable, the possibility of preventing fetal damage by intrauterine treatment should be carefully studied.

Fetal growth retardation can be due to fetal metabolic deficiencies or, probably more often, to placental insufficiency. Although fetal growth retardation is not always easy to diagnose with certainty, various ways to correct the situation must be explored. We have made a modest attempt by giving the mother ethanol daily for a certain period of time in the hope of thereby providing the fetus with additional calories (Fuchs, Beling, Lauersen, and Merkatz, 1970). Of the four cases we have treated, rising maternal estriol excretion indicated an increase of the fetal growth rate in three. In the fourth case, a severe fetal malformation was the cause of the growth retardation and ethanol was of no consequence. Admittedly, estriol excretion is a somewhat uncertain indicator of fetal growth and we hope to use measures of the biparietal diameter of the fetal head by sonography in future cases. Accelerated fetal growth has also been observed in patients treated with a β-adrenergic drug, Ritodrine®,* for threatened premature labor, but it remains to be seen if this can be used in retarded fetal growth.

The effect upon the fetus of pharmacotherapy of maternal disease in pregnancy is the area of greatest concern. We are often faced with diseases which endanger the mother's life and thereby also that of the fetus; the most effective drug may protect the mother but damage the fetus. Malaria is a good example. This can apply both to diseases which are particular to pregnancy and to entities which are incidental to pregnancy. The thalidomide tragedy opened the eyes of pharmaceutical manufacturers, obstetricians, and

---

*Philips-Duphar, Weesp, The Netherlands.

patients, but it came as no great surprise to those engaged in studies of placental transfer. To them it was obvious how woefully inadequate our knowledge of the effects of drugs on the fetus was. Today we know a great deal more, but recent findings have shown that there might still be tragic surprises in store. I am referring to the recent discovery of a high incidence of vaginal carcinoma in young women whose mothers were treated with diethylstilbestrol in pregnancy (Herbst, Ulfelder, and Poskanzer, 1971). The virilizing effect on the female fetus of certain synthetic progestagens is an old story; still to be explored is the possibility that sex steroids taken during pregnancy may influence the sex behavior and fertility of the offspring by programming the central nervous system, as has been shown in rats by Harris (1964) and Levine and Treiman (1969). When steroids are given to prevent abortion, a certain risk is justified if the treatment does what it is supposed to do. There is no evidence, however, that treatment with steroids increases fetal salvage (Fuchs, 1967), and it is saddening that such treatment is not only still used but even advertised by pharmaceutical companies who should at least know better.

From the effects of steroids on the developing central nervous system, whether or not the particular finding turns out to apply to the human, we must learn the lesson that drugs taken during pregnancy may alter not only the structural but also the functional development of the fetus. Thus, teratological studies of new (and old) pharmaca are not enough; behavioral studies must be added. One wonders what effect the psychopharmaca may have on the programming of the fetal central nervous system. Some of them have already been shown to produce behavioral changes in the offspring of laboratory animals.

To go into all the fetal aspects of maternal drug therapy would require too much time, but let me venture at least one prediction. It is very gratifying that it has been possible for patients with kidney transplants to conceive and carry through pregnancies successfully. Although immunosuppression with azathioprine and corticosteroids was continued throughout pregnancy, we have observed no fetal damage (Merkatz, Schwartz, David, Stenzel, Riggio, and Whitsell, 1971). It is not too optimistic to predict that one day patients with heart transplants or even transplanted uteri may carry pregnancies successfully to term in spite of immunosuppressive and other supportive drug therapy.

While the obstetrician may be a therapeutic nihilist—and rightly so—during pregnancy, he does use drugs at parturition, mainly to promote or delay uterine activity and to reduce pain. We have made considerable progress in the protection of the fetus against the direct or indirect effects of such medication, but it is still an area of concern. Of particular interest is the recent progress in the prevention of premature birth with ethanol (Fuchs, Fuchs, Poblete, and Risk, 1967) and certain β-adrenergic drugs (Wesselius-de Casparis, Thiery, Yo Le Sian, Baumgarten, Brosens, Gamisans, Stolk, and Vivier, 1971, and others). Although prematurity is the leading cause of perinatal mortality, and prevention of prematurity therefore is extremely important, the effect of such treatment upon the fetus must be studied with great care.

The pharmacological, toxicological, and teratological studies that are necessary to declare a new drug safe for pregnant women are extremely costly. It is a safe but sad prediction, which has probably already come true, that unless a drug is effective in diseases particular to pregnancy, it may not become subject to such studies. It is so much easier to put a warning on the insert that the drug might not be safe in pregnancy. But this is not satisfactory to the obstetrician, because too often the patient does not know that she has conceived or she may forget to tell her obstetrician about a drug prescribed by someone else. It is quite a dilemma, because if such studies become a requirement for registration, some otherwise extremely useful drug may never be marketed.

The effect upon the fetus of maternal drug abuse has become a problem of great dimensions. Whether or not LSD (lysergic acid diethylamide) causes chromosomal damage in the human fetus is a matter of dispute. Heroin as well as methadone, the compound used in the treatment of heroin addicts, affect the fetus and cause severe withdrawal effects in the newborn. In view of the effects of steroids on the fetal central nervous system, one cannot but speculate about the possible effects on the fetal "mind." If we are to believe the psychoanalysts, the intrauterine experience is of utmost importance for the psychological mechanisms in adult life. Our knowledge in this area is quite limited but we shall have plenty of opportunity to study it in the future. Conceivably, new psychedelic drugs will appear on the scene, sharing with those already in use the potential dangers to the offspring.

In our daily life we are constantly and increasingly exposed to a large variety of pharmacological and chemical compounds, such as sweeteners, preservatives, and other food additives, or smoke, car exhaust fumes, gasoline, perfumes, deodorants, and other air pollutants, or chlorine, fluoride, and other water constituents. We are all subject to a variety of unknown compounds, and some of us are exposed to additional occupational hazards. It was recently shown by Askrog and Harvald (1970) and by Cohen, Bellville, and Brown (1971) that operating-room nurses have a high incidence of fetal wastage, and nurse anesthetists and female anesthesiologists an even higher incidence of miscarriage and fetal loss. This is thought to be due to residual volatile anesthetic agents in the operating-room air. It is important that the influence of all such incidental compounds be studied.

Although we have been presented with a number of quite sophisticated approaches to fetal pharmacology, it is a safe bet that some of them will be developed even further and that even more sophisticated methods will be developed. Now that we have access to human ova through the method of Steptoe and Edwards (1970), the studies of Lutwak-Mann, Fabro, and others can be extended to the human embryo. Undoubtedly, methods will be developed to maintain blastocysts and embryos over a longer span of time for such studies. Ovum transplantation in the human is well within reach, but this will give rise to new problems.

The use of previable fetuses for studies of fetal pharmacology has not been mentioned, although some pioneering work with previable fetuses has taken place in Sweden.

I find the use of amniotic fluid cell cultures, as described by Beling and New, a very promising approach. Amniocentesis can be performed from the 15th week of pregnancy without disturbing the fetal integrity and can be repeated at intervals throughout pregnancy. This method is applicable to a variety of studies of drug metabolism in human fetal cells.

The fetus is definitely coming of age. The term "Fetology" was introduced less than 20 years ago, and now we have Fetal Physiology, Fetal Endocrinology, and so on. If we have witnessed the baptism of Fetal Pharmacology at this Symposium, we can all join in wishing it a bright future.

REFERENCES

Askrog, V., and Harvald, B. (1970): Teratogen effekt af inhalationsanestetika. *Nordisk Medicin*, 83:498-500.

Bevis, D. C. A. (1952): The antenatal prediction of haemolytic disease of the new-born. *Lancet*, I:395-398.

Cohen, E. N., Bellville, J. W., and Brown, B. B., Jr. (1971): Anesthesia, pregnancy, and miscarriage. *Anesthesiology*, 35:343-347.

Fuchs, F. (1967): Causes of spontaneous abortion: Endocrine deficiencies. *Proceedings of the Fifth World Congress of Gynaecology and Obstetrics, Sydney, Australia.* Butterworth, Sydney, pp. 714-721.

Fuchs, F., Beling, C. G., Lauersen, N. H., and Merkatz, I. R. (1970): Effect of ethanol on fetus and newborn. *Proceedings of the International Symposium on Utero-Inhibitory Drugs and Their Effects on Mother, Fetus and Newborn, Punta del Este, Uruguay (in press).*

Fuchs, F., and Cederqvist, L. L. (1970): Recent advances in antenatal diagnosis by amniotic fluid analysis. *Clinical Obstetrics and Gynecology,* 13:178-201.

Fuchs, F., Fuchs, A.-R., Poblete, V. F., Jr., and Risk, A. (1967): Effect of alcohol on threatened premature labor. *American Journal of Obstetrics and Gynecology,* 99:627-637.

Harris, G. W. (1964): Sex hormones, brain development and brain function. *Endocrinology,* 75:627-648.

Herbst, A. L., Ulfelder, H., and Poskanzer, D. C. (1971): Adenocarcinoma of the vagina. *New England Journal of Medicine,* 284:878-881.

Levine, S., and Treiman, L. J. (1969): Role of hormones in programming the central nervous system. *CIBA Foundation Symposium on Foetal Autonomy,* edited by G. E. W. Wolstenholme and M. O'Connor. Churchill, London, pp. 271-281.

Merkatz, I. R., Schwartz, G. H., David, D. S., Stenzel, K. H., Riggio, R. R., and Whitsell, J. C. (1971): Resumption of female reproductive function following renal transplantation. *Journal of the American Medical Association,* 216:1749-1754.

Merril, C. R., Geirer, M. R., and Petricciani, J. C. (1971): Bacterial virus gene expression in human cells. *Nature,* 233:398-400.

Milunsky, A., Littlefield, J. W., Kaufer, J. N., Kolodny, E. H., Shih, V. E., and Atkins, L. (1970): Prenatal genetic diagnosis. *New England Journal of Medicine,* 283:1370-1381, 1441-1447, 1498-1504.

Riis, P., and Fuchs, F. (1960): Antenatal determination of foetal sex in prevention of hereditary diseases. *Lancet,* II:180-182.

Schwartz, A. G., Cook, P. R., and Harris, H. (1971): Correction of a genetic defect in a mammalian cell. *Nature, New Biology,* 230:5-8.

Steptoe, P. C., and Edwards, R. G. (1970): Laparoscopic recovery of preovulatory human oocytes after priming of ovaries with gonadotrophins. *Lancet,* I:683-689.

Wesselius-de Casparis, A., Thiery, M., Yo Le Sian, A., Baumgarten, K., Brosens, I., Gamisans, O., Stolk, J. G., and Vivier, W. (1971): Results of double-blind, multicentre study with Ritodrine in premature labour. *British Medical Journal,* II:144-147.

Fetal Pharmacology, edited by L. Boréus
Raven Press, New York © 1973

Biochemical Pharmacology
of Embryonic Development:
Summary of a Discussion

R. Paoletti

*Institute of Pharmacology and Pharmacognosy, University of Milan,
20129 Milan, Italy*

The Symposium concluded with a discussion among the participants on some biochemical and pharmacological aspects of the developing embryo.

Among the questions put forward were the origin and distribution of neurotransmitters, drug metabolism in the fetus, and the diagnosis and possible treatment of diseases in the fetus. Some relevant points can be summarized as follows.

APPEARANCE AND FUNCTION OF NEUROTRANSMITTERS IN
FETAL DEVELOPMENT

Adrenergic transmitters

The sympathetic neurotransmitters appear quite early in life. Norepinephrine is synthesized in the cell bodies of the sympathetic neurons in chick embryos at the age of 3 to 4 days (Enemar et al., 1965), and the peripheral organs of the chick embryo receive their sympathetic innervation during the 3rd to 8th days of incubation (Hamilton, 1952; Romanoff, 1960). The development of the sympathetic synapse, the maturation of the sympathetic neuron, and the initial appearance and development of the enzymes involved in the inactivation of the transmitter are correlated (Giacobini et al., 1970b). The immediate precursors of norepinephrine, DOPA and dopamine, are present in chick embryo heart by the 4th and 6th days (Ignano and Shideman, 1968b). The enzymes responsible for their transformation into norepinephrine and epinephrine (tyrosine hydroxylase, DOPA-decarboxylase, dopamine-β-oxidase, and phenylethanolamine-N-methyl transferase) are present in the heart and other peripheral organs (Burak and Badge, 1964; Ignano and Shideman, 1968b). DOPA-decarboxylase, unlike the other enzymes of the sequence, continues to increase from the 5th day of incubation in the chick embryo until well after hatching (Giacobini, 1971).

The enzymes involved in the metabolism of norepinephrine and epinephrine, such as monoamine oxidases (MAO) and catechol-O-methyl transferases (COMT), also increase in the chick heart from the 4th to the 10th days of embryonic development. COMT activity then gradually declines, whereas MAO activity continues to increase throughout development (Ignano and Shideman, 1968a). The continuous increase of MAO and DOPA-decarboxylase, the only two enzymes present in the neuronal cell body and efferent fibers (Giacobini et al., 1970a), suggests a correlation with the innervation of the peripheral organs. A peak of activity for the two enzymes immediately after birth coincides with the starting of the function. On the other hand, the different pattern of activities during development for MAO and DOPA-decarboxylase may be explained by the different subcellular localization of the two enzymes: MAOs are localized principally in the mitochondria and DOPA-decarboxylase in the cytoplasm, suggesting different rates of transport from the neuronal body to the periphery during development.

In the central nervous system, the concentrations of norepinephrine are correlated with the degree of physiological maturity at birth (Karki et al., 1962). In guinea pigs fully mature at birth, adult levels of norepinephrine are found at the end of the embryonic period, whereas the levels in rat brain increase for at least 10 days after birth. The progression of some amine levels (norepinephrine and serotonin) is caudal to rostral, since they derive from nuclei of the lower brainstem (Loizou and Salt, 1970).

The changes in monoamine patterns during embryonic development may be explained by the sequential development of the successive enzymatic steps in already mature neurons with fully developed axonal and dendritic systems, such as in chick embryos (Ignano and Shideman, 1968b). The nerve endings receive, through the axonal flow, all the subcellular organelles with the enzymes involved in synthesis, storage, and release of the transmitters. Another possibility is the parallel development of the neuroanatomical connections with all the molecular mechanisms necessary for synaptic transmission already present in growing cell bodies. This second hypothesis is supported by the observations that in the rat monoaminergic neurons still divide at birth and that axonal development takes place during the first 10 days of extrauterine life. Some monoamine concentration values and enzyme activities in brain of fetal or neonatal rats are compared with adult values in Table 1.

Cholinergic transmitter

Acetylcholine is present in the unfertilized egg (Marchisio and Consolo, 1968). However, the question of its function is unresolved. It is probably analogous to the role of acetylcholine present in bacteria. It probably serves transport and metabolic processes, such as that of the incorporation of phosphate groups into membrane phospholipids. Cholineacetylase (ChAc), total cholinesterase (ChE), and acetylcholinesterase (AChE) have also been measured in chick spinal and sympathetic ganglia (Marchisio and Consolo, 1968; Giacobini et al., 1970b). AChE corresponds to practically all the cholinesterase activity, and it increases until the 12th day of life, corresponding to the period of maximal multiplication and active differentiation of the neuroblasts. After this period, AChE drops in the spinal ganglia, but remains at high levels in the sympathetic ganglia, in relation with the maturation of synapses starting around the 8th or 9th day of incubation in the chick embryo (Wechsler and Schmekel, 1967).

The cyclic AMP system

The presence of the second messenger in the fertilized egg has not yet been investigated (C. Lutwak-Mann, *personal communication*). Weiss (1971; *personal communication*) has shown and discussed the enzymes relevant in the formation and metabolism of cyclic AMP, respectively, adenyl cyclase and phosphodiesterase which develop at different rates in the mammalian brain. The responsiveness of the pineal adenyl cyclase to norepinephrine is absent at birth, but it develops after several days (Weiss, 1970). On the other hand, both low and high K_m phosphodiesterase activities are present in 1-day-old rats. Heart cells from embryonic and newborn rats, cultivated *in vitro,* increase the rhythmic beats in response to norepinephrine and N^6-2'-

TABLE 1. *Comparison of brain monoaminergic mechanisms between newborn and adult rats*

Transmitters and activities	Fetal or newborn	Adult	Units	References
5-Hydroxytryptamine	0.24	0.52	$\mu g/g$	Tyce et al. (1964)
Norepinephrine	0.12	0.54		Karki et al. (1962)
Dopamine	0.28	0.67		Agrawal et al. (1966)
Normetanephrine	0.00	0.01		Agrawal et al. (1966)
5-Hydroxyindoleacetic acid	0.38	0.41		Tyce et al. (1964)
Tryptophan in plasma	19.0	12.0	$\mu g/ml$	Tyce et al. (1964)
Tyrosine in plasma	24.6	15.5		
Uptake of tryptophan in brain	51.7[a]	28.2[a]	$\mu g/g/30$ min	Tyce et al. (1964)
Uptake of tyrosine in brain	300.	200.	$\mu g/g/hr$	Guroff and Udenfriend (1964)
Tryptophan in brain	21.6	6.7	$\mu g/g$	Tyce et al. (1964)
Tyrosine in brain	36.6	22.8		
Tryptophan-5-hydroxylase (pineal body)	40.	100	% adult activity	Håkanson et al. (1967)
Tryptophan-5-hydroxylase (brainstem)	3.0	3.6	nmoles/g/hr	Renson (1971)
Tyrosine hydroxylase	3.4	3.1	nmoles/g/hr	McGeer et al. (1967)
Aromatic-L-amino acid (whole brain)	0.31	0.38	mg 5-HT formed/g/hr	Karki et al. (1962)
Decarboxylase (pineal body)	0	100.	% adult activity	Håkanson et al. (1967)
Storage	80.	78	% bound	Bennett and Giarman (1965)
Monoamine oxidase	0.59	1.75	mg 5-HT oxidized/g/hr	Karki et al. (1962)
Catechol-O-methyl transferase	20.	100	% adult activity	Glowinsky et al. (1964)

[a] TRY (66 $\mu g/g$) injected, i.p.

O-dibutyryl cyclic AMP, whereas carbachol and dibutyryl cyclic GMP decrease the heart beat (Krauss et al., 1972), indicating that, even during development in some peripheral tissues, cyclic GMP may act as an antagonist of some metabolic or physiological activities elicited by cyclic AMP, as already shown to be the case in the adult mammal (Ferrendelli et al., 1970).

DRUG METABOLISM IN THE FETUS

Some general concepts concerning drug metabolism in the fetus have been discussed throughout this volume. Distribution may be very different from that in maternal or adult tissues. Some agents may alter the fetal development even without reaching it by modifying the placental metabolism or by many other mechanisms (D. Neubert, *personal communication*). Activation of the microsomal enzymes is not extensive, but the most important difference is the susceptibility of the target cells between the adult organism and the fetus. In fetal pharmacology, both the drug and the cell change with time, and this new dimension has been considered in several cases. For instance, caffeine administered to pregnant rats is rapidly metabolized, but the amount transferred across the placental barrier to the fetus, and particularly to the fetal brain, remains much longer in the tissues, suggesting possible pharmacological or even toxicological effects unknown in the adult animal (*unpublished observations*).

Another problem in studying fetal pharmacology is caused by the difference in placental structure and function among the different species, and by changes in placental activities during the different periods of pregnancy (M. E. Dempsey, *personal communication*).

DIAGNOSIS AND POSSIBLE THERAPY OF FETAL DISEASES

The biochemical pharmacology of mammalian fetuses is studied not only to evaluate the possible effects of drugs or toxic agents during the early stages of development, but also to increase the information leading to early diagnosis and treatment of abnormalities present in fetal metabolism.

Drugs can be absorbed directly by the fetal skin and, therefore, can be administered through the amniotic cavity. This route can be used to administer amino acids directly to the fetus (R. Caldeyro-Barcia, *personal communication*). The fetus receives the foreign compounds by swallowing, through the skin, or through the umbilical vessels and their branches. The administration of drugs in the aorta, via the femoral artery, induces a more rapid accumulation in the uterus than in other locations, and this approach may be used when a therapeutic or diagnostic agent should act in the fetus rather than in the mother. The bioavailability of drugs in these cases is very important, since it is impractical to administer drugs too often during the fetal life.

For these reasons, and in order to ensure a prolonged and predetermined accumulation of the drug in the fetal tissues, the use of synthetic polymers as drug carriers seems advisable (*unpublished observations*).

Many of the areas covered by the discussion clearly deserve intensive experimental work in the immediate future. The role of drugs during fetal life is, however, clearly established as a very significant tool for the evaluation of the developmental processes and for the design of therapeutic treatments specific for the fetus at a certain period of growth or differentiation.

REFERENCES

Agrawal, H. C., Glisson, S. N., and Hunwich, W. A. (1966): *Biochim. Biophys. Acta,* 130:511.

Bennett, D. S., and Giarman, N. J. (1965): *J. Neurochem.,* 12:911.

Burak, W. R., and Badge, A. (1964): *Fed. Proc.,* 23:561.

Enemar, A., Folck, B., and Håkanson, R. (1965): *Devel. Biol.,* 11:268.

Ferrendelli, J. A., Steiner, A. L., McDougal, D. B., and Kipnis, D. M. (1970): *Biochem. Biophys. Res. Comm.,* 41:1061.

Giacobini, E. (1971): In: *Chemistry and Brain Development,* edited by R. Paoletti and A. N. Davison. Plenum Press, New York.

Giacobini, E., Karjalamen, K., Kerjel-Fronius, S., and Ritzén, M. (1970a): *Neuropharmacology,* 9:59.

Giacobini, G., Marchisio, P. C., Giacobini, E., and Koslow, S. (1970b): *J. Neurochem.,* 17:1177.

Glowinsky, J., Axelrod, J., Kajin, I. J., and Wurtman, R. J. (1964): *J. Pharm. Exp. Ther.,* 146:48.

Guroff, G., and Udenfriend, S. (1964): *Prog. Brain Res.,* 9:187.

Håkanson, R., Lombard des Gouttes, M.-N., and Owman, C. (1967): *Life Sci.,* 6:2577.

Hamilton, H. L. (1952): In: *Lillie's Development of the Chick.* Holt, Reinhart and Winston, New York.

Ignano, L. J., and Shideman, F. E. (1968a): *J. Pharmacol. Exp. Ther.,* 159:29.

Karki, N., Kuntzman, R., and Brodie, B. B. (1962): *J. Neurochem.,* 9:53.

Krause, E. G., Halle, W., and Wollenberger, A. (1972): In: *Advances in Cyclic Nucleotide Research,* Vol. 1, *Physiology and Pharmacology of Cyclic AMP,* edited by P. Greengard, R. Paoletti, and G. A. Robison. Raven Press, New York.

Loizou, L. A., and Salt, P. (1970): *Brain Res.,* 20:467.

Marchisio, P. C., and Consolo, J. (1968): *J. Neurochem.,* 15:759.

McGeer, E. G., Gibson, S., Wade, J. A., and McGeer, P. L. (1967): *Canad. J. Biochem.,* 45:1943.

Renson, J. (1971): In: *Chemistry and Brain Development,* edited by R. Paoletti and A. N. Davison. Plenum Press, New York.

Romanoff, A. L. (1960): *The Avian Embryo.* The MacMillan Company, New York.

Tyce, G., Flock, E. V., and Oxen, C. A. (1964): *Progr. Brain Res., 9:*198.

Wechsler, W., and Schmekel, L. (1967): *Acta Neuroveget.* (Wien), 30:427.

Weiss, B. (1970): In: *Biogenic Amines as Physiological Regulators.* Prentice-Hall, Inc., Englewood Cliffs, New Jersey.

Weiss, B. (1971): *J. Neurochem., 18:*469.

Index